ALI and ARD  es and Advance

Guest Editors

KRISHNAN RAGHAVENDRAN, MD
LENA M. NAPOLITANO, MD

CRITICAL CARE CLINICS

www.criticalcare.theclinics.com

Consulting Editor
RICHARD W. CARLSON, MD, PhD

July 2011 • Volume 27 • Number 3

SAUNDERS an imprint of ELSEVIER, Inc.

W.B. SAUNDERS COMPANY
A Division of Elsevier Inc.

Elsevier Inc. • 1600 John F. Kennedy Blvd., • Suite 1800 • Philadelphia, Pennsylvania 19103-2899

http://www.theclinics.com

CRITICAL CARE CLINICS Volume 27, Number 3
July 2011 ISSN 0749-0704, ISBN-13: 978-1-4557-1037-9

Editor: Patrick Manley

Critical Care Clinics (ISSN: 0749-0704) is published quarterly by Elsevier Inc., 360 Park Avenue South, New York, NY 10010-1710. Months of issue are January, April, July, and October. Business and Editorial Offices: 1600 John F. Kennedy Blvd., Suite 1800, Philadelphia, PA 19103-2899. Customer Service Office: 6277 Sea Harbor Drive, Orlando, FL 32887-4800. Periodicals postage paid at New York, NY and additional mailing offices. Subscription prices are $179.00 per year for US individuals, $435.00 per year for US institution, $87.00 per year for US students and residents, $222.00 per year for Canadian individuals, $539.00 per year for Canadian institutions, $257.00 per year for international individuals, $539.00 per year for international institutions and $127.00 per year for Canadian and foreign students/residents. To receive student/resident rate, orders must be accompanied by name of affiliated institution, date of term, and the *signature* of program/residency coordinator on institution letterhead. Orders will be billed at individual rate until proof of status is received. Foreign air speed delivery is included in all *Clinics* subscription prices. All prices are subject to change without notice. POSTMASTER: Send address changes to *Critical Care Clinics*, Elsevier Periodicals Customer Service, 11830 Westline Industrial Drive, St. Louis, MO 63146. **Customer Service: 1-800-654-2452 (US). From outside of the US, call 1-314-447-8871. Fax: 1-314-447-8029. E-mail: journalscustomerservice-usa@elsevier.com (for print support) or journalsonlinesupport-usa@elsevier.com (for online support).**

Reprints. For copies of 100 or more of articles in this publication, please contact the Commercial Reprints Department, Elsevier Inc., 360 Park Avenue South, New York, NY 10010-1710. Tel.: 212-633-3813; Fax: 212-462-1935; E-mail: reprints@elsevier.com.

Critical Care Clinics is also published in Spanish by Editorial Inter-Medica, Junin 917, 1[er] A, 1113, Buenos Aires, Argentina.

Critical Care Clinics is covered in *MEDLINE/PubMed (Index Medicus), EMBASE/Excerpta Medica, Current Concepts/Clinical Medicine, ISI/BIOMED, and Chemical Abstracts*.

Printed and bound by CPI Group (UK) Ltd, Croydon, CR0 4YY

Transferred to Digital Print 2011

Contributors

CONSULTING EDITOR

RICHARD W. CARLSON, MD, PhD
Chairman Emeritus, Department of Medicine, Maricopa Medical Center; Director, Medical Intensive Care Unit; Professor, University of Arizona College of Medicine; Professor, Department of Medicine, Mayo Graduate School of Medicine, Phoenix, Arizona

GUEST EDITORS

KRISHNAN RAGHAVENDRAN, MD, FACS
Associate Professor of Surgery, Division of Acute Care Surgery, Department of Surgery, University of Michigan Health System, Ann Arbor, Michigan

LENA M. NAPOLITANO, MD
Professor of Surgery, Division Chief, Acute Care Surgery [Trauma, Burns, Surgical Critical Care, Emergency Surgery], Department of Surgery, University of Michigan Health System, Ann Arbor, Michigan

AUTHORS

SAMMY ALI, MD
Internal Medicine Program, Department of Medicine, University of Toronto, Toronto, Ontario, Canada

DJILLALI ANNANE, MD, PhD
General Intensive Care Unit, Université de Versailles SQY (UniverSud Paris), Garches, France

NICOLAS BARNETT, MB ChB
Research Fellow, Division of Allergy, Pulmonary and Critical Care Medicine, Department of Medicine, Vanderbilt University, Nashville, Tennessee

ROBERT H. BARTLETT, MD, FACS, FCCM, FCCP
Emeritus Professor, Surgery, Division of Acute Care Surgery, Department of Surgery, University of Michigan Health System, Ann Arbor, Michigan

GORDON R. BERNARD, MD
Melinda Owen Bass Professor of Medicine, Associate Vice Chancellor for Research, Senior Associate Dean for Clinical Sciences, Vanderbilt University Medical Center, Vanderbilt University School of Medicine, Nashville, Tennessee

ROSS BLANK, MD
Clinical Lecturer, Division of Critical Care, Department of Anesthesiology, University of Michigan Health System, Ann Arbor, Michigan

DAVID A. DEAN, PhD
Department of Pediatrics, School of Medicine and Dentistry, University of Rochester, Rochester, New York

RICHARD PHILLIP DELLINGER, MD, FCCP
Professor, Division Head, Critical Care Medicine; Vice-Chair Medicine, Department of Critical Care Medicine; Department of Medicine, Cooper University Hospital Robert Wood Johnson Medical School, Camden, New Jersey

SHARON DICKINSON, RN, MSN, CNS-BC, ANP, CCRN
Clinical Nurse Specialist, SICU, Division of Acute Care Surgery (Trauma, Burn, Critical Care, Emergency Surgery), Department of Surgery, University of Michigan Health System, Ann Arbor, Michigan

NIALL D. FERGUSON, MD, MSc
Interdepartmental Division of Critical Care; Division of Respirology, Department of Medicine, University Health Network and Mount Sinai Hospital, University of Toronto, Toronto, Ontario, Canada

JEFFREY E. GOTTS, MD, PhD
Fellow, Pulmonary and Critical Care Medicine, Departments of Medicine and Anesthesiology, The Cardiovascular Research Institute, University of California, San Francisco, San Francisco, California

CARL F. HAAS, MLS, RRT, FAARC
Educational and Research Coordinator, University Hospital Respiratory Care, University of Michigan Hospitals and Health Centers, Ann Arbor, Michigan

DON HAYES Jr, MD, MS
Assistant Professor, Department of Pediatrics, University of Kentucky College of Medicine, University of Kentucky Medical Center, Lexington, Kentucky

MARGARET S. HERRIDGE, MD, MPH
Associate Professor of Medicine, Division of Respiratory and Interdepartmental Division of Critical Care Medicine, Toronto General Hospital, University of Toronto, Toronto, Ontario, Canada

LEWIS J. KAPLAN, MD, FACS, FCCM, FCCP
Associate Professor of Surgery, Department of Surgery, Section of Trauma, Surgical Critical Care and Surgical Emergencies, Yale University School of Medicine, New Haven, Connecticut

ANNA KRZAK, RD
Nutrition Services, University of Michigan Health System, Ann Arbor, Michigan

XIN LIN, PhD
Department of Pediatrics, School of Medicine and Dentistry, University of Rochester, Rochester, New York

JAMES E. LYNCH, MD
General Surgery Resident, Division of General Surgery, Department of Surgery, University of Kentucky College of Medicine, University of Kentucky Medical Center, Lexington, Kentucky

PAUL E. MARIK, MD, FCCM, FCCP
Division of Pulmonary and Critical Care Medicine, Department of Medicine, Eastern Virginia Medical School, Norfolk, Virginia

THOMAS R. MARTIN, MD
Medical Research Service, Division of Pulmonary and Critical Care Medicine, Department of Medicine, Veterans Affairs Puget Sound Medical Center, University of Washington School of Medicine, Seattle, Washington

MICHAEL A. MATTHAY, MD
Professor, Departments of Medicine and Anesthesiology, The Cardiovascular Research Institute, University of California, San Francisco, San Francisco, California

GUSTAVO MATUTE-BELLO, MD
Medical Research Service, Division of Pulmonary and Critical Care Medicine, Department of Medicine, Veterans Affairs Puget Sound Medical Center, University of Washington School of Medicine, Seattle, Washington

ADRIAN A. MAUNG, MD, FACS
Assistant Professor of Surgery, Department of Surgery, Section of Trauma, Surgical Critical Care and Surgical Emergencies, Yale University School of Medicine, New Haven, Connecticut

G. UMBERTO MEDURI, MD
Division of Pulmonary, Critical Care, and Sleep Medicine, Department of Medicine, University of Tennessee Health Science Center and Memphis Veterans Affairs Medical Center, Memphis, Tennessee

LENA M. NAPOLITANO, MD
Professor of Surgery, Division Chief, Acute Care Surgery [Trauma, Burns, Surgical Critical Care, Emergency Surgery], Department of Surgery, University of Michigan Health System, Ann Arbor, Michigan

R.H. NOTTER, MD, PhD
Professor of Pediatrics and Environmental Medicine, University of Rochester School of Medicine, Rochester, New York

PAULINE K. PARK, MD, FACS, FCCM
Associate Professor; Co-Director, SICU, Division of Acute Care Surgery [Trauma, Burn, Critical Care, Emergency Surgery], Department of Surgery, University of Michigan Health System, Ann Arbor, Michigan

MELISSA PLEVA, PharmD
Department of Pharmacy Services, University of Michigan Health System, Ann Arbor, Michigan

NITIN PURI, MD
Fellow, Pulmonary and Critical Care Medicine, Department of Medicine, Cooper University Hospital, Robert Wood Johnson Medical School, Camden, New Jersey

KRISHNAN RAGHAVENDRAN, MD, FACS
Associate Professor of Surgery, Division of Acute Care Surgery, Department of Surgery, University of Michigan Health System, Ann Arbor, Michigan

PATRICIA R.M. ROCCO, MD, PhD
Laboratory of Pulmonary Investigation, Carlos Chagas Filho Biophysics Institute, Federal University of Rio de Janeiro, Rio de Janeiro, Brazil

B. TAYLOR THOMPSON, MD
Pulmonary Associates, Professor of Medicine, Director, Medical Intensive Care Unit, Harvard Medical School, Massachusetts General Hospital, Boston, Massachusetts

LORRAINE B. WARE, MD
Associate Professor of Medicine, Division of Allergy, Pulmonary and Critical Care Medicine, Department of Medicine, Vanderbilt University, Nashville, Tennessee

D. WILLSON, MD
Professor, Departments of Pediatrics and Anesthesia, University of Virginia Health Services System, Charlottesville, Virginia

JOSEPH B. ZWISCHENBERGER, MD
Johnston-Wright Professor and Chair, Department of Surgery, University of Kentucky College of Medicine, University of Kentucky Medical Center, Lexington, Kentucky

Contents

Preface: ALI and ARDS: Challenges and Advances xiii

Krishnan Raghavendran and Lena M. Napolitano

Definition of ALI/ARDS 429

Krishnan Raghavendran and Lena M. Napolitano

Although acute lung injury (ALI) and acute respiratory distress syndrome (ARDS) are caused by different injuries and conditions, their similar clinical picture makes a compelling case for them to be studied as a single entity. An array of potential specific targets for pharmacologic intervention can be applied to ALI/ARDS as one disease. Although a working definition of ALI/ARDS that includes pulmonary and extrapulmonary causes can have benefit in standardizing supportive care, it can also complicate assessments of the efficacy of therapeutic interventions. In this article, definitions that have been recently used for ALI/ARDS in various clinical studies are discussed individually.

Epidemiology of ARDS and ALI 439

Ross Blank and Lena M. Napolitano

Acute respiratory distress syndrome (ARDS) and acute lung injury (ALI) are distinctly modern clinical entities. Recent epidemiologic research has taken advantage of large cohorts in efforts to better describe these highly lethal syndromes with a focus on differentiation of clinically meaningful subtypes and early prediction in an effort to improve treatment and prevention. This article identifies the most significant studies and systematic reviews of recent years, defining the incidence, mortality, risk and prognostic factors, and etiologic classes of ARDS/ALI.

ARDS Network (NHLBI) Studies: Successes and Challenges in ARDS Clinical Research 459

B. Taylor Thompson and Gordon R. Bernard

To hasten the development of effective therapy for acute respiratory distress syndrome (ARDS), in 1994, the National Heart, Lung, and Blood Institute initiated a clinical network to carry out multicenter clinical trials of ARDS treatments. The ARDS Network is a clinical research network of approximately 42 hospitals, organized into 12 clinical sites. The goal of the Network is to efficiently test promising agents, devices, or management strategies to improve the care of patients with ARDS. Comprehensive information regarding all completed and ongoing ARDSNet clinical trials is available at www.ardsnet.org, but a brief summary is provided in this article.

Mechanical Ventilation with Lung Protective Strategies: What Works? 469

Carl F. Haas

Essentially all patients with acute lung injury or acute respiratory distress syndrome require mechanical ventilatory assistance to support gas exchange and reduce the work of breathing associated with the lung impairment. Unfortunately, this life-sustaining support may actually cause further

reviews clinical studies of surfactant therapy in pediatric and adult patients with ALI/ARDS, focusing on its potential advantages in patients with direct pulmonary forms of these syndromes.

Inhaled Nitric Oxide and Inhaled Prostacyclin in Acute Respiratory Distress Syndrome: What is the Evidence? **561**

Nitin Puri and Richard Phillip Dellinger

The mortality for acute respiratory distress syndrome remains unacceptably high. Two vasodilators, inhaled prostacyclin and inhaled nitric oxide, are reviewed in this article. Knowledge of inhaled prostacyclin has grown substantially in the past 30 years, but less research exists about its utility in acute respiratory distress syndrome. Inhaled prostacyclin and other prostaglandin derivatives are used in acute respiratory distress syndrome with increasing frequency. Currently, only randomized controlled trials exist for inhaled nitric oxide in acute respiratory distress syndrome patients. Randomized controlled trials with consistent dosing methods are needed for both vasodilators to better define their role in the treatment of acute respiratory distress syndrome.

Glucocorticoid Treatment in Acute Lung Injury and Acute Respiratory Distress Syndrome **589**

Paul E. Marik, G. Umberto Meduri, Patricia R.M. Rocco, and Djillali Annane

Experimental and clinical evidence show a strong association between dysregulated systemic inflammation and progression of acute respiratory distress syndrome (ARDS). This article reviews eight controlled studies evaluating corticosteroid treatment initiated before day 14 of ARDS. Available data provide a consistent strong level of evidence for improving outcomes. Treatment was also associated with a markedly reduced risk of death. This low-cost highly effective therapy is well-known, and has a low-risk profile when secondary prevention measures are implemented. The authors recommend prolonged methylprednisolone at 1 mg/kg/d initially in early ARDS, increasing to 2 mg/kg/d after 7 to 9 days of no improvement.

Extracorporeal CO_2 Removal in ARDS **609**

James E. Lynch, Don Hayes Jr, and Joseph B. Zwischenberger

Acute respiratory distress syndrome remains one of the most clinically vexing problems in critical care. As technology continues to evolve, it is likely that extracorporeal CO_2 removal devices will become smaller, more efficient, and safer. As the risk of extracorporeal support decreases, devices' role in acute respiratory distress syndrome patients remains to be defined. This article discusses the functional properties and management techniques of CO_2 removal and intracorporeal membrane oxygenation and provides a glimpse into the future of long-term gas-exchange devices.

Extracorporeal Membrane Oxygenation in Adult Acute Respiratory Distress Syndrome **627**

Pauline K. Park, Lena M. Napolitano, and Robert H. Bartlett

The role of extracorporeal membrane oxygenation (ECMO) in supporting adult refractory respiratory failure continues to evolve. Technical advances and the clinical challenges of H1N1 associated severe ARDS have spurred

systems, and the current status of gene therapy applied to ALI/ARDS-associated pulmonary diseases is reviewed. With the development of more efficient gene therapy vectors, gene therapy is a promising strategy for clinical application.

Mesenchymal Stem Cells and Acute Lung Injury **719**

Jeffrey E. Gotts and Michael A. Matthay

Acute respiratory distress syndrome (ARDS) is a clinical syndrome of acute respiratory failure presenting with hypoxemia and bilateral pulmonary infiltrates, most often in the setting of pneumonia, sepsis, or major trauma. The pathogenesis of ARDS involves lung endothelial injury, alveolar epithelial injury, and the accumulation of protein-rich fluid and cellular debris in the alveolar space. No pharmacologic therapy has so far proved effective. A potential strategy involves cell-based therapies, including mesenchymal stem cells (MSCs). Herein we review basic properties of MSCs, their use in preclinical models of lung injury and ARDS, and potential therapeutic mechanisms.

Experimental Models and Emerging Hypotheses for Acute Lung Injury **735**

Thomas R. Martin and Gustavo Matute-Bello

Acute lung injury (ALI) involves the activation of multiple pathways leading to lung injury, resolution, and repair. Exploration of the roles of individual pathways in humans and animal models has led to a greater understanding of the complexity of ALI and the links between ALI and systemic multiorgan failure. However, there is still no integrated understanding of the initiation, the progression, and the repair of ALI. A better understanding is needed of how pathways interact in the human ALI syndrome and how complementary treatments can be used to modify the onset, severity, and outcome of ALI in humans.

Index **753**

FORTHCOMING ISSUES

October 2011
Venous Thromboembolism in Critical Care
Kenneth Wood, MD, *Guest Editor*

January 2012
Economics of Critical Care
Donald Chalfin, MD and John Rizzo, PhD, *Guest Editors*

April 2012
CPR
Wanchung Tang, MD, *Guest Editor*

RECENT ISSUES

April 2011
Biomarkers in the Critically Ill Patient
Mitchell M. Levy, MD, *Guest Editor*

January 2011
Optimizing Antimicrobial Therapy of Sepsis and Septic Shock
Anand Kumar, MD, *Guest Editor*

October 2010
Critical Care Considerations of the Morbidly Obese
Marilyn Haupt, MD and
Mary Jane Reed, MD, *Guest Editors*

Preface

ALI and ARDS: Challenges and Advances

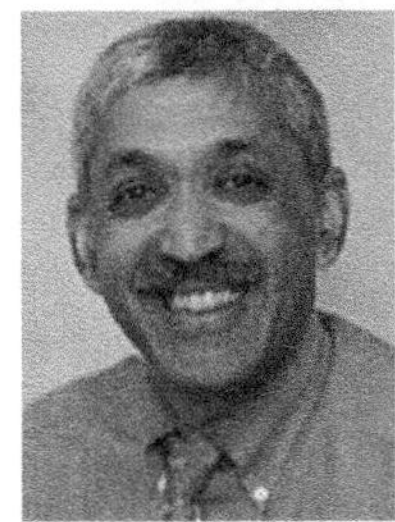
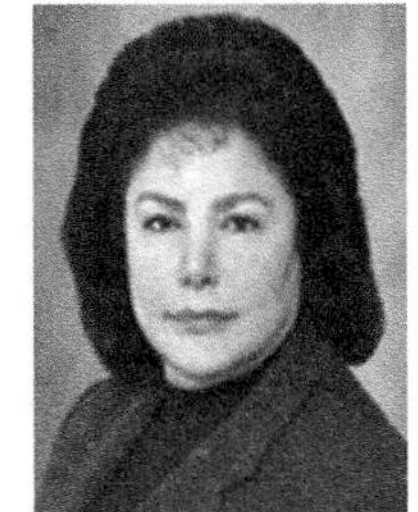

Krishnan Raghavendran, MD   Lena M. Napolitano, MD
Guest Editors

Acute lung injury (ALI) and acute respiratory distress syndrome (ARDS) are life-threatening diseases, and patients with ALI/ARDS require extensive critical care support for treatment of acute respiratory failure with hypoxemia and hypercarbia, and support of other failing organs. This issue of *Critical Care Clinics* is aimed at providing an overview of the significant advances that have been made in the last decade in the understanding and treatment of this disease, and the persistent challenges that still remain.

Since the initial description of ARDS more than 40 years ago by Ashbaugh and colleagues in 1967, much has changed. Epidemiologic data confirm that there has been a significant decline in the incidence of ALI/ARDS over the past decade, related to both direct pulmonary and indirect extrapulmonary causes. Despite this reduced incidence, mortality rates in ARDS are high, at approximately 40%. Severe ARDS due to the 2009 Influenza A (H1N1) virus occurred in young adults and was associated with severe hypoxemia and high mortality rates, and epidemiologic data from this pandemic are still emerging. Our enhanced knowledge of ARDS has uncovered important limitations to the current ARDS definitions that are being used in clinical trials, and we critically evaluate the current ARDS criteria and discuss whether a new ARDS definition should be considered.

The development of the ARDS Network was a groundbreaking advance with the completion of many multicenter clinical trials of ARDS treatments that have now refined our standard therapy for ARDS. The present therapeutic approaches for ALI/ARDS include: (1) identification and treatment of the underlying cause; (2) optimal fluid management–fluid conservative approach; (3) lung protective mechanical ventilation [lower tidal volume, optimal positive end-expiratory pressure (PEEP)]; (4) avoidance of secondary lung injury and infection; and (5) supportive critical care. Despite provision of these standard treatments, some ALI/ARDS patients progress to develop severe hypoxemia, requiring additional "rescue" therapies.

Crit Care Clin 27 (2011) xiii–xiv
doi:10.1016/j.ccc.2011.05.012

Key topics reviewed in this issue include innovative treatment strategies for ARDS including high-frequency oscillatory ventilation (HFOV), airway pressure release ventilation (APRV), extracorporeal membrane oxygenation (ECMO), and extracorporeal carbon dioxide removal ($ECCO_2R$). Potential pharmacologic treatment strategies for ARDS include surfactant therapy, inhaled nitric oxide, prostacyclin, and corticosteroid therapy, and comprehensive reviews of the evidence supporting these treatments are provided. Prone positioning therapy and specialized nutrition support are also discussed fully as adjunct treatments in ALI/ARDS.

Recent data regarding long-term follow-up of ARDS survivors revealed sustained lung recovery with near-normal lung function, but persistent physical functional limitations, advocating for early mobility in ALI/ARDS patients during their intensive care unit stay. Significant progress has been made in the field of biomarkers for prediction, diagnosis, and prognosis in ALI/ARDS. The development and refinement of experimental models for ALI/ARDS will continue to move research forward in this important area. The current state of research in two exciting areas—the potential for gene therapy as an effective treatment for ALI/ARDS and possible cell-based therapy with mesenchymal stem cells—are both reviewed.

We would like to thank the authors for their generous contributions of both their time and their expertise in the preparation of this issue. We would also like to acknowledge Dr Richard Carlson and the Elsevier editorial staff for their tireless support and assistance in bringing this issue to completion.

We hope that this issue of *Critical Care Clinics* provides an up-to-date resource for critical care practitioners regarding the optimal management of patients with ALI/ARDS and also reviews the current areas of active investigation in this life-threatening disease.

Krishnan Raghavendran, MD
Lena M. Napolitano, MD

Division of Acute Care Surgery
Department of Surgery
University of Michigan Health System
1500 East Medical Center Drive
1C340A-UH, SPC 5033
Ann Arbor, MI 48109-5033, USA

E-mail addresses:
kraghave@umich.edu (K. Raghavendran)
lenan@umich.edu (L.M. Napolitano)

Definition of ALI/ARDS

Krishnan Raghavendran, MD*, Lena M. Napolitano, MD

KEYWORDS

- Acute respiratory distress syndrome • Acute lung injury
- Respiratory failure • Terminology

The description of acute respiratory distress syndrome (ARDS) as a distinct entity was first reported by Ashbaugh and colleagues[1] in 1967, defined as a clinical pattern including "severe dyspnea, tachypnea, cyanosis that is refractory to oxygen therapy, loss of lung compliance, and diffuse alveolar infiltration seen on chest x-ray." In their initial report of 12 patients, 7 patients died, and the autopsy finding confirmed striking findings on lung microscopy including the presence of hyaline membranes, diffuse interstitial inflammation, and interstitial and intra-alveolar edema and hemorrhage. Since the initial description of ARDS more than 40 years ago, the optimal definition of acute lung injury (ALI)/ARDS remains a controversial subject.

ALI and ARDS are characterized by rapid-onset respiratory failure following a variety of direct and indirect insults to the parenchyma or vasculature of the lungs. The pulmonary pathology of ALI/ARDS can be divided conceptually into acute and fibroproliferative phases that have distinctive features but vary in detail depending on the cause of injury. Mortality from ALI/ARDS is substantial, and current therapy primarily emphasizes lung-protective mechanical ventilation and a restrictive fluid management strategy plus standard treatment of the initiating insult or underlying disease.

Although ALI/ARDS are "syndromes" caused by different injuries and conditions, the pathobiology of the lung injury and similar clinical picture makes a compelling case for us to study them as a single entity rather than characterize the individual risk factors as separate clinical entities. More importantly, an array of potential specific targets for pharmacologic intervention can be applied to ALI/ARDS as one disease entity.

Clinical presentations consistent with ALI and ARDS can arise in patients of all ages from direct (pulmonary) or indirect (extrapulmonary) insults that induce pulmonary inflammation, damage the cells of the alveolar-capillary membrane, and lead to severe acute respiratory failure. Uniform diagnostic criteria are essential for meaningful clinical studies and therapeutic development for ALI/ARDS. The clinical entities of ALI and

The support of NIH grant HL-102013 (K.R.) and DOD grant HUM 30091 (L.M.N.) are gratefully acknowledged.
Division of Acute Care Surgery, Department of Surgery, University of Michigan Health System, 1500 East Medical Center Drive, 1C340A-UH, SPC 5033, Ann Arbor, MI 48109-5033, USA
* Corresponding author.
E-mail address: kraghave@med.umich.edu

Crit Care Clin 27 (2011) 429–437
doi:10.1016/j.ccc.2011.05.006 **criticalcare.theclinics.com**
0749-0704/11/$ – see front matter

ARDS are syndromes defined by a relatively limited set of descriptive pathophysiologic clinical findings, and patients are included regardless of the specific etiology of acute pulmonary dysfunction.

Although a working definition of ALI/ARDS that includes both pulmonary and extrapulmonary causes can have benefit in standardizing supportive intensive care, it can also complicate assessments of the efficacy of therapeutic interventions. For example, the lack of stratification of patients with ALI/ARDS by etiology has the potential to confound data interpretation in therapeutic trials, because interventions that might benefit one cause of ALI/ARDS may have no benefit or may even be harmful in treating another cause.

In this article, the definitions that have been recently used for ALI/ARDS in various clinical studies are discussed individually.

IMPORTANCE OF DEFINING ALI/ARDS

A precise definition of ARDS is necessary to facilitate research into the pathogenesis and standardize treatment modalities. There is broad recognition that ALI/ARDS has many predisposing risk factors, and the definition merely represents a functional indicator of the severity of the lung injury. Should we be studying individual risk factors/disease that led to this syndrome, such as aspiration-induced lung injury, lung contusion, transfusion-related acute lung injury (TRALI), or lung injury secondary to sepsis? There exist major differences in the pathogenesis of these individual insults, especially when studied in animal model systems. However, there are major advantages of defining a syndrome like ALI/ARDS.

A standardized universal definition for ALI/ARDS has many benefits. Most importantly, it would allow comparison of the findings of various clinical trials in ALI/ARDS with a greater degree of certainty. For the clinician, a functional definition of ALI/ARDS allows early institution of standardized clinical care, that is, certain therapeutic modalities that have been tested and proved to have benefits. For instance, early identification of patients with ALI/ARDS allows the early application of protective lung ventilation with lower tidal volumes based on predicted body weights.[2]

In addition, a standardized definition including ALI and ARDS can assist with outcome prognostication, and is of help especially while discussing the care of the patient with families. For the researcher, it helps to capture a larger patient population for potential recruitment into large clinical studies, as proved by multiple clinical trials conducted under the auspices of the ARDS Network.[2,3] Moreover, it offers a common language of communication between the basic and clinical researcher whereby therapeutic modalities can be constantly tested in the laboratory and brought to the clinical arena.

Moreover, for the public and health care administrators, the many epidemiologic studies reporting on the incidence and outcomes of ALI/ARDS in specific countries and populations helps determine the amount of ever shrinking health care dollars that can be ascribed to this disease and its societal impact.[4–7] Finally, it has to be understood that while combining both ALI and ARDS as one entity offers advantages, the results of the clinical studies with testing of therapeutic modalities have to be carefully interpreted, as many specific discrete disease entities have been examined as one.

DEFINITIONS OF ALI/ARDS

The American-European Consensus Conference Definition

The American-European Consensus Conference (AECC) on ARDS in 1994 defined ALI as respiratory failure of acute onset with a PaO_2/FiO_2 ratio of less than 300 mm Hg (regardless of the level of positive end-expiratory pressure, PEEP), bilateral infiltrates on frontal chest radiograph, and a pulmonary capillary wedge pressure of 18 mm Hg or less (if measured) or no evidence of left atrial hypertension.[8] ARDS was defined identically except for a lower limiting value of less than 200 mm Hg for PaO_2/FiO_2 (**Box 1**).[8]

The AECC definition of ALI/ARDS is in common use and is simple to apply, but also has serious deficiencies in discrimination. There is often not a good correlation between these broad clinical definitions and diffuse alveolar damage (DAD), which is widely considered to be a major characteristic histologic feature of ALI/ARDS.[9] The AECC definitions also do not take into consideration variables such as the mode of ventilation and the level of PEEP, which can significantly influence oxygenation. In addition, with the publication of studies that have shown that routine use of Swan-Ganz catheters can be associated with higher complications, the pulmonary capillary occlusive pressure (PCOP) component of the definition is not commonly measured,[10,11] thus placing significant emphasis on chest radiograph interpretation whereby there is a significant lack of interobserver reliability. However, the AECC definition, particularly with the ARDS component, has proven predictability. For instance, patients with ARDS as per this definition have higher mortality than patients without.[12,13]

The AECC definition of ALI/ARDS has been used in all of the ARDS Network clinical trials (www.ardsnet.org). The important question to consider is: does the ARMA ARDS Network trial (lower [6 mL/kg] vs traditional [12 mL/kg] tidal volumes) with its finding of improved survival (31% vs 39% mortality) for lower tidal volumes using this ALI/ARDS definition lend increased credibility to this definition?[2]

Murray Lung Injury Score

In 1988, Murray and colleagues[14] proposed an expanded definition of ARDS, taking into account various pathophysiological features of the clinical syndrome. The Murray scoring system includes 4 criteria for the development of ALI/ARDS: a "scoring" of hypoxemia, a "scoring" of respiratory system compliance, chest radiographic findings, and level of PEEP. Each criterion receives a score from 0 to 4 according to the severity of the condition. The final score is obtained by dividing the collective score by the number of components used. A score of zero indicates no lung injury, a score of 1 to 2.5 indicates mild to moderate lung injury, and a final score of more than 2.5 indicates the presence of ARDS (**Table 1**).

The AECC definition of ALI/ARDS is frequently supplemented by lung injury or critical care scores such as the Murray score.[14] The major advantage of this scoring system is that it takes into consideration the amount of PEEP and pulmonary

Box 1
The AECC definition of ALI and ARDS developed in 1994

ALI Criteria

Timing: Acute onset

Oxygenation: $PaO_2/FiO_2 \leq 300$ mm Hg (regardless of PEEP level)

Chest radiograph: Bilateral infiltrates seen on frontal chest radiograph

Pulmonary artery wedge: ≤ 18 mm Hg when measured or no clinical evidence of left atrial hypertension

ARDS Criteria

Same as ALI except:

Oxygenation: $PaO_2/FiO_2 \leq 200$ mm Hg (regardless of PEEP level)

Table 1 The Murray Lung Injury Score		
1. Chest roentgenogram score		
No alveolar consolidation		0
Alveolar consolidation confined to 1 quadrant		1
Alveolar consolidation confined to 2 quadrants		2
Alveolar consolidation confined to 3 quadrants		3
Alveolar consolidation in all 4 quadrants		4
2. Hypoxemia score		
PaO_2/FiO_2	>300	0
PaO_2/FiO_2	225–299	1
PaO_2/FiO_2	175–224	2
PaO_2/FiO_2	100–174	3
PaO_2/FiO_2	<100	4
3. PEEP score (when ventilated) (cm H_2O)		
PEEP	≤5	0
PEEP	6–8	1
PEEP	9–11	2
PEEP	12–14	3
PEEP	>15	4
4. Respiratory system compliance score (when available) (mL/cm H_2O)		
Compliance	>80	0
Compliance	60–79	1
Compliance	40–59	2
Compliance	20–39	3
Compliance	<19	4

The final score is calculated by the addition of the component parts.

Abbreviations: Score 0, no lung injury; score 1–2.5, mild to moderate lung injury; score >2.5, severe lung injury.

Data from Murray JF, Matthay MA, Luce JM, et al. An expanded definition of the adult respiratory distress syndrome. Am Rev Respir Dis 1988;138:720–3.

compliance, a sensitive indicator of lung injury. Recent studies such as the CESAR trial[15] (conventional ventilator support vs extracorporeal membrane oxygenation for severe ARDS) incorporated this scoring system as entry criteria for the study, and only patients with a lung injury score greater than 3 were considered for the trial. The main disadvantage of the Murray score, especially in the conducting of large clinical studies, is that pulmonary compliance is not routinely measured. A significant deficiency of the Murray score is that cardiogenic pulmonary edema is not excluded.

Delphi Consensus Panel Definition

An alternative definition of ARDS by a consensus panel of senior investigators using the Delphi method includes PEEP restrictions (≥10) in defining hypoxemia (partial pressure of arterial oxygen/fraction of inspired oxygen, ie, PaO_2/FiO_2 [P/F] ratio of <200), radiographic criteria for air space disease in 2 or more quadrants, and requires either quantitative pulmonary compliance abnormalities (static compliance of <50 cm H_2O pressure with tidal volume of 8 mL/kg) or the presence of a predisposing condition (direct/indirect cause of lung injury).[16] In addition, the panel emphasized the noncardiogenic origin of the pulmonary dysfunction by either pulmonary artery catheter or cardiac echocardiography evaluation. The investigators acknowledged that signs of left atrial hypertension can coexist in patients with ARDS. However, the same investigators reported that although the Delphi definition is more specific than the AECC criteria, it is less sensitive when autopsy findings of DAD were chosen as the gold standard for the diagnosis of ARDS.[17]

Oxygenation Index and P/F Ratio

Oxygenation Index[18] (OI) is the system most widely used to quantify the degree of lung injury and hypoxemia in pediatric critical care. OI specifically takes into account mean airway pressure (MAP), an important determinant of oxygenation. OI is defined as the product of MAP $\times$ FiO_2 $\times$ 100/PaO_2. OI has been associated with outcome in both adults and children with ALI/ARDS. The original study in 2005 reported on the ability of OI to predict the duration of mechanical ventilation but not survival.[18] Since then many adult studies have examined the efficacy of OI as a predictor of both duration of mechanical ventilation and mortality.[19–21] In comparison, measurement of P/F ratio as a predictor of mortality in ALI/ARDS is uncertain. Although there are few differences in outcome based on P/F ratio early in the course of ARDS, it is likely that persistently lower P/F ratios are associated with higher mortality.[22] A summary of the pros and cons of the definitions is listed in **Table 2**.

ACCURACY OF CURRENT ALI/ARDS DEFINITIONS

The diagnostic accuracy of the ALI/ARDS definitions currently in use has been critically examined. A comparison of the AECC definition with autopsy findings of DAD in a series of 382 patients found the sensitivity (75%) and specificity (84%) to be only moderate.[12]

Table 2
Comparative analyses of commonly used definitions for ALI/ARDS

Definition	Pros	Cons
AECC[8]	Simple and easy to use Differentiates ALI and ARDS Prognostic capability based on ARMA study?	Acute onset: not defined PAOP often not measured PEEP/Compliance/MAP not taken into consideration Risk factors not emphasized
Murray score[14]	Takes PEEP/Compliance into consideration Differentiates mild to moderate from severe lung injury Radiologic criteria more specific	Does not include MAP Does not exclude heart failure Does not identify individual risk factors Prognostic ability not validated
Delphi[16]	Defines criteria for onset(<72 h) Risk factor emphasized Takes PEEP into consideration Objectively rules out heart failure	Excludes P/F >200 and <300 Does not include compliance or MAP
Oxygenation Index[18]	Takes MAP into consideration Prognostic ability validated	Does not take PEEP and compliance in consideration Does not exclude heart failure Does not evaluate radiologic signs

Abbreviations: AECC, American-European Consensus Conference; MAP, mean airway pressure; PAOP, pulmonary artery occlusion pressure; PEEP, positive end-expiratory pressure; P/F, Partial pressure of arterial oxygen/Fraction of inspired oxygen.

Of interest, the AECC definition was more accurate for patients with extrapulmonary risk factors than for patients with pulmonary risk factors. The AECC definition has performed poorly in limited reliability testing.[23,24] Furthermore, there is only moderate agreement between the AECC and the Murray Lung Injury Score (LIS) definitions.[25]

A study of 183 intensive care unit (ICU) patients who underwent autopsy after being mechanically ventilated compared the diagnostic accuracy of 3 clinical ARDS definitions (AECC, Murray LIS, and Delphi). Sensitivity and specificity were as follows: AECC

Table 3
Severity of hypoxemia and outcome in ALI/ARDS

Study	n	PaO_2/FiO_2 ratio (mm Hg)	Mortality	
Meade et al,[32] 2008	983		*Hospital Mortality*	
			Lung Open Ventilation	*Control*
		41–106	57 (50%)	77 (58%)
		>106–142	46 (39%)	55 (43%)
		>142–180	43 (33%)	40 (33%)
		>180–250	27 (25%)	33 (26%)
Villar et al,[33] 2011	220		*Hospital Mortality*	—
		<112	47%	
		112–142	30%	
		>142	23%	
Cooke et al,[34] 2008	1113		*Hospital Mortality*	—
		≤100	50%	
		≤100 + shock	58%	
		≤100 + oliguric renal failure	71%	
Villar et al,[35] 2007	170		*ICU Mortality*	*Hospital Mortality*
		<112	45 (45.5%)	45 (45.5%)
		112–142	11 (20%)	11 (20%)
		>142	1 (6.3%)	2 (12.6%)
Rubenfeld et al,[6] 2005	1113		*Hospital Mortality*	—
		<200 (ARDS)	41.1%	
		200–300 (ALI)	38.5%	
		ALI progressed to ARDS on day 3 or day 7	41.0%	
		ALI: no progression to ARDS on day 3 or day 7	28.6%	
Brun-Buisson et al,[36] 2004 ALIVE study	463		*ICU Mortality*	*Hospital Mortality*
		<200 (ARDS)	49.4%	57.9%
		200–300 (ALI)	22.6%	32.7%
Esteban et al,[12] 2002	120		*ICU Mortality*	—
		<100	83%	
		100–149	47%	
		150–199	31%	
		200–300	25%	
		>300	24%	
Taccone et al,[37] 2009 Prone-Supine II	342		*ICU Mortality*	*Hospital Mortality*
		<100 (severe ARDS)	42.0%	50.7%
		100–200 (ARDS)	24.0%	31.8%

0.83, 0.51; Murray LIS 0.74, 0.77; Delphi 0.69, 0.82. Specificity was significantly higher for both the Murray LIS and the Delphi definition than for the AECC definition, but sensitivity was not significantly different. It should be noted that none of the data for the Murray LIS require subjective interpretation, whereas this is not true for the other ARDS definitions.

IS THE SEVERITY OF HYPOXEMIA IMPORTANT?

The traditional thinking with ARDS is that it is the multiorgan dysfunction and not hypoxemia that is responsible for mortality. This assumption was based on several ARDS network trials in which hypoxia was well tolerated (up to saturations of 88%)[2] and improvements in oxygenation did not translate into a survival advantage. A detailed discussion of such studies is provided in the chapter by Thompson and Bernard elsewhere in this issue.

It must be pointed out that some studies after the adoption of lung-protective strategies have suggested a strong correlation between the severity of hypoxemia and ICU or hospital mortality (**Table 3**). In light of this, it is recommended that in future clinical trials of ARDS, severity of hypoxemia should be considered on patient enrollment into the study, and that outcomes should be assessed based on severity of hypoxemia.

What could be the reasons for these observations? One can speculate on the following possibilities. In patients with severe hypoxia, there is perhaps increased incidence of hyperoxia-induced lung injury from increased requirements of FiO_2 to maintain saturations of 88%. Hyperoxia has been implicated as a factor responsible for increased lung injury in many animal models by the generation of reactive oxygen species, increased apoptosis, and necrosis.[26–29]

Second, it is important to consider the pathophysiologic disturbances linking ARDS with multiorgan dysfunction. Is the multiorgan dysfunction as a result of ALI/ARDS or is the ALI/ARDS a result of multiorgan dysfunction? Are these two separate entities? These questions need to be fully explored in additional studies through basic and clinical research.

IS IT TIME TO CHANGE THE DEFINITION OF ALI/ARDS?

Over the past few years many different study groups have raised doubts about the validity of the current ALI/ARDS definitions and have recommended a change.[30,31] The authors believe strongly that it is time to change the definition after 17 years of the predominant use of the AECC definition for ALI/ARDS. Based on available data with various validity studies, it is suggested that the new definition should be standardized as follows. (a) Risk factors: direct (pulmonary) or indirect (extrapulmonary), as most experimental data suggest that these two entities have distinct pathogenic mechanisms. (b) Calculation of P/F ratios with specific and standard ventilator settings (PEEP and MAP). (c) Exclude heart failure objectively (use of echocardiogram). (d) Only include patients with P/F ratio with standard ventilator settings of less than 200.

REFERENCES

1. Ashbaugh DG, Bigelow DB, Petty TL, et al. Acute respiratory distress in adults. Lancet 1967;2:319–23.
2. The Acute Respiratory Distress Syndrome Network. Ventilation with lower tidal volumes as compared with traditional tidal volumes for acute lung injury and the acute respiratory distress syndrome. N Engl J Med 2000;342:1301–8.

3. ARDS Network. Ketoconazole for early treatment of acute lung injury and acute respiratory distress syndrome: a randomized controlled trial. The ARDS Network. JAMA 2000;283(15):1995–2002.
4. Hudson LD, Milberg JA, Anardi D, et al. Clinical risks for development of the acute respiratory distress syndrome. Am J Respir Crit Care Med 1995;151: 293–301.
5. Rubenfeld GD. Epidemiology of acute lung injury. Crit Care Med 2003;31(4 Suppl): S276–84.
6. Rubenfeld GD, Caldwell E, Peabody E, et al. Incidence and outcomes of acute lung injury. N Engl J Med 2005;353(16):1685–93.
7. Erickson S, Schibler A, Numa A, et al. The Paediatric Study Group of the Australian and New Zealand Intensive Care Society (ANZICS). Acute lung injury in pediatric intensive care in Australia and New Zealand: a prospective, multicentre, observational study. Pediatr Crit Care Med 2007;8:317–23.
8. Bernard GR, Artigas A, Brigham KL, et al. The American-European Consensus Conference on ARDS: definitions, mechanisms, relevant outcomes, and clinical trial coordination. Am J Respir Crit Care Med 1994;149:818–24.
9. Esteban A, Fernandez-Segoviano P, Frutos-Vivar F, et al. Comparison of clinical criteria for the acute respiratory distress syndrome with autopsy findings. Ann Intern Med 2004;141:440–5.
10. Stewart RM, Park PK, Hunt JP, et al. Less is more: improved outcomes in surgical patients with conservative fluid administration and central venous catheter monitoring. J Am Coll Surg 2009;208(5):725–35 [discussion: 735–7].
11. Wheeler AP, Bernard GR, Thompson BT, et al. Pulmonary-artery versus central venous catheter to guide treatment of acute lung injury. N Engl J Med 2006; 354(21):2213–24.
12. Esteban A, Anzueto A, Frutos F, et al. Characteristics and outcomes in adult patients receiving mechanical ventilation: a 28-day international study. JAMA 2002;287(3):345–55.
13. Roupie E, Lepage E, Wysocki M, et al. Prevalence, etiologies and outcome of the acute respiratory distress syndrome among hypoxemic ventilated patients. SRLF Collaborative Group on Mechanical Ventilation. Societe de Reanimation de Langue Francaise. Intensive Care Med 1999;25(9):920–9.
14. Murray JF, Matthay MA, Luce JM, et al. An expanded definition of the adult respiratory distress syndrome. Am Rev Respir Dis 1988;138:720–3.
15. Peek GJ, Clemens F, Elbourne D, et al. CESAR: conventional ventilatory support vs extracorporeal membrane oxygenation for severe adult respiratory failure. BMC Health Serv Res 2006;6:163.
16. Ferguson ND, Davis AM, Slutsky AS, et al. Development of a clinical definition for acute respiratory distress syndrome using the Delphi technique. J Crit Care 2005; 20(2):147–54.
17. Ferguson ND, Frutos-Vivar F, Esteban A, et al. Acute respiratory distress syndrome: underrecognition by clinicians and diagnostic accuracy of three clinical definitions. Crit Care Med 2005;33(10):2228–34.
18. Trachsel D, McCrindle BW, Nakagawa S, et al. Oxygenation index predicts outcome in children with acute hypoxemic respiratory failure. Am J Respir Crit Care Med 2005;172:206–11.
19. Monchi M, Bellenfant F, Cariou A, et al. Early predictive factors of survival in the acute respiratory distress syndrome. A multivariate analysis. Am J Respir Crit Care Med 1998;158(4):1076–81.

20. Nuckton TJ, Alonso JA, Kallet RH, et al. Pulmonary dead-space fraction as a risk factor for death in the acute respiratory distress syndrome. N Engl J Med 2002; 346(17):1281–6.
21. Seeley E, McAuley DF, Eisner M, et al. Predictors of mortality in acute lung injury during the era of lung protective ventilation. Thorax 2008;63(11):994–8.
22. Ware LB. Prognostic determinants of acute respiratory distress syndrome in adults: impact on clinical trial design. Crit Care Med 2005;33(3 Suppl):S217–22.
23. Meade MO, Cook RJ, Guyatt GH, et al. Interobserver variation in interpreting chest radiographs for the diagnosis of acute respiratory distress syndrome. Am J Respir Crit Care Med 2000;161(1):85–90.
24. Rubenfeld GD, Caldwell E, Granton J, et al. Interobserver variability in applying a radiographic definition for ARDS. Chest 1999;116(5):1347–53.
25. Meade MO, Guyatt GH, Cook RJ, et al. Agreement between alternative classifications of acute respiratory distress syndrome. Am J Respir Crit Care Med 2001; 163(2):490–3.
26. Bhandari V, Choo-Wing R, Lee CG, et al. Hyperoxia causes angiopoietin 2-mediated acute lung injury and necrotic cell death. Nat Med 2006;12(11):1286–93.
27. Mantell LL, Horowitz S, Davis JM, et al. Hyperoxia-induced cell death in the lung—the correlation of apoptosis, necrosis, and inflammation. Ann N Y Acad Sci 1999; 887:171–80.
28. Ward NS, Waxman AB, Homer RJ, et al. Interleukin-6-induced protection in hyperoxic acute lung injury. Am J Respir Cell Mol Biol 2000;22(5):535–42.
29. Waxman AB, Einarsson O, Seres T, et al. Targeted lung expression of interleukin-11 enhances murine tolerance of 100% oxygen and diminishes hyperoxia-induced DNA fragmentation. J Clin Invest 1998;101(9):1970–82.
30. Phua J, Stewart TE, Ferguson ND. Acute respiratory distress syndrome 40 years later: time to revisit its definition. Crit Care Med 2008;36(10):2912–21.
31. Villar J, Blanco J, Kacmarek RM. Acute respiratory distress syndrome definition: do we need a change? Curr Opin Crit Care 2011;17(1):13–7.
32. Meade MO, Cook DJ, Guyatt GH, et al. Ventilation strategy using low tidal volumes, recruitment maneuvers, and high positive end-expiratory pressure for acute lung injury and acute respiratory distress syndrome: a randomized controlled trial. JAMA 2008;299(6):637–45.
33. Villar J, Perez-Mendez L, Basaldua S, et al. A risk tertiles model for predicting mortality in patients with acute respiratory distress syndrome: age, plateau pressure, and P(aO(2))/F(IO(2)) at ARDS onset can predict mortality. Respir Care 2011;56(4):420–8.
34. Cooke CR, Kahn JM, Caldwell E, et al. Predictors of hospital mortality in a population-based cohort of patients with acute lung injury. Crit Care Med 2008;36(5): 1412–20.
35. Villar J, Perez-Mendez L, Lopez J, et al. An early PEEP/FIO_2 trial identifies different degrees of lung injury in patients with acute respiratory distress syndrome. Am J Respir Crit Care Med 2007;176(8):795–804.
36. Brun-Buisson C, Minelli C, Bertolini G, et al. Epidemiology and outcome of acute lung injury in European intensive care units. Results from the ALIVE study. Intensive Care Med 2004;30(1):51–61.
37. Taccone P, Pesenti A, Latini R, et al. Prone positioning in patients with moderate and severe acute respiratory distress syndrome: a randomized controlled trial. JAMA 2009;302(18):1977–84.

Epidemiology of ARDS and ALI

Ross Blank, MD[a,*], Lena M. Napolitano, MD[b]

KEYWORDS

- Acute respiratory distress syndrome • Acute lung injury
- Epidemiology • Incidence • Mortality • Risk factors
- Prognostic factors • 2009 Influenza A (H1N1)

Acute respiratory distress syndrome (ARDS) and acute lung injury (ALI) are distinctly modern clinical entities. First described in 1967[1] and codified by a consensus of experts in 1994,[2] they are syndromes that require the intensive care unit (ICU) for their very existences. Without arterial blood gas analysis, portable chest radiography, clinical assessment of left atrial hypertension, and (typically) mechanical ventilation, ARDS/ALI cannot be diagnosed. Historically, they simply did not exist, as such degrees of severe hypoxemia were fatal in the absence of supplemental oxygen and positive-pressure ventilation. The same holds in present times for patient populations without ready access to ICU services.

Any effort to understand the epidemiology of ARDS/ALI must take into account the practical challenges of diagnosis. PaO_2/FiO_2 ratios are dynamic and can be greatly influenced by changes in FiO_2 and positive end-expiratory pressure (PEEP),[3] interpretation of chest radiographs is subjective,[4,5] and left atrial pressures are less and less frequently measured in an era of declining use of the pulmonary artery catheter.[6] The finding of diffuse alveolar damage, generally considered to reflect the common histopathologic pathway of ARDS from multiple insults, requires lung biopsy and is not pursued for routine diagnosis. Moreover, a recent autopsy study has shown poor correlation between clinical and pathologic diagnoses in those patients who succumbed to their illnesses.[7] Last, it must be remembered that the experience of any single center will be affected by referral patterns, case mix, and ICU specialization.

In essence, the 1994 American-European Consensus Conference (AECC) definition[2] describes a heterogeneous syndrome with multiple etiologies and degrees of severity. Its inclusivity has facilitated the recruitment of patients for collaborative clinical research, notably the multicenter treatment trials of the ARDS Network[8] and other

---

Conflicts of Interest: The authors have no conflict of interest to declare.

[a] Division of Critical Care, Department of Anesthesiology, University of Michigan Health System, 1500 East Medical Center Drive, SPC 5861, Ann Arbor, MI 48109-5861, USA

[b] Division of Acute Care Surgery, Department of Surgery, University of Michigan Health System, 1500 East Medical Center Drive, 1C340A-UH, SPC 5033, Ann Arbor, MI 48109-5033, USA

* Corresponding author.

E-mail address: rossblan@med.umich.edu

Crit Care Clin 27 (2011) 439–458
doi:10.1016/j.ccc.2011.05.005 **criticalcare.theclinics.com**

groups. Recent epidemiologic research has taken advantage of large prospective cohorts in efforts to better describe these highly lethal syndromes with a focus on differentiation of clinically meaningful subtypes and early prediction in an effort to improve treatment and prevention. This article identifies the most significant studies and systematic reviews of recent years defining the incidence, mortality, risk and prognostic factors, and etiologic classes of ARDS/ALI. Recovery and long-term outcomes are covered in the article by Margaret S. Herridge elsewhere in this issue.

INCIDENCE

Assessments of the incidence of ARDS/ALI in the general population help to define the syndromes from public health and research-funding perspectives. Early incidence studies focused on specific geographic populations[9–14] or retrospectively analyzed administrative databases.[15] Using varying definitions and methodologies, these studies generated a range of low-incidence figures of 1.5 to 34.0 cases per 100,000 person-years, with the higher numbers observed when the AECC definition was used.[12,14]

Recent years have seen more elegant approaches that have yielded higher incidence figures. In 2003, hypothesizing that the rigorous case definitions of clinical trials would improve case-finding, Goss and colleagues[16] reviewed the screening logs from the 20 hospitals participating in the ARDSNet Acute Respiratory Distress Syndrome Management with Lower versus Higher Tidal Volume (ARMA) trial from 1996 to 1999.[17] They were able to identify 7455 patients with ALI, a number far higher than in any previous incidence studies. Using American Hospital Association data, they used various assumptions to extrapolate their figures to all ICUs in the United States and generated national ALI incidence estimates ranging from 17.6 to 64.0 cases per 100,000 person-years.

In 2005, Rubenfeld and colleagues[18] reported the data of the King County Lung Injury Project (KCLIP), a prospective cohort study of all 18 hospitals in King County in the state of Washington, plus 3 hospitals in adjacent counties. King County includes the city of Seattle and is bounded on either side by water and mountains such that the investigators felt confident that their survey would capture all cases of ALI in the population of a large metropolitan area. Meticulous review of all patients undergoing mechanical ventilation in the ICUs was used to determine cases of ALI using AECC criteria. Over a year-long period from 1999 to 2000, they identified 1113 adult cases of ALI and calculated a crude incidence of 78.9 cases per 100,000 person-years. This extrapolates to a national annual incidence of 190,600 cases with an estimated 74,000 deaths from ALI annually in the United States. Of note, 59% of patients with ALI were identified outside of academic centers and represent a significant burden to community hospitals.

Most recently, Li and colleagues[19] published the results of an 8-year retrospective cohort study of ICU patients in the Mayo Clinic, which provides all ICU-level care to the population of Olmsted County, Minnesota. Using an electronic medical record database, all ICU patients from 2001 to 2008 who resided in Olmsted County were electronically screened for the PaO_2/FiO_2 and chest radiograph AECC criteria for ARDS/ALI with subsequent verification of the diagnosis by clinician-researchers. There were a total of 795 episodes (787 new, 8 recurrent) of ARDS/ALI identified. Interestingly, there was a statistically significant trend of decreasing incidence over the 8-year time period with age- and sex-adjusted incidence rates dropping from 81 to 38 cases per 100,000 person-years (**Fig. 1**). Further scrutiny revealed that community-acquired ARDS/ALI rates remained stable while decreases in hospital-acquired ARDS/ALI accounted for the overall decline. The authors hypothesized that changes in Mayo

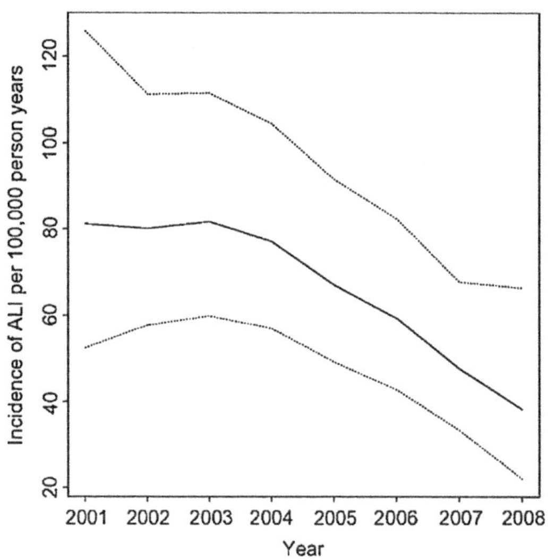

Fig. 1. Trends in incidence of ARDS/ALI from 2001 to 2008 in Olmsted County, Minnesota; dotted lines represent 95% confidence intervals. (*From* Li G, Malinchoc M, Cartin-Ceba R, et al. Eight-year trend of acute respiratory distress syndrome: a population-based study in Olmsted County, Minnesota. Am J Respir Crit Care Med 2011;183:59–66; Reprinted with permission of the American Thoracic Society. Copyright 2011 American Thoracic Society.)

Clinic ICU practice including low tidal volume ventilation for all patients, a restrictive transfusion policy, sepsis and pneumonia treatment protocols, and increased intensivist staffing contributed to the observed decline in hospital-acquired ARDS/ALI.

MORTALITY

In the 1967 initial ARDS case series by Ashbaugh and colleagues,[1] 7 (58%) of 12 patients died and reported mortality rates have remained high ever since. As can be expected in a quite heterogeneous syndrome, mortality rates can vary greatly depending on the specific patient population being studied and the severity of illness. The best available population-based data, from the KCLIP, places in-hospital mortality at 38.5% with significant variation owing to age (**Fig. 2**) and risk factors (see the Risk and Prognostic Factors section).[18]

Considerable controversy exists in the medical literature regarding temporal trends in ARDS/ALI mortality. Single-center retrospective studies[20–25] suggested that mortality decreased throughout the 1980s and 1990s, although a meta-analysis of 101 studies found no change in mortality rates from 1967 to 1994 (mean overall mortality 53%, mean 1994 mortality 51%).[26]

More recent analyses have focused on the post-1994 era of the AECC definition and ensuing ARDS Network trials. The single-center before-and-after study of Kallet and colleagues[27] attributed improved outcomes to the adoption of low tidal volume ventilation. Erickson and colleagues[28] retrospectively analyzed 2451 enrolled patients in the ARMA,[17] Assessment of Low tidal Volume and Elevated End-expiratory Volume to Obviate Lung Injury (ALVEOLI),[29] and Fluid and Catheter Treatment Trial (FACTT)[30] ARDS Network treatment studies from 1996 to 2005 and reported a decrease in crude mortality from 36% in 1996–1997 to 26% in 2004–2005. The change persisted after adjusting for covariates, including low tidal volume ventilation. Adding preliminary

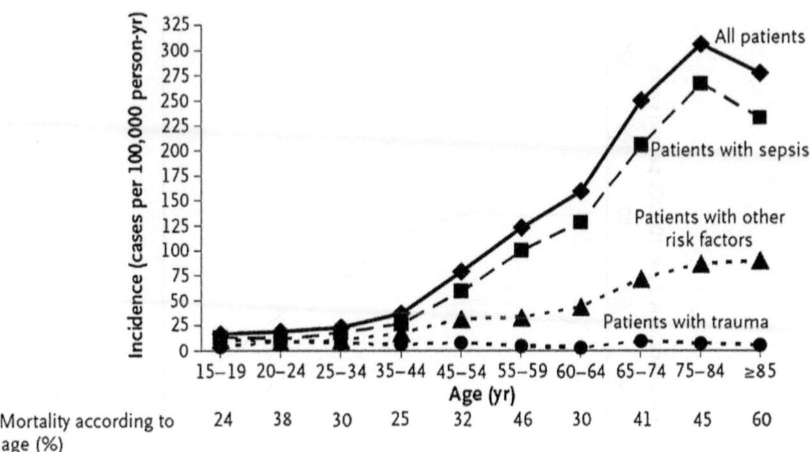

Fig. 2. Age- and risk-specific incidence of and age-specific mortality from acute lung injury. (*From* Rubenfeld GD, Caldwell E, Peabody E, et al. Incidence and outcomes of acute lung injury. N Engl J Med 2005;353:1685–93; with permission. Copyright © 2005 Massachusetts Medical Society.)

data from the more recent Albuterol for the Treatment of ALI (ALTA) and Omega-3 Fatty Acid, Gamma-Linolenic Acid, and Antioxidant Supplementation in the Management of ALI or ARDS (OMEGA) ARDS Network trials suggests that the downward trend in crude mortality has continued, with the most recent rates as low as 20% to 25% (**Fig. 3**).[31]

It must be remembered that such data are obtained from prospective clinical trials in specialized centers. These trials necessarily exclude many patients with high-risk comorbidities. Such low mortality rates have not been consistently reported in observational trials. Of note, the 8-year observational study from the Mayo Clinic revealed no change in mortality rates from 2001 to 2008 despite the noted decrease in ARDS/ALI incidence.[19]

Two recent systematic reviews of published mortality rates have reached opposite conclusions despite including many of the same primary studies. Zambon and Vincent[32] limited their literature search to 1994 to 2006, included 72 studies, and found a pooled mortality of 43% with a significant trend toward decreased mortality over time (**Fig. 4**). Phua and colleagues[33] performed a more extensive meta-analysis, including 89 studies from 1984 to 2006, and found an overall pooled mortality of 44.3%. They reported a decline in mortality in observational studies up to 1994 but no further improvements between 1994 and 2006, contrasting with the conclusion of Zambon and Vincent.[32] For randomized controlled trials (RCTs), they found no change in mortality over time (**Fig. 5**). The discordant conclusions of the 2 recent reviews may in part be because of methodological differences[33,34] and in part because of difficulties of performing meta-analysis on heterogeneous studies on a heterogeneous condition (mortality rates ranged from 15% to 80% in individual studies).[35] Taken together, the current mortality data underscore the persistent unacceptably high mortality rate of approximately 40% for ARDS/ALI outside the setting of an RCT.

RISK AND PROGNOSTIC FACTORS

Patient Risk Factors

The first modern description of ARDS highlighted the fact that the syndrome had multiple etiologies, including severe trauma, pneumonia, and pancreatitis.[1] Subsequent

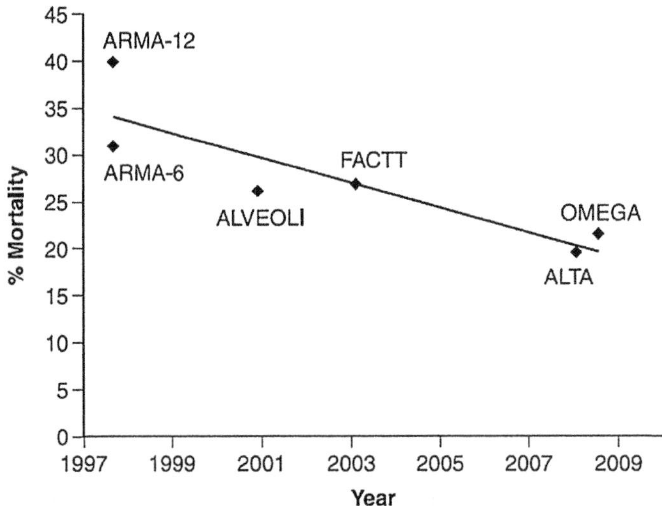

Fig. 3. Observed 60-day mortality reported for the National Heart, Lung, and Blood Institute Acute Respiratory Distress Syndrome Clinical Trials Network studies. Studies included a total of 2944 patients. ARDS Network studies that are not included had significant coenrollment with the studies shown. The reduction in mortality remains significant if ARMA-12 is excluded from the analysis. ARMA, Acute Respiratory Distress Syndrome Management with Lower versus Higher Tidal Volume[17]; ARMA-6 and ARMA-12 are groups receiving 6 or 12 mL tidal volume/kg predicted body weight; ALVEOLI, Assessment of Low tidal Volume and Elevated End-expiratory Volume to Obviate Lung Injury[29]; FACTT, Fluid and Catheter Treatment Trial[30]; ALTA, Albuterol for the Treatment of ALI[126]; OMEGA, Omega-3 Fatty Acid, Gamma-Linolenic Acid, and Antioxidant Supplementation in the Management of ALI or ARDS.[127] (*From* Spragg RG, Bernard GR, Checkley W, et al. Beyond mortality: future clinical research in acute lung injury. Am J Respir Crit Care Med 2010;181(10):1121–7; Reprinted with permission of the American Thoracic Society. Copyright 2010 American Thoracic Society.)

large cohort studies elucidated the most common clinical scenarios in which ARDS/ALI develops, namely sepsis, pneumonia, aspiration, trauma, and multiple transfusions.[36]

It is now accepted that ARDS and ALI can result from 2 general pathophysiologic pathways: (1) from *direct pulmonary causes,* such as pneumonia (bacterial or viral), aspiration pneumonitis, inhalation injury, or lung contusion, or (2) from *indirect extrapulmonary causes,* such as extrapulmonary sepsis, trauma, shock, burn injury, blood transfusion, and others.[37,38] Although some investigators argue that these 2 pathways have implications for ventilator management,[37] it has remained unclear whether this classification of ARDS has an impact on outcomes. A recent meta-analysis of 34 studies with 4311 patients included 2330 patients with a direct pulmonary cause and 1981 patients with an indirect cause. No difference in mortality was identified between the 2 groups (odds ratio [OR] 1.11; 95% confidence interval [CI] 0.88–1.39).[39] A recent retrospective study of ICU patients with bacteremia, pneumonia, or sepsis found a pulmonary site of infection was associated with an increased ARDS incidence but not mortality compared with extrapulmonary sites.[40]

The KCLIP prospectively identified 8 non–mutually exclusive clinical risk factors: severe sepsis (subdivided into pulmonary and extrapulmonary), severe trauma (Injury Severity Score >15), witnessed aspiration, massive transfusion (>15 units of blood in a 24-hour period), drug overdose, pancreatitis, near-drowning, and inhalation injury. By far the most common risk factor was sepsis with 46% and 33% of ALI cases having

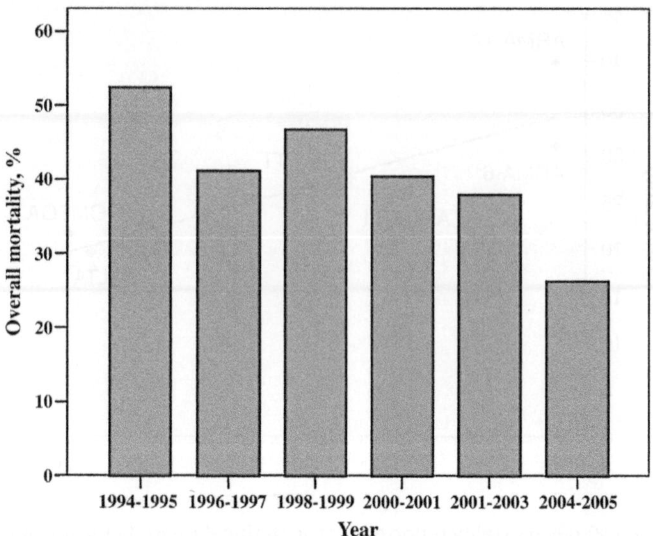

Fig. 4. Pooled mortality rates over time in 72 ARDS/ALI studies. (*From* Zambon M, Vincent JL. Mortality rates for patients with acute lung injury/ARDS have decreased over time. Chest 2008;133:1120–7; with permission.)

pulmonary and extrapulmonary sepsis, respectively. Following sepsis in descending order of frequency were aspiration (11%), trauma (7%), transfusion (3%), drug overdose (3%), and pancreatitis (3%). Cases with another or no risk factor identified constituted 14% of the total. Importantly, KCLIP data also confirmed prior observations that ALI mortality varies considerably depending on clinical risk factor. The highest mortality rates were observed in aspiration-associated (44%) and pulmonary-sepsis–associated ALI (41%) with the lowest rate in trauma-associated ALI (24%).[18] Other specific clinical conditions that have been associated with ALI include cardiopulmonary bypass,[41] nontrauma surgery,[42] burn injury,[43] kidney transplantation,[44] subarachnoid hemorrhage,[45] and recovery from neutropenia.[46]

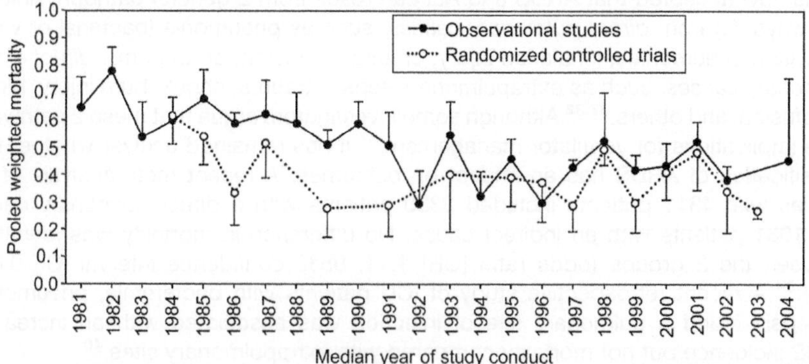

Fig. 5. Annual pooled weighted mortality in 89 ARDS/ALI studies published from 1984 to 2006. (*From* Phua J, Badia JR, Adhikari NK, et al. Has mortality from acute respiratory distress syndrome decreased over time? A systematic review. Am J Respir Crit Care Med 2009;179: 220–7; Reprinted with permission of the American Thoracic Society. Copyright 2009 American Thoracic Society.)

Multiple patient demographic variables, behaviors, and comorbid conditions have been studied as risk modifiers for development of ARDS/ALI and subsequent mortality. Not surprisingly, older patients have consistently higher mortality rates.[18,37,47–49] Incidence also increases with age, although several studies have reported a drop at upper extremes of age.[18,50,51] Both male gender and African American race have been associated with higher mortality rates in a large administrative database.[52] A later study failed to confirm the elevated African American mortality in blunt trauma–associated ARDS but did note higher mortality in patients of Hispanic ethnicity.[53]

Alcohol abuse has been associated with both increased development of ARDS in patients with other risk factors as well as increased mortality from ARDS,[54–57] possibly owing to oxidative stress[58] and/or a relative increase in pulmonary edema formation.[59] Both active cigarette smoking and exposure to second-hand smoke have also been linked to ARDS incidence.[60,61]

The effects of body mass index (BMI) on ARDS development and mortality are complex and may in part reflect the difficulties in diagnosis because of atelectasis affecting PaO_2/FiO_2 ratios and challenging chest radiograph interpretation in obese patients.[62] Higher BMIs have been associated with increased incidence[63,64] but with either no change[63–65] or a decrease[66] in mortality. Lower BMI has been reported as an independent risk factor for mortality.[66] The positive associations between obesity and the severity and mortality of H1N1-associated ARDS stand in contrast to these general findings (see the section ARDS and 2009 Pandemic Influenza A H1N1).

Diabetes mellitus and prehospital antiplatelet therapy also appear to modulate risk. In a prospective study of patients with septic shock[67] and in a recent systematic review,[68] diabetic patients were less likely to develop ARDS than their nondiabetic counterparts. In a recent population-based study at the Mayo Clinic, medical intensive care unit patients at risk for ALI were less likely to develop ALI if they were on antiplatelet medications before hospitalization.[69]

Treatment Risk Factors

Mechanical ventilation

Although it is generally accepted that high tidal volume ventilation increases mortality for patients with established ARDS,[17] the effect of ventilator settings on development of ARDS, the phenomenon of ventilator-induced lung injury (VILI), has recently received increased scrutiny. A retrospective single-center Mayo Clinic study of 332 ventilated patients without ALI by Gajic and colleagues[70] demonstrated tidal volume greater than 6 mL/kg of predicted body weight (PBW) to be an independent risk factor for the subsequent development of ALI in a dose-responsive manner. Gajic and colleagues proceeded to repeat a similar analysis in a larger international multicenter prospectively enrolled cohort[71] of 3261 mechanically ventilated patients and again identified tidal volume and, to lesser extents, peak airway pressure and PEEP level as independent risk factors for development of ARDS.[72] An additional retrospective study of VILI in ICU patients confirmed that peak airway pressure and tidal volume were independently associated with ARDS development. In the same study, nonventilatory risk factors included presence of sepsis, positive fluid balance, and plasma transfusion.[73] A recent RCT of 6 mL/kg versus 10 mL/kg PBW tidal volumes in ICU patients without ALI was terminated early because of higher rates of ALI development, as well as persistent cytokine elevation in the higher tidal volume group.[74]

Transfusion

Transfusion of blood products represents the other major iatrogenic risk factor for ALI. Multiple single-center studies have documented increased risk of ALI in ICU patients receiving packed red blood cells, fresh frozen plasma, and/or platelet transfusions,[75–77] with a National Heart, Lung, and Blood Institute working group publishing a consensus definition of transfusion-related acute lung injury (TRALI) in 2005.[78] Subsequent larger,[79,80] prospective,[81,82] multicenter,[82] and database[83] studies have consistently confirmed the association between blood products, particularly those containing plasma, and ALI development. It must be kept in mind that the diagnosis of TRALI is often confounded by the large volumes of blood products required by individual patients and the concomitant risk of hydrostatic pulmonary edema, so-called transfusion-associated circulatory overload (TACO).

Iatrogenic factors that influence the development of ARDS in susceptible patients are obvious targets of therapeutic intervention. Based in part on the emerging data regarding the risks of VILI and TRALI, the Mayo Clinic has adopted protocols of universal low tidal volume ventilation and a restrictive transfusion policy. Both a before-and-after study[84] and the 8-year longitudinal study[19] that spans the protocol changes have verified marked decreases in ALI incidence.

Sepsis management

Because of the strong association between sepsis and both ALI development and mortality, early treatment of sepsis and septic shock may also positively affect ALI-related outcomes. Focusing on a cohort of Mayo Clinic patients with septic shock without ALI, Iscimen and colleagues[85] identified both delayed antibiotics and delayed goal-directed resuscitation as independent risk factors for ALI. Other risk factors in this cohort included transfusion, alcoholism, diabetes, chemotherapy, and tachypnea.

Prognostic Factors

Clinical risk factors for mortality in ARDS/ALI include advanced age, severity of illness scores, presence of sepsis, and immunosuppression.[62,86–88] Multiple physiologic or laboratory parameters have been studied as prognostic guides in ARDS/ALI. Elevated pulmonary dead-space fraction,[89–91] elevated pulmonary vascular resistance,[92] early air leak,[86] serum hypoproteinemia,[93] serum hyperbilirubinemia,[94] and acidemia[86] have all been reported as independent factors imparting a poor prognosis. Recently, increasingly sophisticated panels of biomarkers[95] have been combined with clinical factors[96–98] in an effort to refine prognostic assessment. Importantly, although degree of impaired oxygenation at diagnosis has been associated with mortality in some studies,[3,71,86,99–102] treatments that improve oxygenation have not generally improved mortality.[17,29,103–106]

SCORING SYSTEMS FOR ALI PREDICTION

The most recent investigations have sought to create scoring systems that identify patients at risk for ALI early and thus create the potential for prospective prevention trials. Once again exploiting the Mayo Clinic database, Trillo-Alvarez and colleagues[107] identified a retrospective derivation cohort of ICU patients at risk for ALI in 2006, derived a lung injury prediction score (LIPS), and validated the score in a prospective cohort of at-risk patients admitted to the Mayo Clinic in 2008–2009. The LIPS includes 8 predisposing conditions and 7 risk modifiers and assigns weighted point values to each. In this initial single-center study, a LIPS of 3 or less discriminated well (specificity 0.84, negative predictive value 0.97) patients in the validation cohort with a low likelihood of developing ALI. Owing to the overall low incidence (0.07) of ALI in the validation cohort, the positive predictive value (0.24) of a LIPS greater than 3 was modest.

The recently formed US Critical Illness and Injury Trials Group (USCIITG) validated and refined the LIPS system by studying 5584 patients from 22 hospitals. This work reduced the predisposing conditions to 6 (shock, aspiration, sepsis, pneumonia, high-risk surgery, and high-risk trauma) and expanded the risk modifiers to 9 (alcohol abuse, obesity, hypoalbuminemia, chemotherapy, FiO_2 >0.35, tachypnea, SpO_2 <95%, acidemia, and diabetes mellitus). Performance of the refined LIPS was as follows for a LIPS greater than 4: area under the curve (AUC) 0.80, sensitivity 0.69, specificity 0.78, positive predictive value 0.18, and negative predictive value 0.97. Thus, a LIPS of 4 or less effectively rules out a serious concern for ALI, although a LIPS greater than 4 is poorly predictive of ALI. Such a scoring system may serve well as a tool for enrollment of patients in a prevention trial, although the present clinical utility of such a system is unclear.[108]

PROGRESSION OF ALI TO ARDS

Few studies have examined the important issue of how many patients presenting with ALI progress to ARDS over time. The Acute Lung Injury Verification of Epidemiology (ALIVE) study[86] was a 2-month inception cohort study performed in 78 ICUs of 10 European countries, in which all patients admitted for more than 4 hours were screened for ALI and followed for 2 months. ALI occurred in 463 (7.1%) of 6522 admissions and 16.1% of all mechanically ventilated patients, with 65.4% of cases present on ICU admission. Among 136 patients initially presenting with ALI, 74 patients (55%) evolved to ARDS within 3 days. The ICU and hospital mortality rates were 22.6% and 32.7% (P <.001) and 49.4% and 57.9% (P = .0005), respectively, for ALI and ARDS. Importantly, this study confirmed that more than half of patients admitted with ALI rapidly evolved to ARDS, and that mortality rates associated with ALI are significantly lower than those of patients with ARDS.

SPECIAL CATEGORIES OF ARDS/ALI

ARDS and 2009 Pandemic Influenza A H1N1

The epidemiology of ARDS owing to 2009 Influenza A (H1N1) infection is an ongoing story, with ICU admissions for patients with severe ARDS caused by H1N1 Influenza continuing in this past influenza season. Most patients diagnosed with H1N1 had a self-limited respiratory illness; however, among patients admitted to hospitals, 20% to 33% required ICU admission because of influenza-associated pneumonia and ARDS. The ICU admission rates recorded in Australasia[109] and Ireland[110] were 28.0 and 22.5 per million population, respectively.

At the University of Michigan, we noted that H1N1 pneumonia in some young healthy patients with no comorbidities evolved quickly to severe ARDS with refractory hypoxemia, necessitating transfer to our ARDS regional referral center. We reported[111] our first 10 patients with severe ARDS caused by H1N1 infection so that clinicians could be aware of the potential for H1N1 to cause severe hypoxemia and severe ARDS. We also noted that obesity was common (9 of 10) in these patients with severe ARDS. A recent meta-analysis (n = 3059) confirmed that severely obese H1N1 patients (body mass index BMI ≥40, n = 804) were twice as likely to be admitted to the ICU or die (OR 2.01, 95% CI 1.29–3.14, P <.002) compared with nonobese patients with H1N1.[112]

A number of worldwide reports of critically ill patients with H1N1 with acute respiratory failure or influenza-associated ARDS documented the severity of pulmonary disease, with fatal outcomes in many patients. Autopsy findings in 8 patients with severe ARDS caused by H1N1 at the University of Michigan confirmed severe hemorrhagic pneumonitis with diffuse alveolar damage in all patients, accompanied by acute bronchopneumonia in 6 patients (**Fig. 6**). Peripheral pulmonary vascular thrombosis was common (5 of 8 patients), and hemophagocytosis was present in all patients.[113]

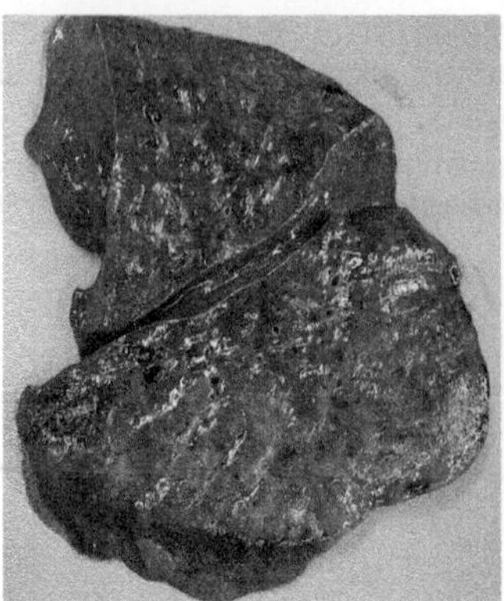
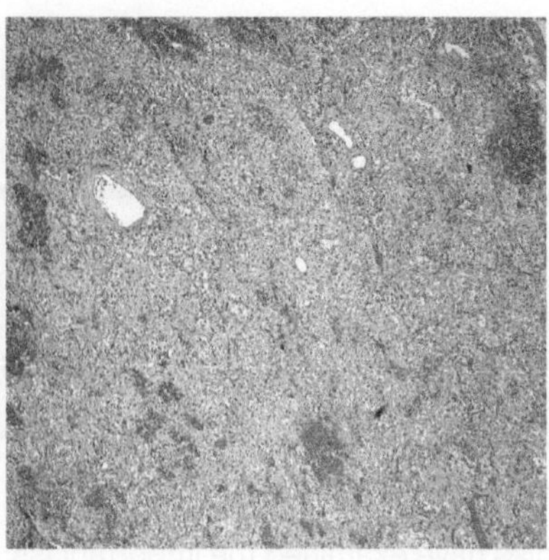

Fig. 6. Gross and microscopic findings at autopsy of a patient with H1N1-associated severe ARDS (from University of Michigan). Hemorrhagic pneumonitis with consolidation, edema, and premortem pulmonary thrombi in distal branches of the pulmonary arteries. Microscopy confirms proliferative organizing diffuse alveolar damage with recent hemorrhage. (Hematoxylin and Eosin (H&E) Stain 100 × Magnification).

Pathologic examination of 100 fatal cases in the United States by the Centers for Disease Control and Prevention confirmed that the most prominent histopathological feature observed was diffuse alveolar damage in the lung in all patients examined. Viral pneumonia and immunolocalization of the viral antigen in alveolar lining cells, including type I and type II pneumocytes, were identified, with bacterial coinfection identified in more than 25% of the patients.[114]

A review of adult mortality from H1N1 in California[115] documented that, of 486 cases hospitalized before death, 441 (91%) required ICU admission, and ICU case-fatality ratios among adults ranged from 24% to 42%, with the highest rates in persons 70 to 79 years old. Interestingly, a total of 425 cases (80%) had no comorbid conditions associated with severe seasonal influenza.

The report from Canada[116] included 168 critically ill patients (adults and children) with 162 confirmed and 6 probable H1N1 infections. All patients were hypoxemic (mean PaO_2/FiO_2 ratio 147, SD 128 mm Hg) at ICU admission, with mechanical ventilation required in 81% of patients, and median duration of ventilation 12 days (interquartile range [IQR] 6–20 days) with ICU length of stay 12 days (IQR 5–20 days), with frequent use of ALI/ARDS rescue strategies. The overall mortality rate was 14.3% at 28 days and 17.3% at 90 days.

Additional reports from other countries documented the high mortality rates of H1N1 patients requiring ICU admission (**Table 1**), ranging from 14% to 39%, although in many reports it is not clear how many of these ICU patients had ALI/ARDS. The variability in these mortality rates are likely related to the severity of the hypoxemia and to the variability and intensity of therapies provided for ARDS treatment. A report from Australia and New Zealand[117] included 68 patients with influenza-associated severe ARDS treated with extracorporeal membrane oxygenation (ECMO; 53 patients with confirmed H1N1, 8 confirmed Influenza A but not subtyped, 7 probable cases) and an additional 133 patients with Influenza A who received mechanical ventilation but no ECMO in the same ICUs. Of the 68 patients who received ECMO, 53 (78%) were weaned from ECMO and 15 (22%) died while receiving ECMO. Of the 53 patients weaned from ECMO, 2 others died in the ICU, with a final ICU and hospital mortality rate of 75%.

Table 1
Characteristics of ICU patients with 2009 influenza A H1N1

	Napolitano[111]	Perez-Padilla[128]	Rello[129]	Jain[130]	Webb[109]	Dominguez-Cherit[131]	Kumar[116]	Miller[132]	Nicolay[110]	Nin[133]
Location	US, Michigan	Mexico	Spain	US	Australia, New Zealand	Mexico	Canada	US, Utah	Ireland	Chile, Uruguay
n	10	18	32	67	722	58	168	47	77	96
PaO_2/FiO_2 ratio, (SD) or [range]	55 (12)	227 (31)	NR	NR	NR	83 [59–145]	147 (128)	122 [52–323]	NR	116 [73–220]
ARDS, n (%)	10 (100%)	7/17 (41%)	NR	24 (36%)	336/689[a] (49%)	NR	NR	30 (64%)	NR	69 (72%)
Age, years (SD) or [range]	46 [21–53]	38 [19–48]	36 [31–52]	29 [1–86]	40 [26–54]	44 [10–83]	32 (21)	34 [15–62]	43 [30–56]	45 (14)
ECMO, n (%)	2 (20%)	NR	0	NR	53 (7%)	0	7 (4%)	0	4 (5%)	0
Mortality, n (%)	3 (30%)	7 (39%)	6 (19%)	19 (28%)	103 (14%)	23 (40%)	24 (14%)	8 (17%)	14 (18%)	48 (50%)

[a] Study gives incidence of "acute respiratory distress syndrome or viral pneumonitis" as 49%.

A recent assessment by Riscilli and colleagues[118] of H1N1 Influenza–associated ARDS compared 23 cases with confirmed H1N1-associated ARDS with patients with non-H1N1 ARDS, reporting that patients with H1N1 were younger with higher body mass index (BMI), worse oxygenation, and increased severity of illness as measured by Sequential Organ Failure Assessment (SOFA) score. They[118] documented more frequent use of rescue therapies for severe ARDS, including prone ventilation, high-frequency oscillatory ventilation (HFOV), and ECMO in patients with H1N1. Furthermore, patients with H1N1 had higher lung injury scores (LIS) at presentation and over the course of the first 6 days of treatment when compared with patients with non–H1N1-associated ARDS, a finding associated with increased duration of mechanical ventilation.

Trauma

ARDS after trauma can have 2 distinct patterns,[119] with *early* postinjury ARDS related to the initial severity of hemorrhagic shock, the consequences of blood and crystalloid resuscitation, and directly to pulmonary contusion,[120] and *late* postinjury ARDS, which is more commonly related to hospital-acquired infections, including pneumonia and sepsis, and multiple organ failure. Interestingly, the development of ARDS in trauma patients has been associated with increased days of mechanical ventilation and increased ICU and hospital length of stay, but not with an increase in hospital mortality.[121,122]

Recent studies[123,124] have confirmed a significant decrease in the incidence of late posttraumatic ARDS. A single-center study from the Los Angeles County University of Southern California Trauma Center confirmed that late ARDS decreased from 14.9% to 3.8% over a 6-year period (**Fig. 7**), and that early transfusions, peak inspiratory pressure of 30 mm Hg or higher, and fluid balance of 2 L or more in the first 48 hours after admission were independently associated with ARDS.[125]

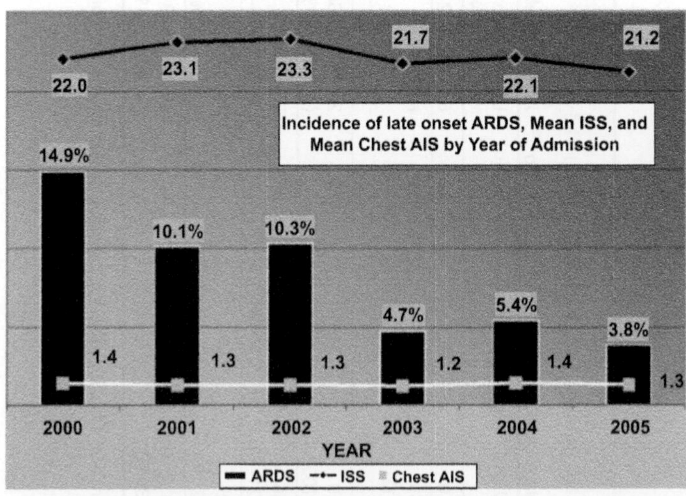

Fig. 7. Incidence of late posttraumatic ARDS (diagnosed after 48 hours of admission) by year of admission. The decrease in the incidence was statistically significant (P <.001 by chi-square) whereas change in Injury Severity Score (ISS) and Chest Abbreviated Injury Scale (AIS) was not significant (P = .2 and .595 by analysis of variance). (*From* Plurad D, Martin M, Green D, et al. The decreasing incidence of late posttraumatic acute respiratory distress syndrome: the potential role of lung protective ventilation and conservative transfusion practice. J Trauma 2007;63:1–7; with permission.)

SUMMARY

There has been a significant decline in the incidence of ARDS/ALI over the past decade. Despite this decline in incidence, ARDS-associated mortality rates remain high at approximately 40%. Increasingly sophisticated large cohort studies are helping to more sharply define risk and prognostic factors in an effort to improve both treatment and prevention protocols. Although ARDS and ALI can be caused by either *direct pulmonary causes* or *indirect extrapulmonary causes*, no difference in mortality has been identified. In trauma, ARDS incidence has also significantly declined, and ARDS has minimal impact on overall outcome. Severe ARDS and critical illness owing to the 2009 Influenza A (H1N1) virus often occurred in young adults, particularly with obesity, and was associated with severe hypoxemia, multisystem organ failure, and high mortality rates. Additional studies are needed to further investigate the epidemiology of ARDS in specific patient populations, because a detailed understanding of the epidemiology and outcomes of ARDS is essential for future research.

REFERENCES

1. Ashbaugh DG, Bigelow DB, Petty TL, et al. Acute respiratory distress in adults. Lancet 1967;2(7511):319–23.
2. Bernard GR, Artigas A, Brigham KL, et al. The American-European Consensus Conference on ARDS. Definitions, mechanisms, relevant outcomes, and clinical trial coordination. Am J Respir Crit Care Med 1994;149(3 Pt 1):818–24.
3. Villar J, Perez-Mendez L, Lopez J, et al. An early PEEP/FIO2 trial identifies different degrees of lung injury in patients with acute respiratory distress syndrome. Am J Respir Crit Care Med 2007;176(8):795–804.
4. Rubenfeld GD, Caldwell E, Granton J, et al. Interobserver variability in applying a radiographic definition for ARDS. Chest 1999;116(5):1347–53.
5. Meade MO, Cook RJ, Guyatt GH, et al. Interobserver variation in interpreting chest radiographs for the diagnosis of acute respiratory distress syndrome. Am J Respir Crit Care Med 2000;161(1):85–90.
6. Wiener RS, Welch HG. Trends in the use of the pulmonary artery catheter in the United States, 1993–2004. JAMA 2007;298(4):423–9.
7. Esteban A, Fernandez-Segoviano P, Frutos-Vivar F, et al. Comparison of clinical criteria for the acute respiratory distress syndrome with autopsy findings. Ann Intern Med 2004;141(6):440–5.
8. NHLBI Ards Network Web site. Available at: http://www.ardsnet.org/. Accessed April 21, 2011.
9. Villar J, Slutsky AS. The incidence of the adult respiratory distress syndrome. Am Rev Respir Dis 1989;140(3):814–6.
10. Lewandowski K, Metz J, Deutschmann C, et al. Incidence, severity, and mortality of acute respiratory failure in Berlin, Germany. Am J Respir Crit Care Med 1995;151(4):1121–5.
11. Thomsen GE, Morris AH. Incidence of the adult respiratory distress syndrome in the state of Utah. Am J Respir Crit Care Med 1995;152(3):965–71.
12. Luhr OR, Antonsen K, Karlsson M, et al. Incidence and mortality after acute respiratory failure and acute respiratory distress syndrome in Sweden, Denmark, and Iceland. The ARF Study Group. Am J Respir Crit Care Med 1999;159(6):1849–61.
13. Arroliga AC, Ghamra ZW, Perez Trepichio A, et al. Incidence of ARDS in an adult population of northeast Ohio. Chest 2002;121(6):1972–6.

14. Bersten AD, Edibam C, Hunt T, et al. Incidence and mortality of acute lung injury and the acute respiratory distress syndrome in three Australian States. Am J Respir Crit Care Med 2002;165(4):443–8.
15. Reynolds HN, McCunn M, Borg U, et al. Acute respiratory distress syndrome: estimated incidence and mortality rate in a 5 million-person population base. Crit Care 1998;2(1):29–34.
16. Goss CH, Brower RG, Hudson LD, et al. Incidence of acute lung injury in the United States. Crit Care Med 2003;31(6):1607–11.
17. Ventilation with lower tidal volumes as compared with traditional tidal volumes for acute lung injury and the acute respiratory distress syndrome. The Acute Respiratory Distress Syndrome Network. N Engl J Med 2000;342(18):1301–8.
18. Rubenfeld GD, Caldwell E, Peabody E, et al. Incidence and outcomes of acute lung injury. N Engl J Med 2005;353(16):1685–93.
19. Li G, Malinchoc M, Cartin-Ceba R, et al. Eight-year trend of acute respiratory distress syndrome: a population-based study in Olmsted County, Minnesota. Am J Respir Crit Care Med 2011;183(1):59–66.
20. Milberg JA, Davis DR, Steinberg KP, et al. Improved survival of patients with acute respiratory distress syndrome (ARDS): 1983–1993. JAMA 1995;273(4):306–9.
21. Abel SJ, Finney SJ, Brett SJ, et al. Reduced mortality in association with the acute respiratory distress syndrome (ARDS). Thorax 1998;53(4):292–4.
22. Jardin F, Fellahi JL, Beauchet A, et al. Improved prognosis of acute respiratory distress syndrome 15 years on. Intensive Care Med 1999;25(9):936–41.
23. Navarrete-Navarro P, Rodriguez A, Reynolds N, et al. Acute respiratory distress syndrome among trauma patients: trends in ICU mortality, risk factors, complications and resource utilization. Intensive Care Med 2001;27(7):1133–40.
24. Rocco TR Jr, Reinert SE, Cioffi W, et al. A 9-year, single-institution, retrospective review of death rate and prognostic factors in adult respiratory distress syndrome. Ann Surg 2001;233(3):414–22.
25. Stapleton RD, Wang BM, Hudson LD, et al. Causes and timing of death in patients with ARDS. Chest 2005;128(2):525–32.
26. Krafft P, Fridrich P, Pernerstorfer T, et al. The acute respiratory distress syndrome: definitions, severity and clinical outcome. An analysis of 101 clinical investigations. Intensive Care Med 1996;22(6):519–29.
27. Kallet RH, Jasmer RM, Pittet JF, et al. Clinical implementation of the ARDS network protocol is associated with reduced hospital mortality compared with historical controls. Crit Care Med 2005;33(5):925–9.
28. Erickson SE, Martin GS, Davis JL, et al. Recent trends in acute lung injury mortality: 1996–2005. Crit Care Med 2009;37(5):1574–9.
29. Brower RG, Lanken PN, MacIntyre N, et al. Higher versus lower positive end-expiratory pressures in patients with the acute respiratory distress syndrome. N Engl J Med 2004;351(4):327–36.
30. Wiedemann HP, Wheeler AP, Bernard GR, et al. Comparison of two fluid-management strategies in acute lung injury. N Engl J Med 2006;354(24):2564–75.
31. Spragg RG, Bernard GR, Checkley W, et al. Beyond mortality: future clinical research in acute lung injury. Am J Respir Crit Care Med 2010;181(10):1121–7.
32. Zambon M, Vincent JL. Mortality rates for patients with acute lung injury/ARDS have decreased over time. Chest 2008;133(5):1120–7.
33. Phua J, Badia JR, Adhikari NK, et al. Has mortality from acute respiratory distress syndrome decreased over time? A systematic review. Am J Respir Crit Care Med 2009;179(3):220–7.

34. Zambon M, Vincent JL. Are outcomes improving in patients with ARDS? Am J Respir Crit Care Med 2009;180(11):1158–9 [author reply: 1159].
35. Brochard L, Rouby JJ. Changing mortality in acute respiratory distress syndrome? Yes, we can! Am J Respir Crit Care Med 2009;179(3):177–8.
36. Garber BG, Hebert PC, Yelle JD, et al. Adult respiratory distress syndrome: a systemic overview of incidence and risk factors. Crit Care Med 1996;24(4): 687–95.
37. Pelosi P, Caironi P, Gattinoni L. Pulmonary and extrapulmonary forms of acute respiratory distress syndrome. Semin Respir Crit Care Med 2001;22(3):259–68.
38. Pelosi P, D'Onofrio D, Chiumello D, et al. Pulmonary and extrapulmonary acute respiratory distress syndrome are different. Eur Respir J Suppl 2003;42:48s–56s.
39. Agarwal R, Srinivas R, Nath A, et al. Is the mortality higher in the pulmonary vs the extrapulmonary ARDS? A meta analysis. Chest 2008;133(6):1463–73.
40. Sheu CC, Gong MN, Zhai R, et al. The influence of infection sites on development and mortality of ARDS. Intensive Care Med 2010;36(6):963–70.
41. Messent M, Sullivan K, Keogh BF, et al. Adult respiratory distress syndrome following cardiopulmonary bypass: incidence and prediction. Anaesthesia 1992;47(3):267–8.
42. Towfigh S, Peralta MV, Martin MJ, et al. Acute respiratory distress syndrome in nontrauma surgical patients: a 6-year study. J Trauma 2009;67(6):1239–43.
43. Dancey DR, Hayes J, Gomez M, et al. ARDS in patients with thermal injury. Intensive Care Med 1999;25(11):1231–6.
44. Shorr AF, Abbott KC, Agadoa LY. Acute respiratory distress syndrome after kidney transplantation: epidemiology, risk factors, and outcomes. Crit Care Med 2003;31(5):1325–30.
45. Kahn JM, Caldwell EC, Deem S, et al. Acute lung injury in patients with subarachnoid hemorrhage: incidence, risk factors, and outcome. Crit Care Med 2006; 34(1):196–202.
46. Rhee CK, Kang JY, Kim YH, et al. Risk factors for acute respiratory distress syndrome during neutropenia recovery in patients with hematologic malignancies. Crit Care 2009;13(6):R173.
47. Suchyta MR, Clemmer TP, Elliott CG, et al. Increased mortality of older patients with acute respiratory distress syndrome. Chest 1997;111(5):1334–9.
48. Ely EW, Wheeler AP, Thompson BT, et al. Recovery rate and prognosis in older persons who develop acute lung injury and the acute respiratory distress syndrome. Ann Intern Med 2002;136(1):25–36.
49. Eachempati SR, Hydo LJ, Shou J, et al. Outcomes of acute respiratory distress syndrome (ARDS) in elderly patients. J Trauma 2007;63(2):344–50.
50. Johnston CJ, Rubenfeld GD, Hudson LD. Effect of age on the development of ARDS in trauma patients. Chest 2003;124(2):653–9.
51. Toba A, Yamazaki M, Mochizuki H, et al. Lower incidence of acute respiratory distress syndrome in community-acquired pneumonia patients aged 85 years or older. Respirology 2010;15(2):319–25.
52. Moss M, Mannino DM. Race and gender differences in acute respiratory distress syndrome deaths in the United States: an analysis of multiple-cause mortality data (1979–1996). Crit Care Med 2002;30(8):1679–85.
53. Ryb GE, Cooper C. Race/ethnicity and acute respiratory distress syndrome: a National Trauma Data Bank study. J Natl Med Assoc 2010;102(10):865–9.
54. Moss M, Bucher B, Moore FA, et al. The role of chronic alcohol abuse in the development of acute respiratory distress syndrome in adults. JAMA 1996; 275(1):50–4.

55. Moss M, Steinberg KP, Guidot DM, et al. The effect of chronic alcohol abuse on the incidence of ARDS and the severity of the multiple organ dysfunction syndrome in adults with septic shock: an interim and multivariate analysis. Chest 1999;116(Suppl 1):97S–8S.
56. Moss M, Parsons PE, Steinberg KP, et al. Chronic alcohol abuse is associated with an increased incidence of acute respiratory distress syndrome and severity of multiple organ dysfunction in patients with septic shock. Crit Care Med 2003; 31(3):869–77.
57. Thakur L, Kojicic M, Thakur SJ, et al. Alcohol consumption and development of acute respiratory distress syndrome: a population-based study. Int J Environ Res Public Health 2009;6(9):2426–35.
58. Yeh MY, Burnham EL, Moss M, et al. Chronic alcoholism alters systemic and pulmonary glutathione redox status. Am J Respir Crit Care Med 2007;176(3):270–6.
59. Berkowitz DM, Danai PA, Eaton S, et al. Alcohol abuse enhances pulmonary edema in acute respiratory distress syndrome. Alcohol Clin Exp Res 2009; 33(10):1690–6.
60. Iribarren C, Jacobs DR Jr, Sidney S, et al. Cigarette smoking, alcohol consumption, and risk of ARDS: a 15-year cohort study in a managed care setting. Chest 2000;117(1):163–8.
61. Calfee CS, Matthay MA, Eisner MD, et al. Active and passive cigarette smoking and acute lung injury following severe blunt trauma. Am J Respir Crit Care Med 2011. [Epub ahead of print].
62. Rubenfeld GD, Herridge MS. Epidemiology and outcomes of acute lung injury. Chest 2007;131(2):554–62.
63. Gong MN, Bajwa EK, Thompson BT, et al. Body mass index is associated with the development of acute respiratory distress syndrome. Thorax 2010; 65(1):44–50.
64. Anzueto A, Frutos-Vivar F, Esteban A, et al. Influence of body mass index on outcome of the mechanically ventilated patients. Thorax 2011;66(1):66–73.
65. O'Brien JM Jr, Welsh CH, Fish RH, et al. Excess body weight is not independently associated with outcome in mechanically ventilated patients with acute lung injury. Ann Intern Med 2004;140(5):338–45.
66. O'Brien JM Jr, Phillips GS, Ali NA, et al. Body mass index is independently associated with hospital mortality in mechanically ventilated adults with acute lung injury. Crit Care Med 2006;34(3):738–44.
67. Moss M, Guidot DM, Steinberg KP, et al. Diabetic patients have a decreased incidence of acute respiratory distress syndrome. Crit Care Med 2000;28(7):2187–92.
68. Honiden S, Gong MN. Diabetes, insulin, and development of acute lung injury. Crit Care Med 2009;37(8):2455–64.
69. Erlich JM, Talmor DS, Cartin-Ceba R, et al. Prehospitalization antiplatelet therapy is associated with a reduced incidence of acute lung injury: a population-based cohort study. Chest 2011;139(2):289–95.
70. Gajic O, Dara SI, Mendez JL, et al. Ventilator-associated lung injury in patients without acute lung injury at the onset of mechanical ventilation. Crit Care Med 2004;32(9):1817–24.
71. Esteban A, Anzueto A, Frutos F, et al. Characteristics and outcomes in adult patients receiving mechanical ventilation: a 28-day international study. JAMA 2002;287(3):345–55.
72. Gajic O, Frutos-Vivar F, Esteban A, et al. Ventilator settings as a risk factor for acute respiratory distress syndrome in mechanically ventilated patients. Intensive Care Med 2005;31(7):922–6.

73. Jia X, Malhotra A, Saeed M, et al. Risk factors for ARDS in patients receiving mechanical ventilation for >48 h. Chest 2008;133(4):853–61.
74. Determann RM, Royakkers A, Wolthuis EK, et al. Ventilation with lower tidal volumes as compared with conventional tidal volumes for patients without acute lung injury: a preventive randomized controlled trial. Crit Care 2010; 14(1):R1.
75. Gajic O, Rana R, Mendez JL, et al. Acute lung injury after blood transfusion in mechanically ventilated patients. Transfusion 2004;44(10):1468–74.
76. Gong MN, Thompson BT, Williams P, et al. Clinical predictors of and mortality in acute respiratory distress syndrome: potential role of red cell transfusion. Crit Care Med 2005;33(6):1191–8.
77. Silverboard H, Aisiku I, Martin GS, et al. The role of acute blood transfusion in the development of acute respiratory distress syndrome in patients with severe trauma. J Trauma 2005;59(3):717–23.
78. Toy P, Popovsky MA, Abraham E, et al. Transfusion-related acute lung injury: definition and review. Crit Care Med 2005;33(4):721–6.
79. Rana R, Fernandez-Perez ER, Khan SA, et al. Transfusion-related acute lung injury and pulmonary edema in critically ill patients: a retrospective study. Transfusion 2006;46(9):1478–83.
80. Khan H, Belsher J, Yilmaz M, et al. Fresh-frozen plasma and platelet transfusions are associated with development of acute lung injury in critically ill medical patients. Chest 2007;131(5):1308–14.
81. Gajic O, Rana R, Winters JL, et al. Transfusion-related acute lung injury in the critically ill: prospective nested case-control study. Am J Respir Crit Care Med 2007;176(9):886–91.
82. Zilberberg MD, Carter C, Lefebvre P, et al. Red blood cell transfusions and the risk of acute respiratory distress syndrome among the critically ill: a cohort study. Crit Care 2007;11(3):R63.
83. Chaiwat O, Lang JD, Vavilala MS, et al. Early packed red blood cell transfusion and acute respiratory distress syndrome after trauma. Anesthesiology 2009; 110(2):351–60.
84. Yilmaz M, Keegan MT, Iscimen R, et al. Toward the prevention of acute lung injury: protocol-guided limitation of large tidal volume ventilation and inappropriate transfusion. Crit Care Med 2007;35(7):1660–6 [quiz: 1667].
85. Iscimen R, Cartin-Ceba R, Yilmaz M, et al. Risk factors for the development of acute lung injury in patients with septic shock: an observational cohort study. Crit Care Med 2008;36(5):1518–22.
86. Brun-Buisson C, Minelli C, Bertolini G, et al. Epidemiology and outcome of acute lung injury in European intensive care units. Results from the ALIVE study. Intensive Care Med 2004;30(1):51–61.
87. Luhr OR, Karlsson M, Thorsteinsson A, et al. The impact of respiratory variables on mortality in non-ARDS and ARDS patients requiring mechanical ventilation. Intensive Care Med 2000;26(5):508–17.
88. Sheu CC, Gong MN, Zhai R, et al. Clinical characteristics and outcomes of sepsis-related vs non-sepsis-related ARDS. Chest 2010;138(3):559–67.
89. Nuckton TJ, Alonso JA, Kallet RH, et al. Pulmonary dead-space fraction as a risk factor for death in the acute respiratory distress syndrome. N Engl J Med 2002; 346(17):1281–6.
90. Lucangelo U, Bernabe F, Vatua S, et al. Prognostic value of different dead space indices in mechanically ventilated patients with acute lung injury and ARDS. Chest 2008;133(1):62–71.

91. Siddiki H, Kojicic M, Li G, et al. Bedside quantification of dead-space fraction using routine clinical data in patients with acute lung injury: secondary analysis of two prospective trials. Crit Care 2010;14(4):R141.
92. Bull TM, Clark B, McFann K, et al. Pulmonary vascular dysfunction is associated with poor outcomes in patients with acute lung injury. Am J Respir Crit Care Med 2010;182(9):1123–8.
93. Mangialardi RJ, Martin GS, Bernard GR, et al. Hypoproteinemia predicts acute respiratory distress syndrome development, weight gain, and death in patients with sepsis. Ibuprofen in Sepsis Study Group. Crit Care Med 2000;28(9):3137–45.
94. Zhai R, Sheu CC, Su L, et al. Serum bilirubin levels on ICU admission are associated with ARDS development and mortality in sepsis. Thorax 2009;64(9): 784–90.
95. Levitt JE, Gould MK, Ware LB, et al. The pathogenetic and prognostic value of biologic markers in acute lung injury. J Intensive Care Med 2009;24(3):151–67.
96. Ware LB. Prognostic determinants of acute respiratory distress syndrome in adults: impact on clinical trial design. Crit Care Med 2005;33(Suppl 3):S217–22.
97. Ware LB, Koyama T, Billheimer DD, et al. Prognostic and pathogenetic value of combining clinical and biochemical indices in patients with acute lung injury. Chest 2010;137(2):288–96.
98. Calfee CS, Ware LB, Glidden DV, et al. Use of risk reclassification with multiple biomarkers improves mortality prediction in acute lung injury. Crit Care Med 2011. [Epub ahead of print].
99. Cooke CR, Kahn JM, Caldwell E, et al. Predictors of hospital mortality in a population-based cohort of patients with acute lung injury. Crit Care Med 2008; 36(5):1412–20.
100. Gajic O, Afessa B, Thompson BT, et al. Prediction of death and prolonged mechanical ventilation in acute lung injury. Crit Care 2007;11(3):R53.
101. Seeley E, McAuley DF, Eisner M, et al. Predictors of mortality in acute lung injury during the era of lung protective ventilation. Thorax 2008;63(11):994–8.
102. Villar J, Perez-Mendez L, Basaldua S, et al. Age, plateau pressure and PaO2/FIO2 at ARDS onset predict outcome. Respir Care 2011;56(4):420–8.
103. Gattinoni L, Tognoni G, Pesenti A, et al. Effect of prone positioning on the survival of patients with acute respiratory failure. N Engl J Med 2001;345(8):568–73.
104. Meade MO, Cook DJ, Guyatt GH, et al. Ventilation strategy using low tidal volumes, recruitment maneuvers, and high positive end-expiratory pressure for acute lung injury and acute respiratory distress syndrome: a randomized controlled trial. JAMA 2008;299(6):637–45.
105. Mercat A, Richard JC, Vielle B, et al. Positive end-expiratory pressure setting in adults with acute lung injury and acute respiratory distress syndrome: a randomized controlled trial. JAMA 2008;299(6):646–55.
106. Taylor RW, Zimmerman JL, Dellinger RP, et al. Low-dose inhaled nitric oxide in patients with acute lung injury: a randomized controlled trial. JAMA 2004; 291(13):1603–9.
107. Trillo-Alvarez C, Cartin-Ceba R, Kor DJ, et al. Acute lung injury prediction score: derivation and validation in a population-based sample. Eur Respir J 2011; 37(3):604–9.
108. Gajic O, Dabbagh O, Park PK, et al. Early identification of patients at risk of acute lung injury: evaluation of lung injury prediction score in a multicenter cohort study. Am J Respir Crit Care Med 2011;183(4):462–70.
109. Webb SA, Pettila V, Seppelt I, et al. Critical care services and 2009 H1N1 influenza in Australia and New Zealand. N Engl J Med 2009;361(20):1925–34.

110. Nicolay N, Callaghan MA, Domegan LM, et al. Epidemiology, clinical characteristics and resource implications of pandemic (H1N1) 2009 in intensive care units in Ireland. Crit Care Resusc 2010;12(4):255–61.
111. Centers for Disease Control and Prevention (CDC). Intensive-care patients with severe novel influenza A (H1N1) virus infection—Michigan, June 2009. MMWR Morb Mortal Wkly Rep 2009;58(27):749–52.
112. Fezeu L, Julia C, Henegar A, et al. Obesity is associated with higher risk of intensive care unit admission and death in influenza A (H1N1) patients: a systematic review and meta-analysis. Obes Rev 2011. [Epub ahead of print].
113. Harms PW, Schmidt LA, Smith LB, et al. Autopsy findings in eight patients with fatal H1N1 influenza. Am J Clin Pathol 2010;134(1):27–35.
114. Shieh WJ, Blau DM, Denison AM, et al. 2009 pandemic influenza A (H1N1): pathology and pathogenesis of 100 fatal cases in the United States. Am J Pathol 2010;177(1):166–75.
115. Louie JK, Jean C, Acosta M, et al. A review of adult mortality due to 2009 pandemic (H1N1) influenza A in California. PLoS One 2011;6(4):e18221.
116. Kumar A, Zarychanski R, Pinto R, et al. Critically ill patients with 2009 influenza A (H1N1) infection in Canada. JAMA 2009;302(17):1872–9.
117. Davies A, Jones D, Bailey M, et al. Extracorporeal membrane oxygenation for 2009 Influenza A(H1N1) acute respiratory distress syndrome. JAMA 2009; 302(17):1888–95.
118. Riscili BP, Anderson TB, Prescott HC, et al. An assessment of H1N1 influenza-associated acute respiratory distress syndrome severity after adjustment for treatment characteristics. PLoS One 2011;6(3):e18166.
119. Croce MA, Fabian TC, Davis KA, et al. Early and late acute respiratory distress syndrome: two distinct clinical entities. J Trauma 1999;46(3):361–6 [discussion: 366–8].
120. Miller PR, Croce MA, Bee TK, et al. ARDS after pulmonary contusion: accurate measurement of contusion volume identifies high-risk patients. J Trauma 2001; 51(2):223–8 [discussion: 229–30].
121. Treggiari MM, Hudson LD, Martin DP, et al. Effect of acute lung injury and acute respiratory distress syndrome on outcome in critically ill trauma patients. Crit Care Med 2004;32(2):327–31.
122. McClintock DE, Matthay MA. Why does acute lung injury have no impact on mortality in patients with major trauma? Crit Care Med 2004;32(2):583–4.
123. Martin M, Salim A, Murray J, et al. The decreasing incidence and mortality of acute respiratory distress syndrome after injury: a 5-year observational study. J Trauma 2005;59(5):1107–13.
124. Ciesla DJ, Moore EE, Johnson JL, et al. Decreased progression of postinjury lung dysfunction to the acute respiratory distress syndrome and multiple organ failure. Surgery 2006;140(4):640–7 [discussion: 647–8].
125. Plurad D, Martin M, Green D, et al. The decreasing incidence of late posttraumatic acute respiratory distress syndrome: the potential role of lung protective ventilation and conservative transfusion practice. J Trauma 2007;63(1):1–7 [discussion: 8].
126. Matthay M, Brower R, Thompson B, et al. Randomized, placebo-controlled trial of an aerosolized beta-2 adrenergic agonist (Albuterol) for the treatment of acute lung injury. Am J Respir Crit Care Med 2009;179:A2166.
127. Rice T, Thompson B, Smoot E, et al. Omega-3 (n-3) fatty acid, gamma-linolenic acid (GLA) and anti-oxidant supplementation in acute lung injury (OMEGA trial). Crit Care Med 2009;37:A408.

128. Perez-Padilla R, de la Rosa-Zamboni D, Ponce de Leon S, et al. Pneumonia and respiratory failure from swine-origin influenza A (H1N1) in Mexico. N Engl J Med 2009;361(7):680–9.
129. Rello J, Rodriguez A, Ibanez P, et al. Intensive care adult patients with severe respiratory failure caused by Influenza A (H1N1)v in Spain. Crit Care 2009; 13(5):R148.
130. Jain S, Kamimoto L, Bramley AM, et al. Hospitalized patients with 2009 H1N1 influenza in the United States, April-June 2009. N Engl J Med 2009;361(20): 1935–44.
131. Dominguez-Cherit G, Lapinsky SE, Macias AE, et al. Critically Ill patients with 2009 influenza A (H1N1) in Mexico. JAMA 2009;302(17):1880–7.
132. Miller RR 3rd, Markewitz BA, Rolfs RT, et al. Clinical findings and demographic factors associated with ICU admission in Utah due to novel 2009 influenza A (H1N1) infection. Chest 2010;137(4):752–8.
133. Nin N, Soto L, Hurtado J, et al. Clinical characteristics and outcomes of patients with 2009 influenza A (H1N1) virus infection with respiratory failure requiring mechanical ventilation. J Crit Care 2011;26(2):186–92.

ARDS Network (NHLBI) Studies: Successes and Challenges in ARDS Clinical Research

B. Taylor Thompson, MD[a,*], Gordon R. Bernard, MD[b]

KEYWORDS

- Acute respiratory distress syndrome • ARDS Network
- Acute lung injury • Clinical trials • Multicenter

HISTORY AND GOAL OF THE ARDS NETWORK

To hasten the development of effective therapy for acute respiratory distress syndrome (ARDS), the National Heart, Lung, and Blood Institute (NHLBI), National Institutes of Health, initiated a clinical network to carry out multicenter clinical trials of ARDS treatments. The ARDS Network was established as a contract program in 1994 following a national competition.

The ARDS Network is a clinical research network of approximately 42 hospitals, organized into 12 clinical sites, and a Clinical Coordinating Center (Massachusetts General Hospital; David Schoenfeld, PhD and B. Taylor Thompson, MD) (**Box 1**). The Principal Investigators from each site together with the NHLBI Project Scientist (Andrea Harabin, PhD) form the Network Steering Committee, the main governing body of the Network. The Steering Committee (Gordon Bernard, MD, Steering Committee Chair) is responsible for identification of promising new agents for the treatment of ARDS, setting Network priorities, developing protocols, facilitating the conduct and monitoring of the trials, and reporting study results. A Protocol Review Committee provides an independent scientific evaluation for the NHLBI on each new protocol. The Data and Safety Monitoring Board (DSMB) monitors the conduct of the trial and advises the NHLBI on the quality of the trial, and may suggest early termination of the study either for unanticipated large beneficial effects or for safety concerns.

[a] Medical Intensive Care Unit, Harvard Medical School, Massachusetts General Hospital, 55 Fruit Street, BUL 148, Boston, MA 02114-2696, USA
[b] Vanderbilt University Medical Center, Vanderbilt University School of Medicine, T-1028 MCN 2650, Nashville, TN 37232, USA
* Corresponding author.
E-mail address: TTHOMPSON1@PARTNERS.ORG

Crit Care Clin 27 (2011) 459–468
doi:10.1016/j.ccc.2011.05.011 **criticalcare.theclinics.com**

Box 1
National Heart Lung and Blood Institute ARDS Clinical Trials Network principal investigators and their associated network centers

Jay Steingrub, MD
 Baystate Medical Center, Massachusetts

Herb Wiedemann, MD
 Cleveland Clinic

Neil McIntyre, MD
 Duke University

Ben Deboisblanc, MD
 Louisiana State University

Michael Matthay, MD
 University of California San Francisco

Marc Moss, MD
 University of Colorado

Roy Brower, MD
 Johns Hopkins, University of Maryland

Alan Morris, MD
 University of Utah

Jon Truwit, MD
 University of Virginia

Terri Hough, MD
 University of Washington

Art Wheeler, MD
 Vanderbilt University

Duncan Hite, MD
 Wake Forest University

Coordinating Center

David Schoenfeld, PhD
 Massachusetts General Hospital

From ARDSNET.org; with permission.

The goal of the Network is to efficiently test promising agents, devices, or management strategies to improve the care of patients with ARDS. The ARDS Network has been a pivotal significant advance in the conduct of groundbreaking clinical research in acute lung injury (ALI) and ARDS, and several important questions regarding optimal clinical care of these patients have been answered while the results of the ongoing trials are awaited.

The significant success of this multicenter clinical trial network for ARDS is documented by the significant number of patients enrolled in the first ARDSNet clinical trials (**Fig. 1**). Comprehensive information, including the clinical study protocols, regarding

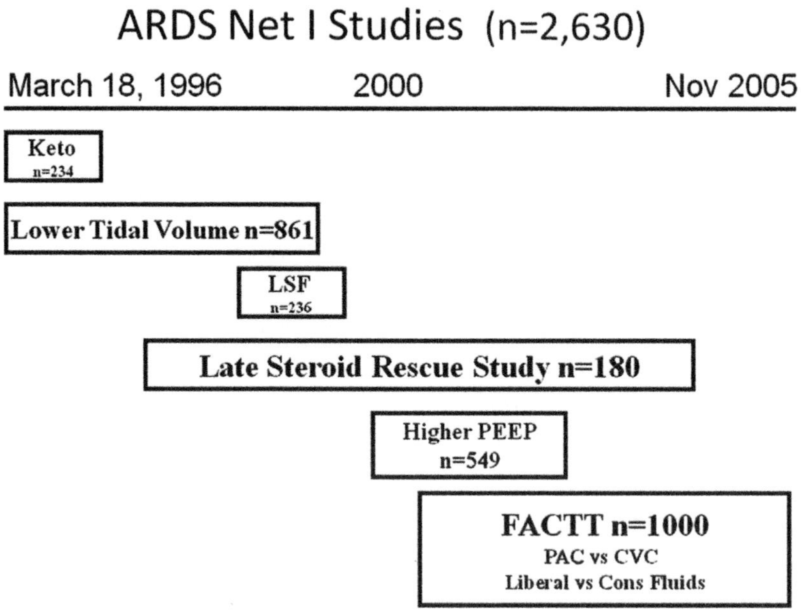

ARDS Net I Studies (n=2,630)

March 18, 1996 — 2000 — Nov 2005

Keto n=234

Lower Tidal Volume n=861

LSF n=236

Late Steroid Rescue Study n=180

Higher PEEP n=549

FACTT n=1000
PAC vs CVC
Liberal vs Cons Fluids

Fig. 1. Patient enrollment in the ARDS Network multicenter clinical trials from 1996 through 2005.

all of the completed and ongoing clinical trials is available on the Web site at www.ardsnet.org, but a brief summary of the ARDSNet clinical trials is provided here.

KETOCONAZOLE FOR ALI/ARDS

Study status: Completed.

Study dates: March 1996 to February 1998.

The first clinical trial completed by the Network was a randomized, controlled trial of ketoconazole versus placebo in patients with ALI and ARDS. Ketoconazole was chosen because of its anti-inflammatory actions noted in the laboratory and because previous phase 2 clinical trials suggested benefit in patients with or at risk for ARDS. This trial was stopped early by the DSMB in January 1997 after finding ketoconazole to be ineffective.[1]

LOWER TIDAL VOLUME TRIAL

Study status: Completed.

Study dates: March 1996 to July 1999.

This landmark third trial examined lower tidal volume ventilation versus a traditionally recommended larger tidal volume approach in patients with ALI. This trial was undertaken because extensive animal studies and 2 small clinical trials suggested lung stretch with larger tidal volumes may injure the lung or prevent recovery. However, 2 other clinical trials raised questions about this hypothesis, and the use of smaller tidal volumes is not always easy to do. The ARMA study was a randomized, controlled multicenter 2 $\times$ 2 factorial study consisting of a drug treatment (ketoconazole vs placebo) and a ventilation strategy (6 mL/kg tidal volume vs 12 mL/kg tidal volume). The ventilator arm of the protocol was designed to compare different ventilator strategies (**Fig. 2**) and their effect on mortality and morbidity. The lower tidal volume

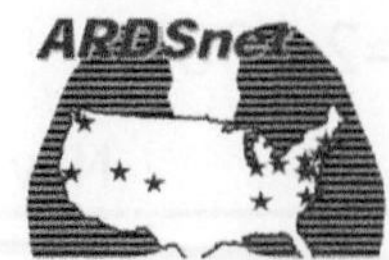

NIH NHLBI ARDS Clinical Network
Mechanical Ventilation Protocol Summary

INCLUSION CRITERIA: Acute onset of

1. $PaO_2/FiO_2 \le 300$ (corrected for altitude)
2. Bilateral (patchy, diffuse, or homogeneous) infiltrates consistent with pulmonary edema
3. No clinical evidence of left atrial hypertension

PART I: VENTILATOR SETUP AND ADJUSTMENT

1. Calculate predicted body weight (PBW)
   Males = 50 + 2.3 [height (inches) - 60]
   Females = 45.5 + 2.3 [height (inches) -60]
2. Select any ventilator mode
3. Set ventilator settings to achieve initial V_T = 8 ml/kg PBW
4. Reduce V_T by 1 ml/kg at intervals ≤ 2 hours until V_T = 6ml/kg PBW.
5. Set initial rate to approximate baseline minute ventilation (not > 35 bpm).
6. Adjust V_T and RR to achieve pH and plateau pressure goals below.

pH GOAL: 7.30-7.45
Acidosis Management: (pH < 7.30)
If pH 7.15-7.30: Increase RR until pH > 7.30 or $PaCO_2$ < 25 (Maximum set RR = 35).
If pH < 7.15: Increase RR to 35.
If pH remains < 7.15, V_T may be increased in 1 ml/kg steps until pH > 7.15 (Pplat target of 30 may be exceeded).
May give $NaHCO_3$
Alkalosis Management: (pH > 7.45) Decrease vent rate if possible.

I: E RATIO GOAL: Recommend that duration of inspiration be ≤ duration of expiration.

PART II: WEANING

A. Conduct a SPONTANEOUS BREATHING TRIAL daily when:

1. $FiO_2 \le 0.40$ and PEEP ≤ 8.
2. PEEP and FiO_2 ≤ values of previous day.
3. Patient has acceptable spontaneous breathing efforts. (May decrease vent rate by 50% for 5 minutes to detect effort.)
4. Systolic BP ≥ 90 mmHg without vasopressor support.
5. No neuromuscular blocking agents or blockade.

OXYGENATION GOAL: PaO_2 55-80 mmHg or SpO_2 88-95%
Use a minimum PEEP of 5 cm H_2O. Consider use of incremental FiO_2/PEEP combinations such as shown below (not required) to achieve goal.

Lower PEEP/higher FIO2

FIO_2	0.3	0.4	0.4	0.5	0.5	0.6	0.7	0.7
PEEP	5	5	8	8	10	10	10	12

FIO_2	0.7	0.8	0.9	0.9	0.9	1.0
PEEP	14	14	14	16	18	18-24

Higher PEEP/lower FIO2

FIO_2	0.3	0.3	0.3	0.3	0.3	0.4	0.4	0.5
PEEP	5	8	10	12	14	14	16	16

FIO_2	0.5	0.5-0.8	0.8	0.9	1.0	1.0
PEEP	18	20	22	22	22	24

PLATEAU PRESSURE GOAL: ≤ 30 cm H_2O
Check Pplat (0.5 second inspiratory pause), at least q 4h and after each change in PEEP or V_T.
If Pplat > 30 cm H_2O: decrease V_T by 1ml/kg steps (minimum = 4 ml/kg).
If Pplat < 25 cm H_2O and V_T< 6 ml/kg, increase V_T by 1 ml/kg until Pplat > 25 cm H_2O or V_T = 6 ml/kg.
If Pplat < 30 and breath stacking or dys-synchrony occurs: may increase V_T in 1ml/kg increments to 7 or 8 ml/kg if Pplat remains ≤ 30 cm H_2O.

B. SPONTANEOUS BREATHING TRIAL (SBT):
If all above criteria are met and subject has been in the study for at least 12 hours, initiate a trial of UP TO 120 minutes of spontaneous breathing with FiO2 ≤ 0.5 and PEEP ≤ 5:

1. Place on T-piece, trach collar, or CPAP ≤ 5 cm H_2O with PS ≤ 5
2. Assess for tolerance as below for up to two hours.
   a. $SpO_2 \ge 90$: and/or $PaO_2 \ge 60$ mmHg
   b. Spontaneous $V_T \ge 4$ ml/kg PBW
   c. RR ≤ 35/min
   d. pH ≥ 7.3
   e. No respiratory distress (distress= 2 or more)
      - HR > 120% of baseline
      - Marked accessory muscle use
      - Abdominal paradox
      - Diaphoresis
      - Marked dyspnea
3. If tolerated for at least 30 minutes, consider extubation.
4. If not tolerated resume pre-weaning settings.

Definition of UNASSISTED BREATHING
(Different from the spontaneous breathing criteria as PS is not allowed)

1. Extubated with face mask, nasal prong oxygen, or room air, OR
2. T-tube breathing, OR
3. Tracheostomy mask breathing, OR
4. CPAP less than or equal to 5 cm H_2O **without pressure support or IMV assistance.**

Fig. 2. Lower tidal volume/higher PEEP reference card for ARMA and ALVEOLI studies. (*From* ARDSNET.org; with permission.)

strategy (6 mL/kg) improved survival, and the study was stopped early after enrollment of 861 subjects.[2]

LATE STEROID RESCUE STUDY: LASRS

Study status: Completed.

Study dates: August 1997 to November 2003.

The late phase of ARDS is often characterized by excessive fibroproliferation leading to gas exchange and compliance abnormalities. Although corticosteroids are not effective in early ARDS, several case reports and uncontrolled case series and one small randomized, controlled trial suggest that corticosteroids may be useful in the management of late-phase ARDS. To test this hypothesis a randomized, double-blinded trial comparing corticosteroids with placebo in severe, late-phase ARDS after 7 days was conducted. The objective of the LaSRS study was to determine whether the administration of corticosteroids, in the form of methylprednisolone sodium succinate, in severe late-phase ARDS would have a positive effect on this fibroproliferation, thereby reducing mortality and morbidity. In addition, bronchoalveolar lavage and serum were collected during the first week of the study to search for inflammatory markers of fibroproliferation. The study enrolled 180 subjects. The study was completed in November of 2003.[3] Although an increase in ventilator-free days was noted during the first 28 days of the study, safety concerns around neuromuscular and hyperglycemic side effects blunted enthusiasm for recommending steroids for the routine treatment of persistent ARDS.

LYSOFYLLINE FOR ALI/ARDS

Study status: Completed.

Study dates: February 1998 to June 1999.

The LARMA study was a randomized, double-blind, placebo-controlled multicenter 2×2 factorial study wherein each patient was randomized between lisofylline and placebo. It was designed to test whether the administration of lisofylline early after the onset of ALI or ARDS would reduce mortality and morbidity. The study was stopped by the DSMB for futility at the first scheduled interim analysis. The decision was based on predetermined criteria, which required a positive trend toward improvement in day-28 survival among the lisofylline recipients for the trial to continue as a phase 3 trial. The results of this study were published in January 2001.[4]

ALVEOLI STUDY

Study status: Completed.

Study dates: November 1999 to March 2002.

Prospective, Randomized, Multi-Center Trial of Higher End-Expiratory Lung Volume/Lower FiO_2 versus Lower End-expiratory Lung Volume/Higher FiO_2 Ventilation in Acute Lung Injury and Acute Respiratory Distress Syndrome.

This study was a prospective, randomized, controlled multicenter trial. The objective was to compare clinical outcomes of patients with ALI and ARDS treated with a higher end-expiratory lung volume/lower FiO_2 versus a lower end-expiratory lung volume/higher FiO_2 ventilation strategy. The study was named ALVEOLI and was based on a phase 2 study of patients with ARDS showing a remarkable improvement in survival when managed with this open lung approach.[5] This approach involved both low tidal volumes and higher positive end-expiratory pressure (PEEP), among other interventions, to keep the lung open, and it was not clear whether the lower tidal volumes or the higher PEEP levels, or both, contributed to the marked improvement. The ALVEOLI study tested lower tidal volumes with higher PEEP (see **Fig. 2**) and, after enrolling 549 patients, found no further improvement in survival with higher PEEP.[6]

In the absence of data proving superiority of lower or higher PEEP for survival, clinicians may elect to use lower PEEP levels to avoid ventilator-induced lung injury from overdistension in patients whose airway pressures are high. Lower levels may also be preferable when there is overt barotrauma or when higher PEEP levels cause hypotension. Higher PEEP levels may be preferable in patients who do not have these limiting factors, especially if there is a clear indication of improved oxygenation, reduced dead space, or improved lung compliance when higher PEEP levels are applied.

FLUID AND CATHETER TREATMENT TRIAL: FACTT

Study status: Completed.

Study dates: June 2000 to October 2005.

Prospective, Randomized, Multi-Center Trial of Pulmonary Artery Catheter (PAC) versus Central Venous Catheter (CVC) for Management of Acute Lung Injury (ALI) and Acute Respiratory Distress Syndrome (ARDS) and Prospective, Randomized, Multi-Center Trial of "Fluid Conservative" versus "Fluid Liberal" Management of Acute Lung Injury (ALI) and Acute Respiratory Distress Syndrome (ARDS).

This study examined two different strategies for managing intravenous fluids and fluid balance in patients with ALI. During ARDS, the lung is vulnerable to the accumulation of fluid in the airspaces. There is considerable variation in current recommendations about how to best use and adjust intravenous fluids, and there were no large randomized clinical trials available to guide clinicians. This trial tested a fluid liberal strategy (that would be expected to improve the overall state of the circulation) against a fluid conservative strategy (that would potentially avoid excess lung fluid accumulation). A second goal of this trial was to determine whether a pulmonary artery catheter (PAC) is superior to a smaller, and less invasive central venous catheter (CVC) in the management of patients with ARDS. This important question arose from a retrospective examination of practice at 6 hospitals that suggested the pulmonary artery catheter, which has been widely used to guide management of patients with ARDS for many years, may actually be harmful.[7] A subsequent consensus conference reviewed this and numerous other studies of PAC effectiveness, and concluded that randomized controlled trials in patients with ARDS and sepsis were urgently needed.[8]

This trial attempted to answer two important questions in a single trial using a 2 × 2 factorial design. The goals of the studies were: (1) to assess the safety and the efficacy of PAC versus CVC-guided management in reducing mortality, need for mechanical ventilation, and morbidity in patients with ALI and ARDS; and (2) to assess the safety and efficacy of "fluid conservative" versus "fluid liberal" management strategies on lung function, nonpulmonary organ function, as well as mortality and the need for mechanical ventilation. Patients were treated with the specific fluid management strategy (to which they were randomized) for 7 days or until unassisted ventilation, whichever occurred first. The study enrolled 1000 patients and showed no benefit with PAC-guided fluid therapy over the less invasive CVC-guided therapy. The study also showed that the liberal approach, which resulted in fluid balance that mirrored traditional intensive care unit practices (**Fig. 3**), was inferior to the new conservative approach. The conservative approach improved the number of days free from mechanical ventilation and the intensive care unit without harming other organ functions, including kidney function or the need for dialysis. The survival was similar with both approaches, but survivors managed with the conservative approach were liberated from the mechanical ventilator 3.2 days faster (**Fig. 4**). In addition, the need for transfusions was reduced by using the conservative approach whether guided by a CVC or a PAC (**Fig. 5**). The conservative approach to fluid management did not increase the incidence of hypotension (**Fig. 6**) or need for vasopressors. To realize the benefits from this approach, most clinicians will need to substantially change their fluid management practices.[9,10]

ALBUTEROL FOR THE TREATMENT OF ALI: ALTA

Study status: Closed.

Study dates: August 2007 to September 2008.

ALTA was a prospective, randomized trial of aerosolized albuterol versus placebo to test the safety and efficacy of aerosolized β2-adrenergic agonist therapy for improving clinical outcomes in patients with ALI. Aerosolized β2-agonist therapy was anticipated to diminish the formation of lung edema, enhance clearance of lung edema, and

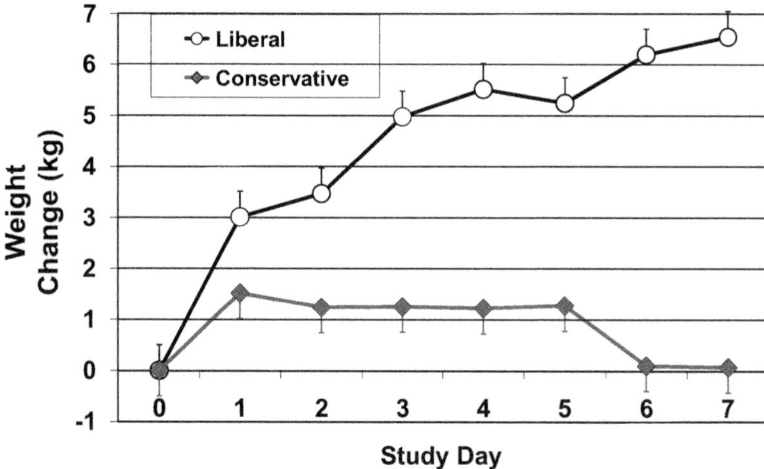

Fig. 3. Change in body weight over the first 7 days of conservative versus liberal fluid management in ALI patients in FACTT. Differences were statistically different from day 1 through day 7. After 7 days, patients in the liberal arm had gained approximately 7 kg whereas those in the conservative arm were near their baseline weight.

decrease pulmonary inflammation in patients with ALI. Because β2-agonists have been shown to reduce permeability-induced lung injury, it was anticipated that the severity of lung injury would be reduced by aerosolized β2-agonist therapy. The therapy may work by enhancing resolution of pulmonary edema by upregulating alveolar epithelial fluid transport mechanisms that will in turn enhance the clearance of alveolar edema. A reduction in the severity of lung injury and the quantity of alveolar edema should result in earlier extubation and more ventilator-free days, improved pulmonary oxygen uptake, and improved lung compliance.

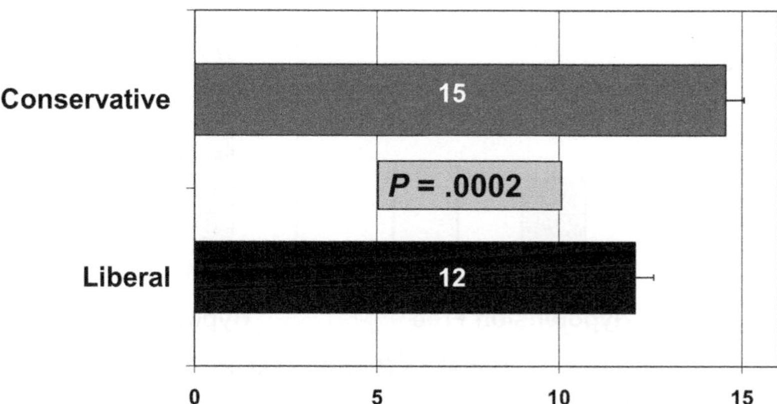

Fig. 4. Patients in FACTT who received conservative fluid management had approximately 3 more days alive and free of mechanical ventilation requirement (ventilator-free days) during the first 28 days of study.

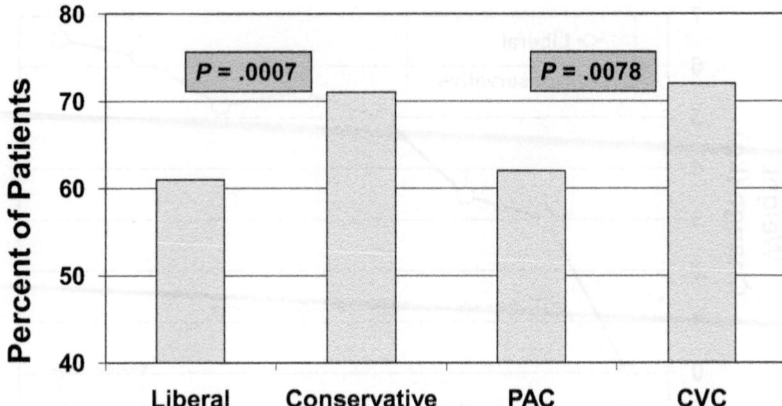

Fig. 5. Whether managed with a central venous catheter (CVC) or a pulmonary artery catheter (PAC), patients receiving conservative fluid management required significantly fewer red cell transfusions. The bars illustrate the percentage of patients who did not require any red cell transfusions during the first 7 days of study.

The study design was a phase 2/3 prospective, randomized, double-blind, placebo-controlled trial (http://clinicaltrials.gov/ct2/show/NCT00434993):

- In phase 2, patients were treated with aerosolized albuterol, 5.0 mg versus normal saline (n = 40–50) administered every 4 hours for 10 days following randomization or until 24 hours following extubation, whichever occurred first. The protocol stipulated that the 5.0-mg dose be reduced to 2.5 mg if patients exceeded defined heart rate limits.

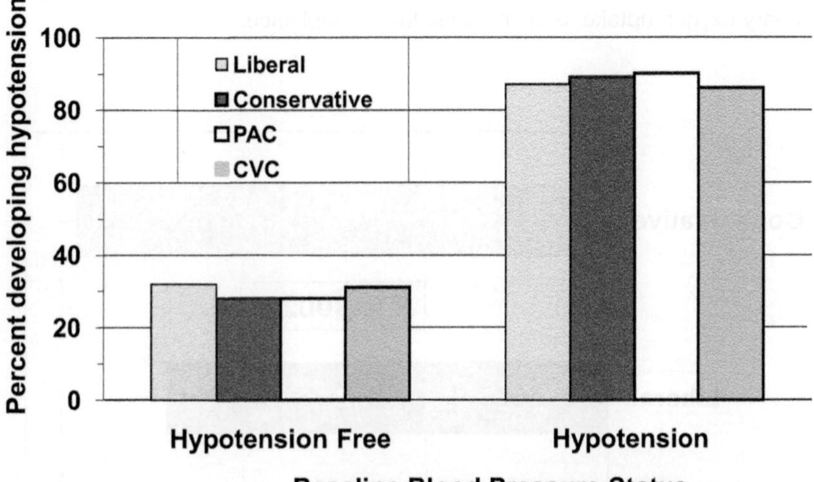

Fig. 6. Bars show percentage of patients who never developed hypotension versus those who developed hypotension during the first 7 days of study in FACTT. There was no difference in the incidence of hypotension whether management was with a PAC or a CVC, nor was there a difference whether managed in the fluid conservative arm or the fluid liberal arm.

- In phase 3, the 5.0-mg dose was used unless there was evidence that this dose had an unacceptable safety profile or dose reductions for tachycardia occurred in a large fraction of patients. In that case, a lower dose of 2.5 mg was to be used.
- Patients were followed for 90 days or until discharge from the hospital to home with unassisted breathing, whichever occurred first.

This study was stopped for futility by the DSMB, and the study results have been submitted for publication.[11]

EDEN-OMEGA STUDY

Study status: Open.

Study dates: November 2006.

Prospective, Randomized Trial of Initial Trophic Enteral Feeding Followed by Advancement to Full-Calorie Enteral Feeding Versus Early Advancement to Full-Calorie Enteral Feeding (http://clinicaltrials.gov/ct2/show/NCT00609180).

This trial ran simultaneously with a trial of omega-3 fatty acid, γ-linolenic acid, and antioxidant supplementation versus a comparator. The ARDSNet trial used an omega-3 and antioxidant supplement added to "usual" feeding (not any specifically commercially available product). The study stopped for futility. "Futility" means there was no realistic chance that the intervention could be proved to be beneficial with the size of trial planned. It would not be appropriate to make any conclusions about any other feeding product based on this study, as it would also be inappropriate to conclude that the treatment was "harmful." The database for this study has been analyzed, and the report has been submitted for publication. (See also the article elsewhere in this issue on nutrition in ALI/ARDS.)

The EDEN portion of the 2×2 factorial design continues, as it has not been terminated by the DSMB. This portion of the trial was recently completed to determine whether early aggressive full feeding of patients with ALI will result in improved outcome as compared with a more conservative feeding strategy that provides only "token" calories for the first 6 days followed by full feeding in both arms thereafter. This study was completed in the spring of 2011 with a study report available by the fall of 2011.

STATINS FOR ACUTELY INJURED LUNGS FROM SEPSIS: SAILS

Study status: Open.

Study dates: March 2010.

The SAILS study is a trial of rosuvastatin versus placebo comparator for the treatment of patients with ALI or ARDS. The objective is to assess the efficacy and safety of oral rosuvastatin in patients with sepsis-induced ALI. The hypothesis of this study is that pleiotropic anti-inflammatory effects of rosuvastatin therapy will improve mortality in patients with sepsis-induced ALI.

This study is a prospective, randomized, controlled multicenter trial. On admission to the intensive care unit, rosuvastatin or placebo will be administered through an enteral feeding tube or administered orally following extubation when patients are able to safely take oral medications. The type and placement of the enteral feeding tube (nasogastric, nasoenteric, PEG, orogastric, oroenteric, and so forth) and the ability to safely take oral medications will be determined by the patient's primary team. The study drug will be blinded with an identical-appearing placebo. The first study drug dose (rosuvastatin or placebo) will be administered within 4 hours of randomization as a loading dose of 40 mg followed by maintenance doses of 20 mg per day. The primary efficacy measure is hospital mortality to day 60. The estimated study completion date is September 2012 with an estimated patient enrollment of 1000 patients (http://clinicaltrials.gov/ct2/show/NCT00979121).

REFERENCES

1. Ketoconazole for early treatment of acute lung injury and acute respiratory distress syndrome. A randomized controlled trial. JAMA 2000;283:1995–2002.
2. ARDS Clinical Trials Network. The Acute Respiratory Distress Syndrome Network. Ventilation with lower tidal volumes as compared with traditional tidal volumes for acute lung injury and the acute respiratory distress syndrome. N Engl J Med 2000;342:1301–8.
3. Steinberg KP, Hudson LD, Goodman RB, et al; NIH/NHLBI ARDSNet. Efficacy and safety of corticosteroids for persistent acute respiratory distress syndrome. N Engl J Med 2006;354(16):1671–84.
4. Randomized, placebo-controlled trial of lisofylline for early treatment of acute lung injury and acute respiratory distress syndrome. Crit Care Med 2002; 30(1):1–6.
5. Amato MB, Barbas CS, Medeiros DM, et al. Effect of a protective-ventilation strategy on mortality in the acute respiratory distress syndrome. N Engl J Med 1998;338:347–54.
6. Brower RG, Lanken PN, MacIntyre N, et al. ARDS Clinical Trials Network. Higher vs. lower positive end-expiration pressures in patients with the acute respiratory distress syndrome. N Engl J Med 2004;351(4):327–36.
7. Connors AF Jr, Speroff T, Dawson NV, et al. The effectiveness of right heart catheterization in the initial care of critically ill patients. JAMA 1996;276:889–97.
8. Bernard GR, Sopko G, Cerra F, et al. Pulmonary artery catheterization and clinical outcomes: National Heart, Lung, and Blood Institute and Food and Drug Administration workshop report. Consensus statement. JAMA 2000;283(19):2568–72.
9. Wiedemann HP, Wheeler AP, Bernard GR, et al; The National Heart, Lung, and Blood Institute Acute Respiratory Distress Syndrome (ARDS) Clinical Trials Network. Comparison of two fluid-management strategies in acute lung injury. N Engl J Med 2006;354:2564–75.
10. Wheeler AP, Bernard GR, Thompson BT, et al; The National Heart, Lung, and Blood Institute Acute Respiratory Distress Syndrome (ARDS) Clinical Trials Network. Pulmonary-artery versus central venous catheter to guide treatment of acute lung injury. N Engl J Med 2006;354:2213–24.
11. Matthay MA, Brower RG, Carson S, et al; National Heart, Lung, and Blood Institute ARDS Clinical Trials Network. Randomized, placebo-controlled clinical trial of an aerosolized beta-2 agonist for treatment of acute lung injury. Am J Respir Crit Care Med 2011. [Epub ahead of print].

Mechanical Ventilation with Lung Protective Strategies: What Works?

Carl F. Haas, MLS, RRT

KEYWORDS

- Lung protective ventilation • Positive end-expiratory pressure
- Recruitment maneuver

Essentially all patients with acute lung injury (ALI) or acute respiratory distress syndrome (ARDS) require mechanical ventilatory assistance to support gas exchange and reduce the work of breathing associated with the lung impairment. Unfortunately, this life-sustaining support may actually cause further lung damage and possibly lead to increased mortality. This article reviews strategies that may help minimize ventilator-induced lung injury (VILI). Some strategies that might be considered lung protective, such as airway pressure release ventilation, prone positioning, high-frequency oscillatory ventilation, and inhaled vasodilators are addressed separately in other articles in this issue.

VENTILATOR-INDUCED LUNG INJURY

Several types of lung injury are associated with mechanical ventilation. High levels of inspired oxygen can cause oxidant injury in the airways and lung parenchyma of animals, and oxygen toxicity is a concern in humans.[1,2] The toxic threshold is still debated and may be variable depending on many factors, including preexisting lung disease that may offer some protection.[2,3] High alveolar oxygen concentrations can also result in absorption atelectasis.[1] It is generally desirable to reduce fraction of inspired oxygen (FiO_2) to below 0.60, and it is assumed that an FiO_2 of 0.40 can be safely tolerated for extended periods, but FiO_2 should be reduced to the lowest level that maintains acceptable oxygenation. In patients with ARDS, other triggers of VILI are likely more important in causing pulmonary damage.[1]

Gross extra-alveolar air (barotrauma) is associated with high ventilating pressure and alveolar overdistension, although it can occur at modest pressures in the

---

The author has nothing to disclose.
University Hospital Respiratory Care, University of Michigan Hospitals and Health Centers, 1500 East Medical Center Drive, Ann Arbor, MI 48109-5024, USA
E-mail address: chaas@med.umich.edu

Crit Care Clin 27 (2011) 469–486
doi:10.1016/j.ccc.2011.05.008 **criticalcare.theclinics.com**

presence of preexisting lung injury.[4] This air can find its way to the pleural space and subcutaneous tissue, as well as to the mediastinal, pericardial, and vascular spaces. The incidence of barotrauma appears to be low when alveolar inflation pressures are kept below 35 cm H_2O.[5]

The parenchymal lung injury and gas distribution associated with ALI/ARDS is heterogenic in nature. Using computed tomography of the chest, Gattinoni and colleagues[6] described 3 general lung "regions": a region of normal lung tissue, primarily in the nondependent areas; a region of densely consolidated, fluid-filled, or atelectatic tissue, primarily in the dependent areas; and a region that is collapsed during expiration but recruitable during inspiration. In severe ARDS, the healthy lung areas that receive most of the tidal ventilation may be reduced to one-third of normal or more, resulting in the term "baby lung" to describe the adult ARDS lung.[6]

The mammalian lung is maximally inflated to total lung capacity at a transpulmonary pressure of 30 to 35 cm H_2O. Animal studies have demonstrated that regional overinflation can result in a stretch injury (volutrauma), which does not manifest as an air leak but rather as diffuse alveolar damage, similar to what is seen in ARDS.[7–9] This injury is most likely to occur in the normal lung regions, as delivered volume goes to the area of least resistance and elastance. Injury can also occur when lung units are allowed to repeatedly open and collapse with tidal ventilation (atelectrauma).[9] Both volutrauma and atelectrauma can trigger release of inflammatory mediators and bacterial translocation, which may incite end-organ failure (biotrauma) and possibly increased mortality.[10–13]

LUNG PROTECTIVE VENTILATION

Protecting the lung from injury is a balancing act between opening and maintaining patency of as many lung units as possible to support oxygenation while ventilating (stretching) the lung units as gently as possible to support carbon dioxide removal and blood pH balance. **Fig. 1** shows the inflation and deflation pressure-volume (PV) relationship of an ARDS lung.[14] Initially modest pressure is required to overcome the critical opening pressure of lung units and allow volume to inflate the lung. As pressure continues to be applied the slope of the inflation curve becomes steeper,

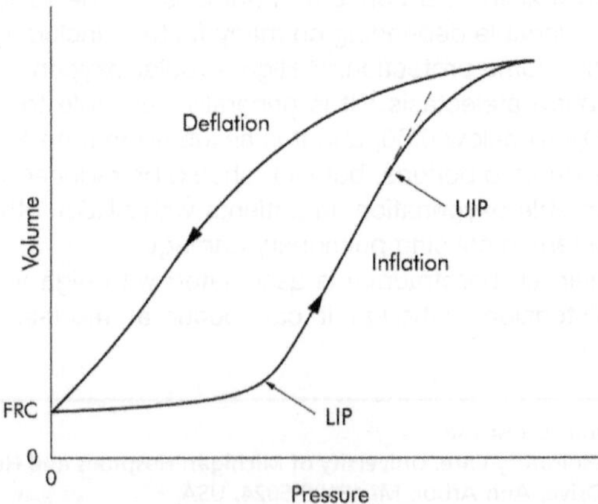

Fig. 1. Pressure-volume curve derived from a patient with ARDS. FRC, functional residual capacity; LIP, lower inflection point; UIP, upper inflection point. (*Adapted from* Whitehead T, Slutsky AS. The pulmonary physician in critical care, 7: ventilator induced lung injury. Thorax 2002;57:636; with permission.)

suggesting better compliance and easier inflation. When the lung is near maximal inflation the slope of the curve becomes flatter, suggesting the end of tidal recruitment and then overdistension. Note that for a given pressure, the lung is at a higher volume on deflation than it was during inflation. This volume difference (hysteresis) is to a large degree dependent on surfactant function, the degree of lung impairment, and recruitability; less hysteresis is seen with more normal function and/or less recruitment potential. Two goals and management strategies during mechanical ventilation are to (1) avoid overdistending lung units by limiting the inflation volume and pressure, and (2) avoid repetitive opening and collapse by applying adequate positive end-expiratory pressure (PEEP).[15] Ideally, ventilation would take place in a "zone of safety" on the deflation limb of the PV curve. The challenge is how to accomplish this.

INITIAL VENTILATORY SUPPORT IN ALI/ARDS

It is generally accepted that the primary ventilator strategy for patients with ALI/ARDS should be the one reported in 2000 by the National Institutes of Health ARDS Network, which to date is the only ventilator-related therapy showing a benefit regarding mortality.[16] **Figs. 2** and **3** are algorithms describing the ventilation and oxygenation strategies of this ARDSnet study.[17] Tidal volume (VT) is targeted to 6 mL/kg of predicted body weight (PBW) (see **Box 1** for formulas). Volume-controlled ventilation (VCV) in the continuous mandatory ventilation (assist-control) mode was used in the study and is generally recommended, but pressure control ventilation (PCV) can be used provided VT is monitored and maintained at approximately 6 mL/kg PBW.[18] End-inspiratory plateau pressure (Pplat) should be maintained at 30 cm H_2O or less. If necessary, VT is reduced as low as 4 mL/kg with a commensurate increase in rate, up to a maximum of 35 breaths/min. The set rate is adjusted to maintain a ventilation pH goal of 7.30 to 7.45, but care must be made to minimize auto-PEEP.[19] Administering a buffering agent might be necessary to maintain pH greater than 7.15 so that VT and Pplat can be kept within target, particularly when allowing permissive hypercapnia.

Initially an FiO_2 of 1.0 and PEEP of 8 to 12 cm H_2O are used, and then adjusted according to one of the tables in **Fig. 3**. The lower-PEEP and higher-PEEP tables were used in the ARDSnet ARMA[16] and ALVEOLI[20] trials, respectively. Oxygenation targets are a partial pressure of oxygen (PaO_2) of 55 to 80 mm Hg or oxygen saturation (SpO_2) of 88% to 95%. The Pplat threshold of 30 cm H_2O can be exceeded if: (1) FiO_2 is 1.0 and VT is 4 mL/kg, to allow further increases in PEEP, and (2) pH is less than 7.15 despite buffering, to allow a larger VT. VT can also be increased as high as 8 mL/kg to address ventilator asynchrony, provided Pplat is below threshold; otherwise sedation might be considered.

REFRACTORY HYPOXEMIA

Some patients remain hypoxemic despite this initial management strategy. Depending on the degree of blood gas derangement, clinicians may feel compelled to try alternative strategies rather than "waiting it out." **Fig. 4** shows an abbreviated version of an ARDS ventilator management strategy used at the University of Michigan, which begins with the ARDSnet low-VT management and proceeds through several strategies before ultimately considering extracorporeal membrane oxygenation.

In addition to increasing FiO_2, the ventilator response to hypoxemia is generally to increase mean airway pressure (Pmean) by increasing PEEP, lengthening inspiratory time (with an inspiratory pause in volume control ventilation or preferably directly using PCV), and increasing ventilating pressure. Establishing an adequate PEEP level should

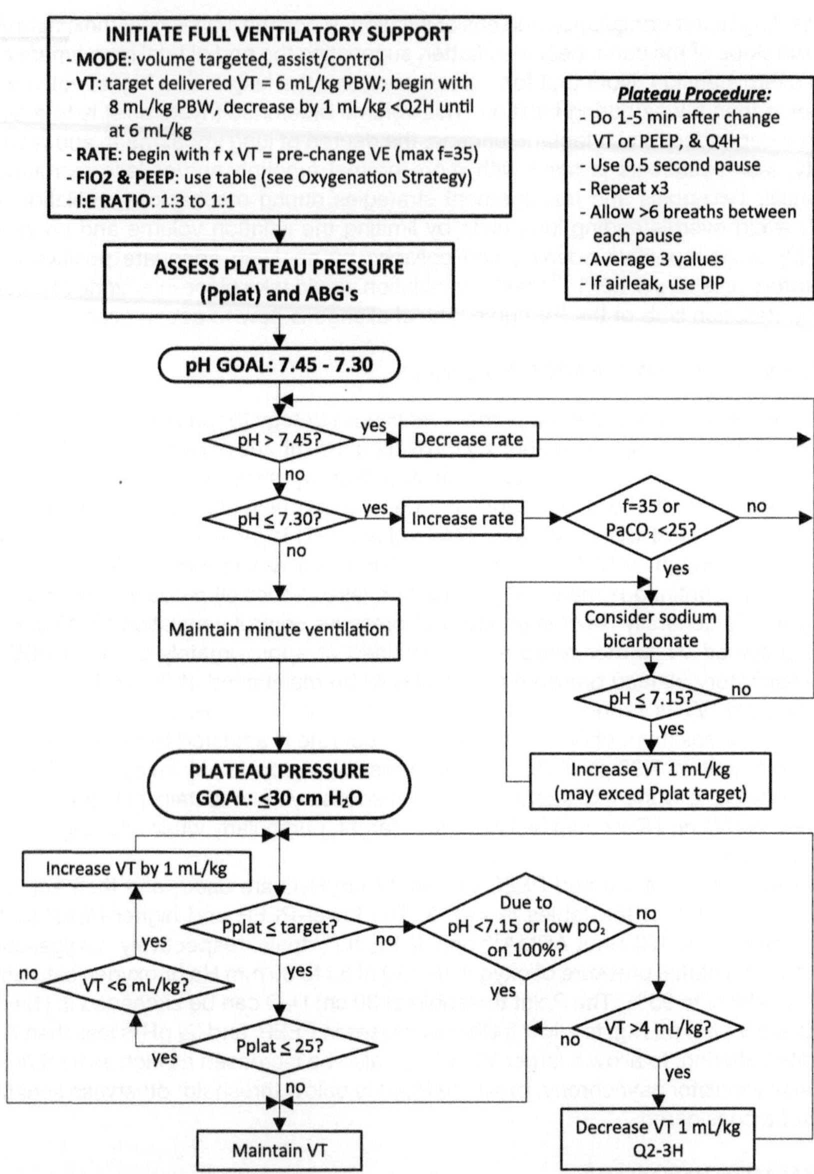

Fig. 2. Ventilation algorithm using the ARDSnet Strategy. (*Modified from* Haas CF. Lung protective mechanical ventilation in acute respiratory distress syndrome. Respir Care Clin N Am 2003;9(3):363–96; with permission.)

be the first step, because minimizing atelectrauma should be as high a priority as improving oxygenation.

SETTING PEEP

Some clinicians prefer to set PEEP per the ARDSnet tables, and others to individualize the PEEP titration. When using tables, Ramnath and colleagues[21] suggested that it be

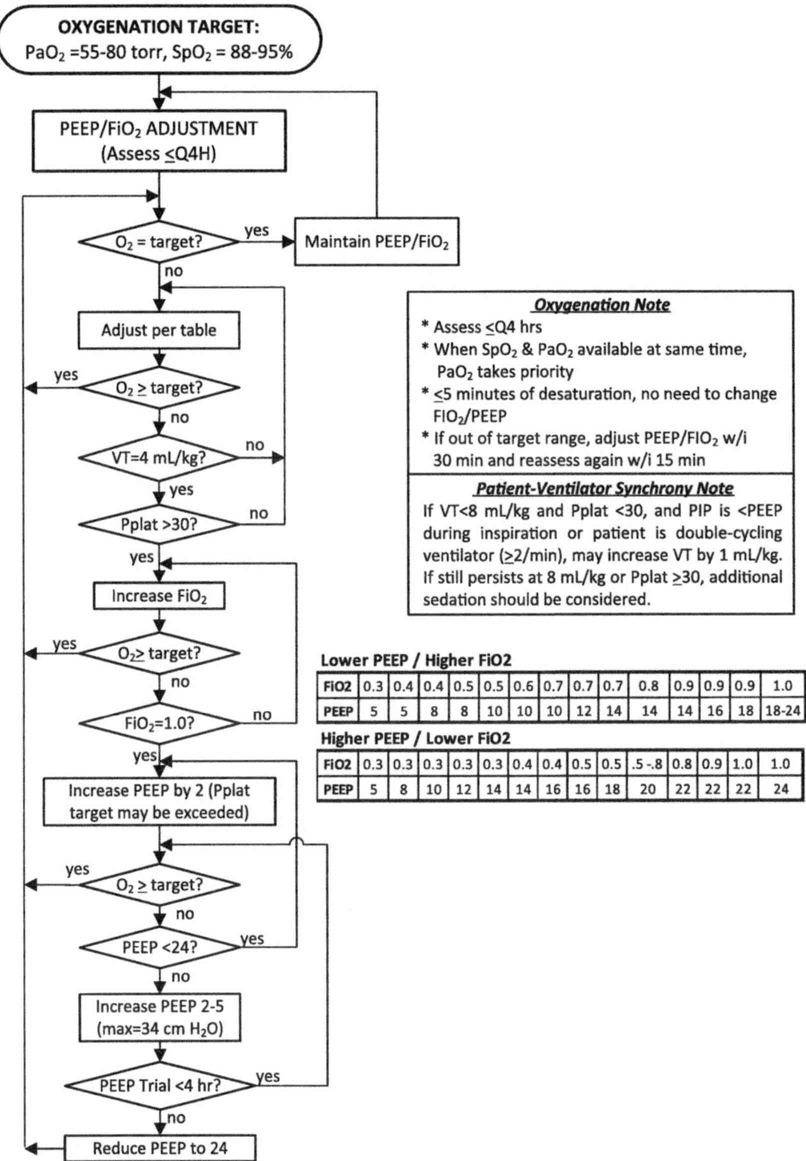

Lower PEEP / Higher FiO2

FiO2	0.3	0.4	0.4	0.5	0.5	0.6	0.7	0.7	0.7	0.8	0.9	0.9	0.9	1.0
PEEP	5	5	8	8	10	10	10	12	14	14	14	16	18	18-24

Higher PEEP / Lower FiO2

FiO2	0.3	0.3	0.3	0.3	0.3	0.4	0.4	0.5	0.5	.5-.8	0.8	0.9	1.0	1.0
PEEP	5	8	10	12	14	14	16	16	18	20	22	22	22	24

Fig. 3. Oxygenation algorithm using the ARDSnet Strategy. (*Modified from* Haas CF. Lung protective mechanical ventilation in acute respiratory distress syndrome. Respir Care Clin N Am 2003;9(3):363–96; with permission.)

determined whether the patient has recruitable lung units by increasing PEEP from 5 cm H_2O to 15 cm H_2O, and observing response in dynamic compliance and dead space fraction. If the patient responds favorably one should use the higher-PEEP table, if there is minimal or no response the lower-PEEP table should be used. Both ARDSnet PEEP tables list 24 cm H_2O as the upper limit, but the actual ARDSnet study protocol allowed a brief "PEEP challenge." **Fig. 3** shows that if oxygenation was below

Box 1
Calculation of predicted body weight (PBW) in kg

- Male: 50.0 + 2.3(height in inches−60)
- Female: 45.5 + 2.3(height in inches−60)

target with PEEP of 24 cm H_2O and a FiO_2 of 1.0, PEEP could be increased by 2 to 5-cm H_2O increments to a maximum of 34 cm H_2O. If oxygenation does not improve within 4 hours, PEEP should be reduced to 24 cm H_2O. This additional management element may apply to a very small subset of severely hypoxemic patients with altered chest wall compliance, such as those reported during the H1N1 influenza outbreak.[22,23]

An individualized approach to setting PEEP is encompassed in the Open Lung (OL) concept.[24,25] The OL procedure attempts to place the patient on the expiratory limb of the PV curve using 4 steps (**Fig. 5**): (1) opening the lung by increasing inflation pressure to above the critical opening pressure of a significant number of lung units via a recruitment maneuver (RM); (2) gradually reducing the end-expiratory pressure from

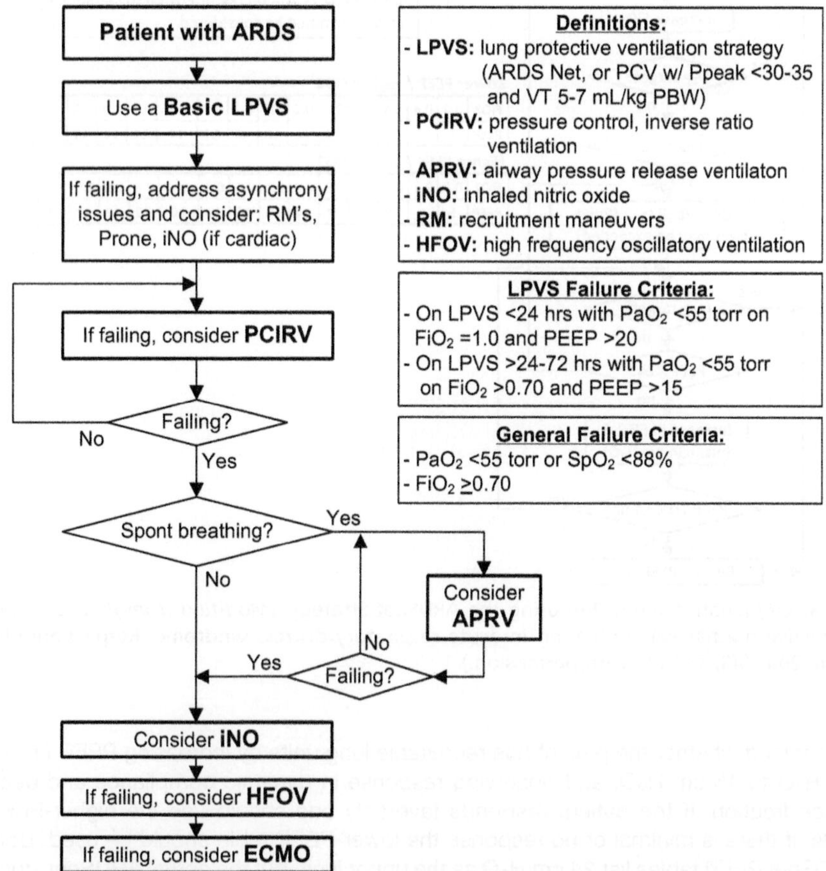

Fig. 4. Abbreviated version of the ARDS ventilator management strategies.

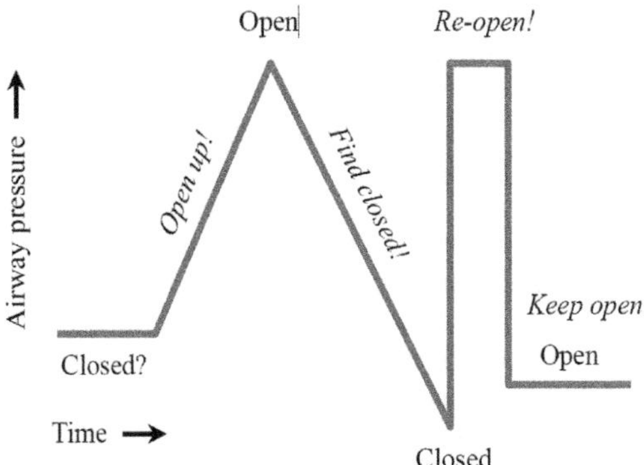

Fig. 5. The opening procedure for collapsed lungs. Note: the imperatives (!) mark the treatment goal of each specific intervention. The non-italic words mark the achieved state of the lung. At the beginning, the precise amount of collapsed lung tissue is not known. (*Reprinted from* Lachmann B. Open lung in ARDS. Minerva Anesthesiol 2002;68(9):637–8; with permission.)

a modest level, via a decremental PEEP trial, until the critical closing pressure point is reached indicating lung derecruitment; (3) performing another RM to take the lung to total lung capacity; and (4) keeping the lung open by setting PEEP to 2 cm H_2O above the PEEP associated with the critical closing pressure.[25] Various methods to open the lung have been reported. Using a constant pressure of 35 to 45 cm H_2O for 30 to 40 seconds is common[26–29]; however, PCV and maintaining a constant drive pressure as PEEP is incrementally increased is currently a popular method, as it appears to be better tolerated.[29–32] When the recruitment step is complete, the end-inspiratory pressure should be sufficiently high to open as many lung units as possible, generally 40 to 45 cm H_2O, although some groups have reported using pressures as high as 55 to 60 cm H_2O.[32,33] Some choose an arbitrary upper limit target pressure, such as 40 cm H_2O, whereas others monitor a surrogate of lung recruitment such as dynamic compliance (Cdyn),[34,35] the volume of carbon dioxide exhaled per breath ($VTCO_2$),[34,36] the sum of PaO_2 and $PaCO_2$,[33] or oxygenation.[32] A theoretical advantage of applying pressure based on response is that a patient may not require as much pressure as the arbitrary target or more likely a higher pressure, as many patients may require pressure of greater than 40 cm H_2O to fully recruit.[33] Of importance, complete recruitment may occur at the expense of significant hyperinflation of normal lung tissue.[37] $VTCO_2$ has been shown in animal studies to correlate with lung recruitment when compared with computed tomography.[34] Once the RM is accomplished, optimal PEEP is determined by incrementally reducing PEEP while monitoring for a reduction in Cdyn or oxygenation to suggest lung unit collapse and identify the closing pressure. A change in respiratory mechanics should occur before the oxygenation response, especially if SpO_2 is high at baseline.

Three other individualized PEEP approaches include PV curves, esophageal balloon manometry, and the stress index. Many ventilators have the ability to perform a slow-flow (<10 L/min constant flow) or pressure-step change PV loop to assess lower (LIP) and upper (UIP) inflection points on the inspiratory limb of the curve. It has been suggested that PEEP be set to 2 cm H_2O above LIP and that inflation pressure remain below UIP.[38–40] Because PEEP is an antiderecruitment pressure, keeping open the lung units that were opened during inspiration, the expiratory limb of the PV loop may be more informative.[6,41–43] Several ventilators control expiratory flow during the PV loop procedure and provide information, such as the point of maximum curvature[42] or the pressure at the point of maximum hysteresis,[43–46] which may prove helpful. Unfortunately, the patient must be sedated or at least passive while the procedure is being performed, which limits the tool's applicability.

A criticism of using the PV loop is that it is influenced by increased pleural and abdominal pressure (ie, altered chest wall compliance). Although evidence of improved outcome is lacking, there is much interest in using esophageal pressure (Pes) manometry to calculate transpulmonary pressure (Ptp = Palv - Pes) at end-exhalation to set PEEP, as well as at end-inspiration to provide a rationale for using higher than recommended plateau pressures.[47–52] It has been suggested that relying on Pplat to set ventilation may result in underventilating patients with increased abdominal pressure and overdistending those with atelectasis, and that Ptp should be considered when interpreting Pplat.[53]

The stress index uses the shape of the ventilator pressure-time waveform, during constant inspiratory flow, to reflect tidal recruitment and overdistension.[54–57] **Fig. 6** shows the 3 basic shapes: the downward sloping convex shape suggesting continuing tidal recruitment, the straight line suggesting no continuing recruitment or overdistension, and the upward sloping concave shape suggesting overdistension. Ventilators may incorporate such a feature in the future, although the waveforms may also be influenced by chest wall mechanics and therefore must be interpreted with caution, as with the PV curve.[58]

The Evidence for PEEP

There have been 5 recent meta-analyses attempting to determine whether a high-PEEP strategy has better outcomes than a low-PEEP strategy.[59–63] One is a patient-level analysis[63] and the others are study-level analyses. Each study has a slightly different approach; although they basically reviewed the same core randomized controlled trials (RCTs). The 3 core RCTs include the ARDSnet ALVEOLI study reported by Brower and colleagues,[20] the Canadian/Australian LOVS trial reported by Meade and colleagues,[64] and the French EXPRESS trial reported by Mercat and

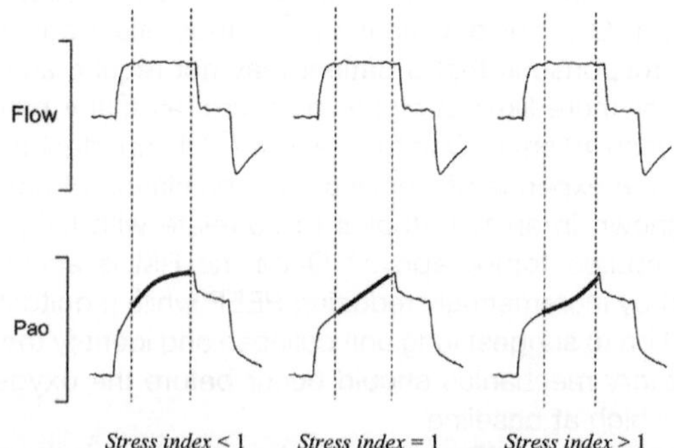

Fig. 6. Stress index concept. The shape of airway opening pressure (Pao) waveform during constant flow volume control ventilation is used to calculate the stress index (SI). An SI value of less than 1 (curve presents downward concavity) suggests a continuous decrease in elastance and tidal recruitment. An SI value of 1 (curve is straight) suggests absence of variation in elastance. An SI value of greater than 1 (curve presents an upward concavity) suggests a continuous increase in elastance and overdistension. (*Reprinted from* Grasso S, Stripoli T, De Michele M, et al. ARDSnet ventilatory protocol and alveolar hyperventilation: role of positive end-expiratory pressure. Am J Respir Crit Care Med 2007;176:761–7; with permission.)

colleagues.[65] Each is a large multicenter trial that used high-PEEP versus low-PEEP strategy combined with a low-VT strategy. The Brower and Meade studies used the same PEEP/FiO_2 table, although the Meade trial allowed Pplat up to 40 cm H_2O and RMs in the high-PEEP group. The Mercat study used a similar low-PEEP table but individualized high-PEEP by increasing PEEP to attain a Pplat of 28 to 30 cm H_2O. None of these studies reported a mortality difference; the studies by the Brower and Mercat groups were stopped early for reasons of futility. Two other smaller RCTs were included in several of the meta-analyses. The studies by Amato and colleagues[38] and Villar and colleagues[39] set high PEEP above the lower inflection point on the PV curve and used a low VT in the study group, although both used a larger VT in the low-PEEP control group. Both studies reported a fairly large benefit regarding mortality when using the high-PEEP, low-VT strategy.

Putensen and colleagues[59] included the 5 RCTs[20,38,39,64,65] in their meta-analysis. These investigators found that higher PEEP did not reduce hospital mortality, although it did reduce the need for rescue therapies to prevent life-threatening hypoxemia and death in those receiving rescue therapies. Oba and colleagues[62] included the same 5 studies and concluded that a small but significant mortality benefit of high PEEP may exist, and that the effects of high PEEP are greater in patients with higher intensive care unit (ICU) severity scores. Phoenix and colleagues[61] included the same 5 studies, as well as the small study by Ranieri and colleagues.[40] Ranieri's group set VT and PEEP in the high-PEEP group to the PV curve (VT below UIP, PEEP above LIP) and reported lower concentrations of inflammatory mediators, reduced 28-day mortality, and more ventilator-free-days in the high-PEEP group. When all 6 studies were included in the analysis, there was a reduction in 28-day mortality in the high-PEEP group, but the 3 smaller studies created a disproportionate effect. Analysis with just the 3 large RCTs (Brower, Meade, Mercat) showed a nonsignificant trend toward mortality benefit in the high-PEEP group (number needed to treat = 28), although the risk of barotrauma favored the low-PEEP group (number needed-to-treat = 75). Phoenix and colleagues concluded that the potential benefit of high PEEP outweighed the risk.

Dasenbrook and colleagues[63] included the 3 large RCTs,[20,64,65] as well as a recent study by Talmor and colleagues[47] Talmor and colleagues set PEEP in the study group to Ptp as assessed by esophageal balloon manometry; otherwise the patients were managed per the ARDSnet strategy. The investigators reported improved oxygenation and a nonsignificant trend toward improved mortality in the Ptp-guided PEEP group. The study-level meta-analysis of 2360 patients found a nonsignificant trend toward reduced mortality in the higher PEEP group and no difference in barotrauma.

Briel and colleagues[60] analyzed the actual data of the 2299 patients from the 3 large RCTs. For all patients there was no difference in hospital mortality, although higher PEEP was associated with reduced ICU mortality, total rescue therapies, and death after rescue therapy. There was a significant interaction for the presence of ARDS at baseline. **Table 1** is a table from the Briel study that shows the outcomes stratified by those with ARDS and without ARDS at baseline. In addition to those significant outcomes already mentioned, reduced hospital mortality (34.4% vs 39.1%) and more ventilator-free days at day 28 (12 vs 7 days) were observed in the higher PEEP group. There was no difference in the incidence of barotrauma or use of vasopressors. Of note, there was a nonsignificant trend toward improved mortality in the lower-PEEP group without ARDS at baseline.

In summary, it appears that for patients with less severe lung injury the low-PEEP table from the ARDSnet study is most appropriate. In patients with severe ARDS and refractory hypoxemia, either the higher-PEEP table or individualizing the PEEP to respiratory mechanics may be beneficial.

Table 1
Meta-analysis by Briel and colleagues,[60] reporting clinical outcomes in all patients and stratified by presence of ARDS at baseline

	All Patients				With ARDS				Without ARDS			
	No. (%)				No. (%)				No. (%)			
Outcomes	Higher PEEP (n = 1136)	Lower PEEP (n = 1163)	Adjusted RR (95% CI)[a]	*P* Value	Higher PEEP (n = 951)	Lower PEEP (n = 941)	Adjusted RR (95% CI)[a]	*P* Value	Higher PEEP (n = 184)	Lower PEEP (n = 220)	Adjusted RR (95% CI)[a]	*P* Value
Death in hospital	374 (32.9)	409 (35.2)	0.94 (0.86–1.04)	.25	324 (34.1)	368 (39.1)	0.90 (0.81–1.00)	.049	50 (27.2)	44 (19.4)	1.37 (0.98–1.92)	.07
Death in ICU[b]	324 (28.5)	381 (32.8)	0.87 (0.78–0.97)	.01	288 (30.3)	344 (36.6)	0.85 (0.76–0.95)	.001	36 (19.6)	37 (16.8)	1.07 (0.74–1.55)	.71
Pneumothorax between days 1 and 28[c]	87 (7.7)	75 (6.5)	1.19 (0.89–1.60)	.24	80 (8.4)	64 (6.8)	1.25 (0.94–1.68)	.13	7 (3.8)	11 (5.0)	0.72 (0.37–1.39)	.33
Death after pneumothorax[c]	43 (3.8)	40 (3.5)	1.11 (0.73–1.69)	.63	41 (4.3)	35 (3.7)	1.20 (0.79–1.81)	.39	2 (1.1)	5 (2.3)	0.44 (0.08–2.35)[d]	.34
Days with unassisted breathing between days 1 and 28, median (IQR)[e]	13 (0–22)	11 (0–21)	0.64 (−0.12–1.39)[f]	.10	12 (0–21)	7 (0–20)	1.22 (0.39–2.05)[f]	.004	17 (0–23)	19 (5.5–24)	−1.74 (−3.60–0.11)[f]	.07

Total use of rescue therapies[g]	138 (12.2)	216 (18.6)	0.64 (0.54–0.75)	<.001	130 (13.7)	200 (21.3)	0.63 (0.53–0.75)	<.001	8 (4.4)	16 (7.3)	0.60 (0.25–1.43)[d]	.25
Death after rescue therapy[g]	85 (7.5)	132 (11.3)	0.65 (0.52–0.80)	<.001	82 (8.6)	124 (13.2)	0.66 (0.52–0.82)	<.001	3 (1.6)	8 (3.6)	0.37 (0.10–1.46)[d]	.15
Use of vasopressors	722 (63.6)	759 (65.3)	0.93 (0.75–1.14)[d]	.49	627 (65.9)	647 (68.8)	0.90 (0.72–1.13)[d]	.37	95 (51.6)	111 (50.5)	0.92 (0.56–1.50)[d]	.72

Abbreviations: ARDS, acute respiratory distress syndrome; CI, confidence interval; ICU, intensive care unit; IQR, interquartile range; PEEP, positive end-expiratory pressure; RR, relative risk.

[a] Multivariable regression with the outcome of interest as dependent variable; PEEP group, age, probability of dying in hospital derived from prognostic scores at baseline, severe sepsis at baseline, and trial as independent variables; and hospital as a random effect.

[b] Patients who died before being discharged from the intensive care unit for the first time up to day 60.

[c] Defined as the need for chest tube drainage.

[d] Adjusted odds ratio substitutes for relative risk, because the corresponding log-binomial model did not converge.

[e] Median number of days of unassisted breathing to day 28 after randomization, assuming a patient survives and remains free of assisted breathing for at least 2 consecutive calendar days after initiation of unassisted breathing.

[f] Coefficient from a corresponding linear regression model using the same independent variables and random effect as the above-described log-binomial model; for example, a coefficient of 1.22 means that patients in the group treated with higher PEEP have, on average, 1.22 days more of unassisted breathing during the first 28 days compared with patients in the group treated with lower PEEP.

[g] As defined in each trial; rescue therapies included in the Assessment of Low Tidal Volume and Elevated End-Expiratory Pressure to Obviate Lung Injury and the Lung Open Ventilation to Decrease Mortality in the Acute Respiratory Distress Syndrome studies: inhaled nitric oxide, prone ventilation, high-frequency oscillation, high-frequency jet ventilation, extracorporeal membrane oxygenation, partial liquid ventilation, and surfactant therapy. Rescue therapies included in the Expiratory Pressure Study: prone ventilation, inhaled nitric oxide, and almitrine bismesylate.

Reprinted from Briel M, Meade M, Mercat A, et al. Higher vs lower positive end-expiratory pressure in patients with acute lung injury and acute respiratory distress syndrome. JAMA 2010;303(9):865–73; with permission.

RECRUITMENT MANEUVERS

A recent systematic review analyzed 40 studies that evaluated RMs; 4 were RCTs, 32 prospective studies, and 4 retrospective cohort studies.[66] The sustained inflation method (ie, continuous positive airway pressure [CPAP] of 35–50 cm H_2O for 20–40 seconds) was used most often (45%), followed by high pressure control (23%), incremental PEEP (20%), and a high VT/sigh (10%). Oxygenation was significantly increased after an RM (106 vs 193 mm Hg) but was generally short lived. Adverse events during the RM included hypotension (12%) and desaturation (8%), which were generally transient, returning to normal shortly after the RM, and rarely caused the RM to be prematurely discontinued. Serious adverse events, such as barotrauma (1%) and arrhythmias (1%), were infrequent. The investigators concluded that given the uncertain benefit of transient oxygenation improvement, routine use of RMs could not be recommended nor discouraged, and that they be considered on an individualized basis in patients with ALI who have life-threatening hypoxemia.

It has been suggested that most studies showing oxygenation improvement with short duration of benefit may not have set PEEP to an adequate level following the RM, and that those showing no benefit used relatively low recruiting pressures or applied them late in the disease course.[67] Iannuzzi and colleagues[68] recently demonstrated that the pressure control method (45 cm H_2O peak airway pressure [Ppeak], 16 cm H_2O PEEP for 2 minutes) compared with the sustained inflation method (CPAP 45 cm H_2O for 40 seconds) improved oxygenation to a larger degree and was better tolerated hemodynamically.

Current evidence suggests that that RMs should not be routinely used on all ARDS patients unless severe hypoxemia persists. RMs might be used as a rescue maneuver to overcome severe hypoxemia, to open the lung when setting PEEP, or following evidence of acute lung derecruitment such as a ventilator circuit disconnect.[69]

PRESSURE CONTROL VENTILATION

PCV is time cycled and pressure limited. When inspiration begins, flow pressurizes the circuit and lungs to achieve the set target pressure. As target pressure is reached, flow decays while the lungs continue to inflate. If the inspiratory time is long enough to allow flow to return to baseline, the lung is maximally inflated for that pressure and at this static pressure point, Ppeak equals Pplat.

When not used as the initial ventilator strategy, PCV is often initiated when Pplat becomes excessive, the patient is asynchronous with VCV, or when oxygenation is inadequate and lengthening inspiratory time is desired to increase Pmean.[18] When Pplat is excessive during VCV and the patient is switched to PCV, a reduced inspiratory pressure is only possible if a smaller VT is delivered, so reducing the VT in VCV might be considered first. A potential protective feature of PCV is that VT will automatically be reduced as respiratory mechanics become worse, and a disadvantage is that VT may become excessive as mechanics improve. The variable flow available in PCV may be more comfortable to patients exhibiting significant respiratory effort who are asynchronous with the fixed flow in VCV. This approach may result in less use of sedation, and possibly reduced breathing work.[70]

Regarding oxygenation, PCV is the preferred method of lengthening inspiratory time (Ti) to increase Pmean. The longer Ti may help to recruit lung units with longer respiratory time constants (ie, increased compliance and/or increased resistance). As Ti is gradually lengthened, the expiratory flow waveform should be monitored to detect the creation of auto-PEEP. Focusing on specific I:E ratios (ie, going from 1:2, 1:1, 2:1, and so forth) may work for the first few steps, but the Ti should be lengthened up to the point of creating auto-PEEP and stopped, regardless of the ratio, unless the intent is to create auto-PEEP. A concern with auto-PEEP is that it is not uniformly distributed throughout the lung, particularly a diseased lung with many different time constants.[71,72] For example, if 7 cm H_2O auto-PEEP is measured, it may be 3 in the low-compliance lung units and 11 cm H_2O in the high-compliance lung units. One may surmise that if 7 cm H_2O PEEP was added to the system, the lung units that may require more PEEP (the stiff ARDS units) might be receiving less than desired, whereas the more normal lung units may be more prone to overdistension. As auto-PEEP is created, VT will be reduced in PCV, as the effective driving pressure is reduced, which may reduce minute ventilation but will protect the lung from increased inspiratory pressure. When auto-PEEP occurs with VCV, Ppeak and Pplat will increase, putting the lung at risk of overinflation.

PATIENT-VENTILATOR ASYNCHRONY

When gas delivery from the ventilator does not match the patient's respiratory center neural output, patient-ventilator asynchrony may occur.[73] Asynchrony can occur in 3 major areas as the patient desires: not turning on (trigger), not keeping up (flow), and not turning off (cycle). There is no specific ventilator manipulation that works for all patients, nor for a given patient in all situations, and it becomes a matter of trial and error at the bedside. Obvious asynchrony is apparent in the patient who uses accessory muscles, is tachypneic, tachycardic, and diaphoretic, has nasal flaring or sternal retractions, or shows other signs of respiratory distress. More subtle asynchrony can be detected by observing the ventilator waveforms, particularly the pressure and flow scalars.

Trigger asynchrony can occur in the presence of auto-PEEP, as the patient has to pull down to a pressure equal to the auto-PEEP plus the set trigger threshold to initiate a breath. Adjustments to minimize auto-PEEP may help. Conversely, the ventilator may auto-cycle from too sensitive a set trigger, leaks in the system, and cardiac oscillation.[67,74,75]

Flow asynchrony may be present when the ventilator either pushes faster or slower than the patient is pulling. In VCV, increasing the set flow rate may help match the patient's flow demand, and using a decelerating flow pattern (if the ventilator provides it) will allow a faster initial flow for the same inspiratory time, but unfortunately the flow in VCV is fixed and does not adjust with changing demands of the patient. Pressure control and pressure support allow a variable flow that may be more comfortable. Another approach is to use a volume-targeted variable flow mode, such as pressure-regulated volume control. This mode allows flow to be influenced by patient demand and automatically adjusts inspiratory pressure based on the previous exhaled VT to maintain target volume. A challenge with this mode in patients with a low target VT is that inspiratory pressure is reduced if the patient exceeds the set VT target, which will provide less support when the patient may need more support.

Cycle asynchrony is present when the ventilator inspiratory (Ti-vent) and expiratory times are different to the patient's neural inspiratory (Ti-pt) and expiratory times. Double cycling in VCV suggests that the patient is still inspiring when the ventilator is turned off (Ti-pt >Ti-vent). Lengthening inspiratory time by adding an inspiratory pause or reducing flow may help, as might increasing VT depending on the current level. An end-inspiratory spike in the pressure-time waveform may suggest that the patient is trying to exhale while the ventilator is still pushing (Ti-pt <Ti-vent); increasing the set flow or reducing VT might alleviate this. PCV may be helpful in this situation, but the inspiratory time is still constant and may not be comfortable. Some new ventilators

allow PCV to be flow cycled (to function like pressure support with a back-up rate); otherwise a trial of high-level pressure support might be attempted.

For the tachypneic patient, increasing the ventilator rate may override the patient and reduce their respiratory drive, but it may also create auto-PEEP. When the ventilator adjustments do not seem to help, sedation and/or neuromuscular blockade may be indicated, particularly if the asynchrony is compromising hemodynamics or oxygenation. Studies suggest that sedation administration is not necessarily higher when using the low-volume strategy, contrary to many perceptions, and that sedation needs are more related to clinical factors other than the ventilator.[76,77] It is interesting, and somewhat paradoxic to current thought, that neuromuscular blocking agents given early in ARDS have been shown to reduce 90-day mortality and increase the time off the ventilator.[78]

Although it is imperative that patients should be made as comfortable as possible, concern for patient-ventilator asynchrony should not force clinicians to abandon lung-protective ventilation strategies.[79]

SUMMARY

Because ventilator management is associated with causing lung injury, preventing VILI should be a major goal of mechanical ventilation in addition to maintaining gas exchange. Limiting tidal stretch and transpulmonary end-inspiratory pressure are important, as well as minimizing tidal recruitment and collapse. The major components of the ARDSnet low tidal volume strategy are currently the most evidence-based concepts for managing ALI/ARDS patients. Various tools are being considered to help identify whether a patient has recruitable lungs, to help predict who might benefit from particular therapies and to aid in bedside management. Further research is required to determine their place in routine management.

REFERENCES

1. Carvalho CR, de Paula Pinto Schettino G, Maranhao B, et al. Hyperoxia and lung disease. Curr Opin Pulm Med 1998;4(5):300–4.
2. Durbin CG, Wallace KK. Oxygen toxicity in the critically ill patient. Respir Care 1993;93(7):739–50.
3. Capellier G, Maupoil V, Boussat S, et al. Oxygen toxicity and tolerance. Minerva Anestesiol 1999;65(6):388–92.
4. Parker JC, Hernandez LA, Peevy KJ. Mechanisms of ventilator-induced lung injury. Crit Care Med 1993;21(1):131–43.
5. Boussarsar M, Thierry G, Jaber S, et al. Relationship between ventilatory settings and barotrauma in the acute respiratory distress syndrome. Intensive Care Med 2002;28(4):406–13.
6. Gattinoni L, Caironi P, Pelosi P, et al. What has computed tomography taught us about the acute respiratory distress syndrome? Am J Respir Crit Care Med 2001; 164(9):1701–11.
7. Webb HH, Tierney DF. Experimental pulmonary edema due to intermittent positive pressure ventilation with high inflation pressures. Protection by positive end-expiratory pressure. Am Rev Respir Dis 1974;110(5):556–65.
8. Dreyfuss D, Soler P, Basset G, et al. High inflation pressure pulmonary edema: respective effects of high airway pressure, high tidal volume, and positive end-expiratory pressure. Am Rev Respir Dis 1988;137(5):1159–64.
9. Dreyfuss D, Saumon G. Ventilator-induced lung injury: lessons from experimental studies. Am J Respir Crit Care Med 1998;157(1):294–323.

10. Murphy DB, Cregg N, Tremblay L, et al. Adverse ventilatory strategy causes pulmonary-to-systemic translocation of endotoxin. Am J Respir Crit Care Med 2000;162(1):27–33.
11. Slutsky AS, Tremblay LN. Multiple system organ failure: is mechanical ventilation a contributing factor? Am J Respir Crit Care Med 1998;157(6):1721–5.
12. Tremblay L, Valenza F, Ribeiro SP, et al. Injurious ventilatory strategies increase cytokines and c-*fos* m-RNA expression in an isolated rat lung model. J Clin Invest 1997;99(5):944–52.
13. Tremblay LN, Slutsky AS. Ventilator-induced injury: from barotrauma to biotrauma. Proc Assoc Am Physicians 1998;110(6):482–8.
14. Whitehead T, Slutsky AS. The pulmonary physician in critical care, 7: ventilator induced lung injury. Thorax 2002;57(7):635–42.
15. Gattinoni L, Pelosi P, Crotti S, et al. Effects of positive end-expiratory pressure on regional distribution of tidal volume and recruitment in adult respiratory distress syndrome. Am J Respir Crit Care Med 1995;151(6):1807–14.
16. Brower RG, Matthay MA, Morris A, et al. Ventilation with lower tidal volumes as compared with traditional tidal volumes for acute lung injury and the acute respiratory distress syndrome. N Engl J Med 2000;342(18):1301–8.
17. Haas CF. Lung protective mechanical ventilation in acute respiratory distress syndrome. Respir Care Clin N Am 2003;9(3):363–96.
18. MacIntrye NR, Sessler CN. Are there benefits or harm from pressure targeting during lung-protective ventilation? Respir Care 2010;55(2):175–80.
19. Vieillard-Baron A, Prin S, Augarde R, et al. Increasing respiratory rate to improve CO_2 clearance during mechanical ventilation is not a panacea in acute respiratory failure. Crit Care Med 2002;30(7):1407–12.
20. Brower RG, Lanken PN, MacIntryre N, et al. Higher versus lower positive end-expiratory pressures in patients with the acute respiratory distress syndrome. N Engl J Med 2004;351(4):327–36.
21. Ramnath VR, Hess DR, Thompson BT. Conventional mechanical ventilation in acute lung injury and acute respiratory distress syndrome. Clin Chest Med 2006;27(4):601–13.
22. Ramsey CD, Funk D, Miller RR III, et al. Ventilator management for hypoxemic respiratory failure attributable to H1N1 novel swine origin influenza virus. Crit Care Med 2010;38(Suppl 4):e58–65.
23. Centers for Disease Control and Prevention. Intensive-care patients with severe influenza A (H1N1) virus infection—Michigan, June 2009. Morb Mortal Wkly Rep 2009;58(27):749–52.
24. Lachmann B. Open the lung and keep the lung open. Intensive Care Med 1992; 18(6):319–21.
25. Lachmann B. Open lung in ARDS. Minerva Anestesiol 2002;68(9):637–42.
26. Suh GY, Yoon JW, Park SJ, et al. A practical protocol for titrating "optimal" PEEP in acute lung injury: recruitment maneuver and PEEP decrement. J Korean Med Sci 2003;18(3):349–54.
27. Tugrul S, Akinci O, Ozcan PE, et al. Effects of sustained inflation and postinflation positive end-expiratory pressure in acute respiratory distress syndrome: focusing on pulmonary and extrapulmonary forms. Crit Care Med 2003;31(3):738–44.
28. Toth I, Leiner T, Mikor A, et al. Hemodynamic and respiratory changes during lung recruitment and descending optimal positive end-expiratory pressure titration in patients with acute respiratory distress syndrome. Crit Care Med 2007;35(3):787–93.
29. Takeuchi M, Imanaka H, Tachibana K, et al. Recruitment maneuver and high positive end-expiratory pressure improve hypoxemia in patients after pulmonary

thromboendarterectomy for chronic pulmonary thromboembolism. Crit Care Med 2005;33(9):2010–4.
30. Gernoth C, Wagner G, Pelosi P, et al. Respiratory and haemodynamic changes during decremental open lung positive end-expiratory pressure titration in patients with acute respiratory distress syndrome. Crit Care 2009;13(2):R59.
31. Povoa P, Almeida E, Fernandes A, et al. Evaluation of a recruitment maneuver with positive inspiratory pressure and high PEEP in patients with severe ARDS. Acta Anaesthesiol Scand 2004;48(3):287–93.
32. Hodgson CL, Tuxen DV, Bailey MJ, et al. A positive response to a recruitment maneuver with PEEP titration in patients with ARDS, regardless of transient oxygen desaturation during the maneuver. J Intensive Care Med 2011;26(1):41–9.
33. Borges JB, Okamoto VN, Matos GF, et al. Reversibility of lung collapse and hypoxemia in early acute respiratory distress syndrome. Am J Respir Crit Care Med 2006;174(3):268–78.
34. Hanson A, Gothberg S, Nilsson K, et al. $VTCO_2$ and dynamic compliance-guided lung recruitment in surfactant-depleted piglets: a computed tomography study. Pediatr Crit Care Med 2009;10(6):687–92.
35. Maisch S, Reissmann H, Fuellekrug B, et al. Compliance and dead space fraction indicate an optimal level of positive end-expiratory pressure after recruitment in anesthetized patients. Anesth Analg 2008;106(1):175–81.
36. Tusman G, Bohm SH, Suarez-Sipman F, et al. Lung recruitment and positive end-expiratory pressure have different effects on CO_2 elimination in healthy and sick lungs. Anesth Analg 2010;111(4):968–77.
37. Carvalho AR, Jandre FC, Pinto AV, et al. Positive end-expiratory pressure at minimal respiratory elastance represents the best compromise between mechanical stress and lung aeration in oleic induced lung injury. Crit Care 2007;11(4):R86.
38. Amato MB, Barbas CS, Medeiros DM, et al. Effect of a protective-ventilation strategy on mortality in the acute respiratory distress syndrome. N Engl J Med 1998;338(6):347–54.
39. Villar J, Kacmarek RM, Perez-Mendez L, et al, ARIES Network. A high positive end-expiratory pressure, low tidal volume ventilation strategy improves outcome in persistent acute respiratory distress syndrome: a randomized, controlled trial. Crit Care Med 2006;34(5):1311–8.
40. Ranieri VM, Suter PM, Tortorella C, et al. Effect of mechanical ventilation on inflammatory mediators in patients with acute respiratory distress syndrome: a randomized controlled trial. JAMA 1999;282(1):54–61.
41. Caramez MP, Kacmarek RM, Helmy M, et al. A comparison of methods to identify open-lung PEEP. Intensive Care Med 2009;35(4):740–7.
42. Albaiceta GM, Luyando LH, Parra D, et al. Inspiratory vs expiratory pressure-volume curves to set end-expiratory pressure in acute lung injury. Intensive Care Med 2005;31(10):1370–8.
43. Koefoed-Nielsen J, Andersen G, Barklin A, et al. Maximal hysteresis: a new method to set positive end-expiratory pressure in acute lung injury? Acta Anaesthesiol Scand 2008;52(5):641–9.
44. Koefoed-Nielsen J, Nielsen ND, Kjaergaard AJ, et al. Alveolar recruitment can be predicted from airway pressure-lung volume loops: an experimental study in a porcine acute lung injury model. Crit Care 2008;12(1):R7.
45. Demory D, Arnal JM, Wysocki M, et al. Recruitability of the lung estimated by the pressure volume curve hysteresis in ARDS patients. Intensive Care Med 2008;34(11):2019–25.

46. Henzler D, Hochhausen N, Dembinski R, et al. Parameters derived from the pulmonary pressure-volume curve, but not the pressure-time curve, indicate recruitment in experimental lung injury. Anesth Analg 2007;105(4):1072–8.
47. Talmor D, Sarge T, Malhotra A, et al. Mechanical ventilation guided by esophageal pressure in acute lung injury. N Engl J Med 2008;359(20):2095–104.
48. Talmor DS, Fessler HE. Are esophageal pressure measurements important in clinical decision-making in mechanically ventilated patients? Respir Care 2010;55(2): 162–72.
49. Loring SH, O'Donnell CR, Behazin N, et al. Esophageal pressures in acute lung injury: do they represent artifact or useful information about transpulmonary pressure, chest wall mechanics, and lung stress? J Appl Physiol 2010;108(3):515–22.
50. Hubmayer RD. Is there a place for esophageal manometry in care of patient with injured lungs? J Appl Physiol 2010;108(3):481–2.
51. Talmor D, Sarge T, O'Donnell CR, et al. Esophageal and transpulmonary pressures in acute respiratory failure. Crit Care Med 2006;34(5):1389–94.
52. Gattinoni L, Carlesso E, Brazzi L, et al. Positive end-expiratory pressure. Curr Opin Crit Care 2010;16(1):39–44.
53. Kubiak BD, Gatto LA, Jimenez EJ, et al. Plateau and transpulmonary pressure with elevated intra-abdominal pressure or atelectasis. J Surg Res 2010;159(1): e17–24.
54. Ranieri VM, Zhang H, Mascia L, et al. Pressure-time curve predicts minimally injurious ventilatory strategy in an isolated rat lung model. Anesthesiology 2000; 93(5):1320–8.
55. Terragni PP, Rosboch GL, Lisi A, et al. How respiratory system mechanics may help in minimizing ventilator-induced lung injury in ARDS patients. Eur Respir J 2003;22(Suppl 42):15s–21s.
56. Grasso S, Terragni P, Mascia L, et al. Airway pressure-time curve profile (stress-index) detects tidal recruitment/hyperinflation in experimental acute lung injury. Crit Care Med 2004;32(4):1018–27.
57. Grasso S, Stripoli T, De Michele M, et al. ARDSnet ventilatory protocol and alveolar hyperinflation. Am J Respir Crit Care Med 2007;176(8):761–7.
58. Formenti P, Graf J, Santos A, et al. Non-pulmonary factors strongly influence the stress index. Intensive Care Med 2011;37(4):594–600.
59. Putensen C, Theuerkauf N, Zinderling J, et al. Meta-analysis: ventilation strategies and outcomes of the acute respiratory distress syndrome and acute lung injury. Ann Intern Med 2009;151(8):566–76.
60. Briel M, Meade M, Mercat A, et al. Higher vs lower positive end-expiratory pressure in patients with acute lung injury and acute respiratory distress syndrome. JAMA 2010;303(9):865–73.
61. Phoenix SI, Paravastu S, Columb M, et al. Does a higher positive end expiratory pressure decrease mortality in acute respiratory distress syndrome? A systematic review and meta-analysis. Anesthesiology 2009;110(5):1098–105.
62. Oba Y, Thameen D, Zaza T. High levels of PEEP may improve survival in acute respiratory distress syndrome: a meta-analysis. Respir Med 2009;103(8):1174–81.
63. Dasenbrook EC, Needham DM, Brower RG, et al. Higher positive end-expiratory pressure in patients with acute lung injury: a systematic review and meta-analysis. Respir Care 2011;56(5):568–75.
64. Meade MO, Cook DJ, Guyatt GH, et al. Ventilation strategy using low tidal volumes, recruitment maneuvers, and high positive end-expiratory pressure for acute lung injury and acute respiratory distress syndrome. A randomized clinical trial. JAMA 2008;299(6):637–45.

65. Mercat A, Richard JC, Vielle B, et al. Positive end-expiratory pressure setting in adults with acute lung injury and acute respiratory distress syndrome. A randomized controlled trail. JAMA 2008;299(6):646–55.
66. Fan E, Wilcox ME, Brower RG, et al. Recruitment maneuvers for acute lung injury. Am J Respir Crit Care Med 2008;178(11):1156–63.
67. Kacmarek RM, Villar J. Lung recruitment maneuvers during acute respiratory distress syndrome: is it useful? Minerva Anestesiol 2011;77(1):85–9.
68. Iannuzzi M, De Sio A, De Robertis E, et al. Different patterns of lung recruitment maneuvers in primary acute respiratory distress syndrome: effects on oxygenation and central hemodynamics. Minerva Anestesiol 2010;76(9):692–8.
69. Rocco PR, Pelosi P, de Abreu P. Pros and cons of recruitment maneuvers in acute lung injury and acute respiratory distress syndrome. Expert Rev Respir Med 2010;4(4):479–89.
70. Kallet RH, Campbell AR, Alonso JA, et al. The effects of pressure control versus volume control assisted ventilation on patient work of breathing in acute lung injury and acute respiratory distress syndrome. Respir Care 2000;45(9):1085–96.
71. Kacmarek RM, Kirme M, Nishimura M, et al. The effects of applied vs auto-PEEP on local lung unit pressure and volume in a four-unit lung model. Chest 1995; 108(4):1075–9.
72. Kurahashi K, Ohtsuka M, Usuda Y. Central airway occlusion underestimates intrinsic positive end-expiratory pressure: a numerical and physical simulation. Exp Lung Res 2009;35(9):756–69.
73. Kondili E, Prinianakis G, Georgopoulos D. Patient-ventilator interaction. Br J Anaesth 2003;91(1):106–19.
74. Arbour R. Cardiogenic oscillation and ventilator autotriggering in brain-dead patients: a case series. Am J Crit Care 2009;18(5):488–95.
75. Imanaka H, Nishimura M, Takeuchi M, et al. Autotriggering caused by cardiogenic oscillation during flow-triggered mechanical ventilation. Crit Care Med 2000;28(2):402–7.
76. Arroliga AC, Thompson BT, Ancukiewicz M, et al. Use of sedatives, opioids, and neuromuscular blocking agents in patients with acute lung injury and acute respiratory distress syndrome. Crit Care Med 2008;36(4):1083–8.
77. Cheng IW, Eisner MD, Thompson BT, et al, Acute Respiratory Distress Syndrome Network. Acute effects of tidal volume strategy on hemodynamics, fluid balance, and sedation in acute lung injury. Crit Care Med 2005;33(1):63–70.
78. Papazin L, Forel JM, Gacouin A, et al. Neuromuscular blockers in early acute respiratory distress syndrome. N Engl J Med 2010;363(12):1107–16.
79. Hess DR, Thompson BT. Patient-ventilator dyssynchrony during lung protective ventilation: what's a clinician to do? Crit Care Med 2006;34(1):231–3.

High-Frequency Oscillatory Ventilation in ALI/ARDS

Sammy Ali, MD[a], Niall D. Ferguson, MD, MSc[b,c,*]

KEYWORDS

- Acute respiratory distress syndrome
- Acute lung injury
- High-frequency oscillatory ventilation
- Mechanical ventilatory support

In the last 2 decades our goals for mechanical ventilatory support in patients with acute respiratory distress syndrome (ARDS) or acute lung injury (ALI) have changed dramatically. Moving from attempts to maintain normal blood gases,[1] several randomized controlled trials (RCT) have built on a substantial body of preclinical work to demonstrate that the way in which we employ mechanical ventilation has a large impact on important patient outcomes, including mortality.[2–5] Avoiding, or at least limiting, ventilator-induced lung injury (VILI) is, therefore, now a major focus when clinicians are considering which ventilatory strategy to employ in patients with ALI/ARDS. Armed with this knowledge, physicians are now searching for methods that may further limit VILI, while still being able to achieve adequate gas exchange.

One such potential method is high-frequency oscillatory ventilation (HFOV).[6,7] HFOV is one of several ventilatory modes, together termed high frequency ventilation (HFV), that employ frequencies greater than 60 breaths per minute (1 Hz) that deliver small tidal volumes that are often lower than the anatomic dead space. HFOV has properties that make it a theoretically ideal mode for avoiding VILI,[8] and this, as well as an overview of its history, physiology, and practical implementation, is reviewed in this article.

Funding: Dr Ferguson is supported by a New Investigator Award from the Canadian Institutes of Health Research (Ottawa, Canada).

[a] Internal Medicine Program, Department of Medicine, University of Toronto, Toronto, Ontario, Canada

[b] Interdepartmental Division of Critical Care, University of Toronto, Toronto, Ontario, Canada

[c] Division of Respirology, Department of Medicine, University Health Network and Mount Sinai Hospital, University of Toronto, Toronto, Ontario, Canada

* Corresponding author. Mount Sinai Hospital, 600 University Avenue, Suite 18-206, Toronto, ON, Canada M5G 1X5.

E-mail address: n.ferguson@utoronto.ca

Crit Care Clin 27 (2011) 487–499
doi:10.1016/j.ccc.2011.04.006 **criticalcare.theclinics.com**
0749-0704/11/$ – see front matter

HISTORY OF HFOV

Although HFOV is a recent arrival in the adult critical care unit, it has been used and studied extensively in the neonatal intensive care unit over the past 20 years. Indeed, almost 100 years ago the physiologic possibilities of HFOV were made in observations of panting dogs.[9] Moving to the early 1970s, Lunkenheimer and colleagues[10] published their findings showing the surprising finding that they could achieve adequate CO_2 clearance using an electromagnetic vibrator at high respiratory frequencies of up to 40 Hz. Around the same time, Bryan and colleagues,[11] in Toronto, noted similar phenomenon while measuring lung impedance during anesthesia. Over the next decade, a series of experiments on animals and healthy human subjects helped develop HFOV into a viable treatment option for neonates with respiratory distress syndrome.[12–16]

From this point, numerous randomized controlled trials of HFOV in neonatal respiratory distress have been conducted, which in turn have lead to its widespread use in this setting.[17–23] In the last 15 years, the appearance of HFOV in the adult critical care world was facilitated by the development of a commercial ventilator with sufficient power to oscillate adults. Initially used as rescue therapy for patients failing conventional ventilation,[24,25] HFOV is now showing promise as a ventilatory mode for patients with severe ARDS, which may reduce VILI further and lower mortality.[26,27]

PHYSIOLOGY OF HFOV

HFOV works differently than conventional ventilation (CV). In place of large tidal changes in inspiratory pressure seen with CV, during HFOV, the mean airway pressure is held constant and pressure waves in the ventilatory circuit are generated by a diaphragm that oscillates at frequencies between 3 and 15 Hz (180–600 breaths per minute) (**Fig. 1**). In HFOV, the ventilator creates both inspiratory and expiratory

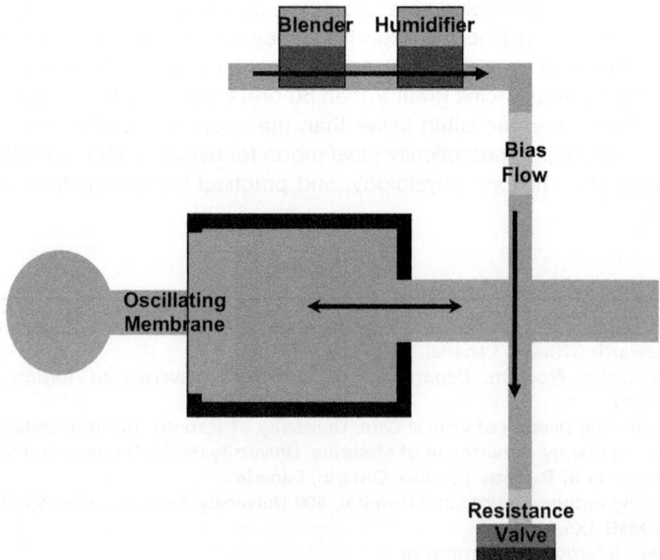

Fig. 1. An HFOV circuit. (*From* Ferguson ND, Stewart TE. New therapies for adults with acute lung injury. High-frequency oscillatory ventilation. Crit Care Clin 2002;18(1):91–6; with permission.)

pressure waves because the diaphragm is actively driven in both directions. Therefore, expiration is also active, which differentiates HFOV from CV and from other modes of high-frequency ventilation where expiration is passive and dependent on the elastic recoil of the respiratory system. Active expiration may be beneficial in preventing hyperinflation and controlling CO_2 elimination.

The ventilator circuit schematic for HFOV is shown in **Fig. 2**. Oxygenated, humidified gas (bias flow) passes in front of the oscillating membrane that generates small tidal volumes (V_T) at high rates. A clinical advantage of HFOV is the decoupling of the management of oxygenation and ventilation. A patient's oxygenation for a given F_IO_2 is usually proportional to the mean airway pressure (mP_{AW}) and resultant lung volume.[15,28] Clinicians can alter the mP_{AW} primarily by adjusting the resistance valve at the end of the bias-flow circuit (see **Fig. 2**). Changes in the rate of bias flow will also affect mP_{AW}. In contrast, alveolar ventilation during HFOV is influenced by the power with which the diaphragm moves (which generates delta P, the peak-to-peak pressure gradient), the frequency of oscillations, and the inspiratory/expiratory (I/E) ratio.[16] CO_2 elimination is proportional to the frequency and the square of the tidal volume ($V_{CO_2}\ \alpha = f \times V_T^2$).[29] Ventilation is enhanced by increases in delta P giving higher V_T. However, because tidal volume decreases with increasing respiratory frequency (because of a shorter inspiratory time), when clinicians want to lower $PaCO_2$, they will often *decrease* frequency (the opposite response usually taken with conventional ventilation). In addition, because humidified gas is simply passed in front of the oscillator, the difficulties with humidification and subsequent risk of tracheobronchitis are less of an issue with HFOV than with other HFV modes, such as high-frequency jet ventilation.

Tidal volumes generated with HFOV are often smaller than anatomic dead space. Therefore, unlike conventional ventilation, which relies principally upon bulk flow of gas to the alveoli, ventilation during HFOV is accomplished largely by enhanced gas mixing within the lung. The numerous mechanisms that account for the ability to achieve adequate ventilation with HFOV are outlined in **Fig. 3** and include bulk convection, cardiac oscillations, Taylor dispersion, asymmetric velocity profiles, pendelluft, and diffusion.[30]

Changes in alveolar pressure are minimized by small excursions of the piston. It should be noted here that although the delta P generated are typically large numbers

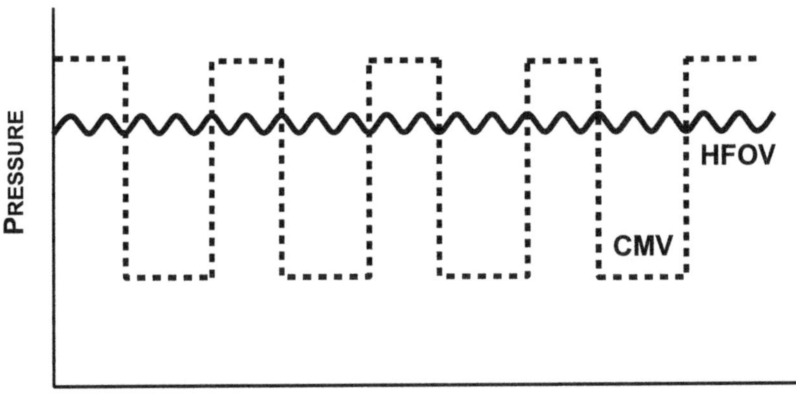

Fig. 2. Pressure-time curve contrasting tidal variations with CV *(dashed line)* with HFOV *(solid line)*. (*From* Ferguson ND, Stewart TE. New therapies for adults with acute lung injury. High-frequency oscillatory ventilation. Crit Care Clin 2002;18(1):91–6; with permission.)

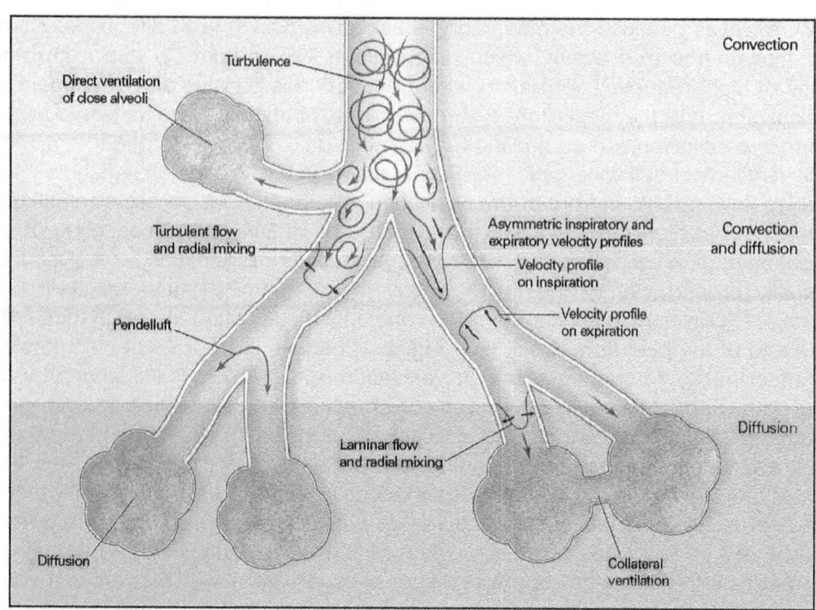

Fig. 3. Alternative mechanisms of gas exchange with HFO. (*From* Slutsky AS, Drazen JM. Ventilation with small tidal volumes. N Engl J Med 2002;347(9):630–1; with permission.)

in the range of 60 to 90 cm H_2O, this is the peak-to-peak pressure range, so inspiratory pressures in the circuit are roughly only half of this. In addition, because of oscillatory harmonics, the delta P is greatly dissipated as the pressure waves enter the lung, with delta P 90 in the ventilator circuit resulting in delta P of 9 to 18 in the trachea, with even smaller dispersions at the alveolar level.[31–33] Because the incremental tidal alveolar stretch in HFOV is minimal, mean airway pressure in HFOV is physiologically and clinically similar to positive end-expiratory pressure (PEEP) in CV.

Another technical note, however, is that when HFOV is used with an inspiratory/expiratory ratio of 1:2 (as is typically applied in many adults), the mP_{AW} in the lung is typically 5 to 6 cm H_2O lower than that measured in the circuit and displayed on the ventilator (which is not the case with CV or with HFOV at a 1:1 I/E ratio).[34] These factors allow clinicians to set this mean airway pressure significantly higher than they are safely able to set PEEP on conventional ventilation because they do not have to allow for a large inspiratory increase in pressure.

RATIONALE FOR HFOV

Over the past few decades we have advanced our understanding that mechanical ventilation can have harmful effects on the lung, specifically describing the process of ventilator-induced lung injury.[35,36] VILI is a consequence of injurious mechanical forces generated during mechanical ventilation. On pathophysiological grounds, this lung injury results from a combination of cyclic alveolar overdistention (volutrauma)[37,38] and repeated cycles of recruitment and derecruitment (atelectrauma),[39,40] both of which contribute to injury from local and systemic release of inflammatory mediators from the lung (biotrauma).[41,42]

As the authors previously mentioned, VILI is not merely a theoretical concern or a disease only in laboratory animals. In the last 10 to 15 years, several clinical trials have demonstrated the impact of ventilator settings to minimize VILI on outcomes in adults with ALI/ARDS. The most convincing evidence of this is the landmark study from the ARDS Network in 2000, which demonstrated a 9% absolute mortality reduction in patients with acute lung injury ventilated with 6 compared with 12 mL/kg predicted body weight (PBW).[2] Despite the impact of these findings, it is important to realize that the ARDS Network low tidal volume protocol does not necessarily represent the final word in lung protective ventilation. Recent data strictly employing this protocol and performing computed tomography (CT) scans at end inspiration and end expiration suggest that in up to one-third of patients with ALI/ARDS (those with the worst degree of lung injury), tidal volumes of 6 mL/kg may still be causing significant overdistention.[43]

The small tidal volumes that HFOV delivers are the key to its lung-protective potential. By delivering these small tidal volumes, HFOV produces minimal variation around the mean airway pressure and mean lung volume during tidal breathing (see **Fig. 1**), and this can clearly limit volutrauma. Additionally, because of this minimal tidal variation in airway pressure, clinicians can set higher mean airway pressures than can be safely applied with conventional ventilation. The lung recruitment that results from this higher mP_{AW} can directly reduce repetitive opening and closing injury: *atelectrauma*.[44] Also, *volutrauma* may be reduced by increasing the size of the baby lung and reducing the tidal stretch that any individual alveolus has to accommodate.[45] This theoretical benefit for HFOV is also supported by numerous preclinical animal data demonstrating that even in comparison to lung-protective conventional ventilation, HFOV is superior in terms of gas exchanges, markers of inflammation, and lung pathology scores.[46–49] Finally, because higher mean airway pressures can be employed without the same risk of tidal overdistention seen with CV, HFOV can be highly effective at improving oxygenation. This improved oxygenation may allow a faster reduction in F_IO_2 and a reduced total exposure to potentially toxic levels of oxygen.[50]

CLINICAL DATA WITH HFOV

As previously mentioned, HFOV has been subjected to the most rigorous evaluation and has undergone the longest clinical experience in the neonatal respiratory distress setting. The results of an initial large RCT of neonatal HFOV raised concerns of increased cerebral hemorrhages and periventricular leucomalacia.[17] However, this study did not use a systematic open-lung approach and, in addition, limited experience in monitoring patients in some centers may have driven adverse neurologic outcomes as a consequence of overventilation leading to low $PaCO_2$ and reduced cerebral perfusion.[51] This result is contrasted by subsequent RCTs employing an open-lung approach with recruitment maneuvers that showed HFOV to be safe in neonates, improving oxygenation, and likely reducing risk of death or chronic lung disease.[52] Interpretation of the neonatal literature is challenging because of differences in study populations (preterm vs term); timing of HFOV (immediately after birth vs delayed); and co-interventions, such as surfactant.[23] Although the neonatal experience increases our understanding of the physiologic mechanism of HFOV and the importance of recruitment maneuvers, these findings can obviously not be directly applied to adults.

Whether or not HFOV impacts outcomes in adult patients with ARDS still remains unclear. Until recently, HFOV has mostly been investigated as a rescue therapy for patients with ARDS who were failing conventional ventilation. The first published case series of this type was by Fort and colleagues,[24] who found improvements in oxygenation with HFOV as rescue therapy in 17 patients with severe ARDS (lung injury score = 3.81 ± 0.23, PaO_2/FiO_2 ratio = 68.6 ± 21.6). Similarly, in 2 case series of

HFOV in patients with ARDS, Mehta and colleagues[25,53] studied patients failing conventional ventilation and found that HFOV achieved an improved PaO_2/FiO_2 ratio within 8 hours. These 3 studies all suggested improved mortality in patients with fewer ventilator days before initiating rescue therapy with HFOV. Based on these and similar case series, most experts agree that HFOV appears safe and effective at improving oxygenation, thereby making it a potentially useful tool in the setting of the rescue therapy for patients with severe hypoxemia.

Subsequent to these initial case series, HFOV has been subjected to randomized controlled trials in the adult intensive care unit (ICU). The largest of these completed to date is the Multicenter Oscillatory Ventilation for Acute Respiratory Distress Syndrome Trial (MOAT), which randomized 150 patients with ARDS to HFOV or conventional ventilation using pressure control targeting a tidal volume of 6 to 10 mL/kg actual body weight.[54] Study patients were ventilated conventionally for an average of 2 to 4 days before randomization. There was no significant difference between groups in the primary outcome measure of survival without need for mechanical ventilation at 30 days. However, there was a nonsignificant trend toward lower mortality at 30 days with HFOV compared with CV (37% vs 52%, $P = .102$). There was also a significant improvement in PaO_2/FiO_2 ratio ($P = .008$) with HFOV in the first 24 hours. Consistent with previous uncontrolled trials, HFOV appeared to be safe with no increased rates of barotrauma or hemodynamic instability. It should be noted that the CV control arm of this trial, which was conceived approximately 15 years ago, does not represent the gold standard of lung-protective CV in ARDS today. However, as discussed later, the HFOV arm from the mid-1990s is also not what would be considered state-of-the-art HFOV today.

A recent meta-analysis has combined all of the published RCTs comparing the use of HFOV in adult and children with ARDS versus conventional ventilation. A total of 8 RCTs (n = 419 patients) were included.[27] On average, trials had enrolled patients within 48 hours of diagnosis of ARDS, and had a median baseline PaO_2/FiO_2 of 112 (range 80–122). In patients randomized to HFOV, mortality was significantly reduced (relative risk [RR] 0.77, 95% confidence interval [CI] 0.61–0.98, $P = .03$, **Fig. 4**) and treatment failure (refractory hypoxemia, hypercapnia, hypotension, or barotraumas) resulting in discontinuation of assigned therapy was also less likely (RR 0.67, 95%

	High frequency oscillation	Conventional mechanical ventilation	Risk ratio (95% CI)	Weight (%)	Risk ratio (95% CI)
Arnold 1994	10/29	12/29		13.0	0.83 (0.43 to 1.62)
Derdak 2002	28/75	38/73		42.6	0.72 (0.50 to 1.03)
Shah 2004	6/15	6/13		7.9	0.87 (0.37 to 20.4)
Bollen 2005	16/37	8/24		12.5	1.30 (0.66 to 2.55)
Mentzelopoulus 2007	11/27	18/27		20.6	0.61 (0.36 to 1.04)
Samransamruajkit 2005	2/6	5/10		3.4	0.67 (0.18 to 2.42)
Total (95% CI)	73/189	87/176		100.0	0.77 (0.61 to 0.98)

Test for heterogeneity: $\tau^2=0.00$, $\chi^2=3.36$, df=5, P=0.64, $I^2=0\%$

Test for overall effect: z=2.12, P=0.03

0.1 0.2 0.5 1 2 5 10

Favours HFO — Favours CMV

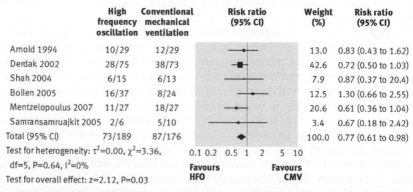

Fig. 4. Hospital or 30-day mortality in patients with ALI/ARDS allocated to HFOV or conventional mechanical ventilation. (*From* Sud S, Sud M, Friedrich JO, et al. High frequency oscillation in patients with acute lung injury and acute respiratory distress syndrome (ARDS): systematic review and meta-analysis. BMJ 2010;340:c2327; with permission.)

CI 0.46–0.99, $P = .04$). At 24, 48, and 72 hours, HFOV increased PaO_2/FiO_2 ratio by 16% to 24% compared with conventional mechanical ventilation (**Fig. 5**).

It should be noted, however, that the mortality benefit of HFOV might have been overestimated because the control group in 3 studies was exposed to higher tidal volumes (>6–8 mL/kg PBW) than currently recommended as part of a lung-protective strategy. Additionally, the mortality data is based on few patients and outcome events, and demonstrates a wide-confidence interval. With this in mind, the authors consider the findings of this meta-analysis, which are consistent with previous

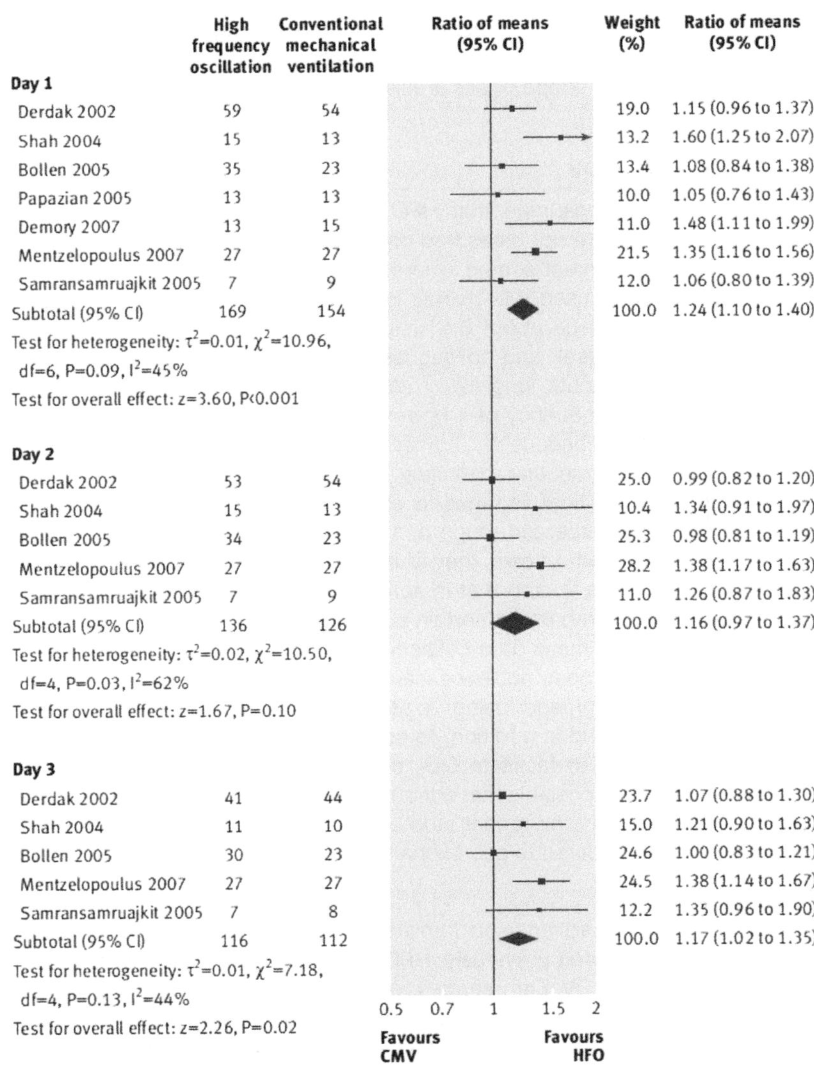

Fig. 5. PaO_2/FiO_2 ratio on days 1 to 3. Ratio of means is mean PaO_2/FiO_2 in HFOV group divided by mean PaO_2/FiO_2 in conventional mechanical ventilation group. *Abbreviation:* CMV, controlled mechanical ventilation. (*From* Sud S, Sud M, Friedrich JO, et al. High frequency oscillation in patients with acute lung injury and acute respiratory distress syndrome (ARDS): systematic review and meta-analysis. BMJ 2010;340:c2327; with permission.)

observational studies and animal data, to be hypothesis generating; HFOV appears to improve oxygenation and may be associated with improvements in mortality, but more studies are needed. To this end, the authors are aware of 2 ongoing, large, prospective, randomized clinical trials: OSCILLation for ARDS treated early (OSCILLATE) (ISRCTN87124254) and OSCAR (ISRCTN10416500). Although they are using different protocols, both of these trials are currently enrolling patients with target sample sizes of 1200 and 1006, respectively, and will compare HFOV with conventional ventilation.

Current Application of HFOV in Adults

Clinical application of HFOV has evolved over the years. With sparse clinical trial evidence to guide therapy, detailed recommendations have been proposed at a recent expert roundtable report on HFOV use.[55] A full discussion about protocols to implement HFOV is beyond the scope of this article; instead, the authors briefly summarize some key aspects.

Optimal Frequency in HFOV

For many years it was assumed that HFOV always delivered low tidal volumes. However, tidal volumes are not measured on the commercially available adult oscillator, and unlike the neonatal setting where either fixed-volume oscillators or high frequencies are routinely used (10–15 Hz), lower frequencies were commonly used in adults (3–6 Hz). The issue about the size of tidal volumes in adults became an area of debate when Sedeek and colleagues[56] measured tidal volumes in a sheep saline-lavage model of acute lung injury using a pneumotachograph. They found that HVOF applied at a frequency of 4 Hz resulted in a tidal volume of 4 mL/kg, not as small as anticipated. Subsequently, however, Hager and colleagues[57,58] performed a potentially more accurate and definitely more relevant study using a hot-wire anemometer to measure tidal volumes in adults with ARDS. They found volumes that were usually in the expected range of 1 to 2 mL/kg PBW. When they adjusted delta P and frequency up and down, they found that frequency had a dominant effect on tidal volume over delta P, and that in some patients tidal volumes that were not negligible could be delivered under certain conditions.

The key message from these data collectively is that HFOV can deliver small tidal volumes in adults, but it does not necessarily happen automatically in every case. Therefore, experts recommend using a strategy whereby the highest tolerated frequency is employed, and in addition, to consider implementing a partial cuff leak in the endotracheal tube to facilitate CO_2 clearance when the frequency is below 6 Hz.[55] Indeed, it appears possible that adequate ventilation can be achieved at higher frequencies in adults, with one recent study demonstrating that frequencies greater than 6 Hz can maintain adequate gas exchange.[59]

When to initiate HFOV

There have been efforts to advance our knowledge regarding the optimal timing of initiation of HFOV. As mentioned previously, HFOV has most often been used as rescue therapy for patients failing CV. Early studies typically initiated HFOV at 5 days following the start of CV. However, the findings of several observational studies have demonstrated improved outcomes if HFOV is initiated earlier before harmful effects of CV take hold. One such observational study by David and colleagues[60] demonstrated a several-fold lower mortality in patients in which HFOV was initiated within 3 days of CV in comparison to after 3 days (20% vs 64%).

Despite the findings of a meta-analysis evaluating the determinants of mortality in adults with ARDS, which found no clear relationship between timing of HFOV and mortality after adjusting for other factors,[61] most experts still agree that HFOV should ideally be used earlier rather than later, and certainly before prolonged exposure to injurious levels of CV. This approach is certainly being employed in the ongoing trials of HFOV versus CV.

Open-Lung Approach

The neonatal experience with HFOV has highlighted the importance of an open-lung approach, with use of lung recruitment maneuvers.[62] Indeed, because of the small tidal volumes used in HFOV, recruitment maneuvers may be more important because of the lack of tidal recruitment seen with CV. In adults with ARDS, there remain 2 schools of thought about how aggressive one should be with higher mean airway pressures trying to achieve lung recruitment, with some experts suggesting that airway pressures be limited and higher FiO2 used.[55] The authors, and others, favor an approach that attempts to open the lung and oscillate on the deflation limb of the volume pressure curve. In a physiologic study, the authors showed that that the combination of recruitment maneuvers and a decremental adjustment of mP_{AW} with HFOV appears safe and results in rapid and sustained improvement in oxygenation, presumably through lung recruitment.[63]

A key point about targeting lung recruitment with HFOV is to select patients that may benefit from this, which means identifying patients with a significant amount of collapsed, consolidated, or derecruited lung who may benefit from increases in mean airway pressure.[64] Because routine CT scanning in these sick patients is often not feasible, the authors recommend an approach where patients with significant airspace disease on chest radiograph and significant hypoxemia be targeted for HFOV use, not those with mild acute lung injury.

In addition to potentially identifying those who may benefit from recruitment, this strategy of targeting patients with more severe ARDS also seems reasonable because the use of intravascular volume loading and heavy sedation with or without neuromuscular blockade are more justified in these patients. Hemodynamic instability can result from the higher mean airway pressure applied during HFOV, because increased intrathoracic pressure leads to reductions in venous return, similar to that seen when high levels of PEEP are used with CV. This factor highlights the importance of ensuring adequate intravascular volume with appropriate volume administration before transition from CV to HFOV. Sedation, and sometimes paralysis, are required to suppress respiratory efforts in adults during HFOV to ensure that inspiratory flow demand does not outstrip the provided bias flow. Risks associated with sedatives and paralytics should be considered when determining whether patients are sick enough to justify their use. Short-term use of neuromuscular blocking agents in patients with ARDS has been reported to improve survival, although their long-term effects remain a question for further study.[65]

SUMMARY

HFOV appears to be theoretically ideal for patients with ARDS, conforming to the new goals of mechanical ventilation: the maintenance of adequate gas exchange without causing further injury to the lung. HFOV appears to be a useful tool in our armamentarium for the treatment of refractory hypoxemia. The authors think that, currently, HFOV should be used in the adult ICU as 1 of several ancillary therapies available for the treatment of these extremely ill, hypoxemic patients with ARDS. The effect of HFOV on other important endpoints, such as mortality, duration of ICU/hospital stay, organ dysfunction, and long-term quality of life, needs to be addressed. To determine whether HFOV should be considered as a more routine strategy for preventing VILI, the authors are awaiting the results of 2 ongoing, large, multicenter, randomized controlled trials: the OSCILLATE trial and OSCAR.

REFERENCES

1. Tobin MJ. Mechanical ventilation. N Engl J Med 1994;330(15):1056–61.
2. The Acute Respiratory Distress Syndrome N. Ventilation with lower tidal volumes as compared with traditional tidal volumes for acute lung injury and the acute respiratory distress syndrome. N Engl J Med 2000;342(18):1301–8.
3. Amato MB, Barbas CS, Medeiros DM, et al. Effect of a protective-ventilation strategy on mortality in the acute respiratory distress syndrome. N Engl J Med 1998;338(6):347–54.
4. Villar J, Kacmarek RM, Perez-Mendez L, et al. A high positive end-expiratory pressure, low tidal volume ventilatory strategy improves outcome in persistent acute respiratory distress syndrome: a randomized, controlled trial. Crit Care Med 2006;34(5):1311–8.
5. Briel M, Meade M, Mercat A, et al. Higher vs lower positive end-expiratory pressure in patients with acute lung injury and acute respiratory distress syndrome: systematic review and meta-analysis. JAMA 2010;303(9):865–73.
6. Ferguson ND, Stewart TE. New therapies for adults with acute lung injury. High-frequency oscillatory ventilation. Crit Care Clin 2002;18(1):91–106.
7. Ferguson ND, Slutsky AS. Point: high-frequency ventilation is the optimal physiological approach to ventilate ARDS patients. J Appl Physiol 2008;104(4):1230–1.
8. Froese AB. High-frequency oscillatory ventilation for adult respiratory distress syndrome: let's get it right this time. Crit Care Med 1997;25(6):906–8.
9. Henderson Y, Chillingsworth F, Whitney J. The respiratory dead space. Am J Physiology 1915;38:1–19.
10. Lunkenheimer PP, Rafflenbeul W, Keller H, et al. Application of transtracheal pressure oscillations as a modification of "diffusion respiration". Br J Anaesth 1972;44:627.
11. Bryan AC. The oscillations of HFO. Am J Respir Crit Care Med 2001;163:816–7.
12. Bryan AC, Slutsky AS. Long volume during high frequency oscillation. Am Rev Respir Dis 1986;133(5):928–30.
13. McCulloch PR, Forkert PG, Froese AB. Lung volume maintenance prevents lung injury during high frequency oscillatory ventilation in surfactant-deficient rabbits. Am Rev Respir Dis 1988;137(5):1185–92.
14. Hamilton PP, Onayemi A, Smyth JA, et al. Comparison of conventional and high-frequency oscillatory ventilation. J Appl Physiol 1983;55:131–8.
15. Kolton M, Cattran CB, Kent G, et al. Oxygenation during high-frequency ventilation compared with conventional mechanical ventilation in two models of lung injury. Anesth Analg 1982;61(4):323–32.
16. Slutsky AS, Kamm RD, Rossing TH, et al. Effects of frequency, tidal volume, and lung volume on CO2 elimination in dogs by high frequency (2-30 Hz), low tidal volume ventilation. J Clin Invest 1981;68(6):1475–84.
17. Group HS. High-frequency oscillatory ventilation compared with conventional mechanical ventilation in the treatment of respiratory failure in preterm infants. N Engl J Med 1989;320(2):88–93.
18. Plavka R, Kopecky P, Sebron V, et al. A prospective randomized comparison of conventional mechanical ventilation and very early high frequency oscillatory ventilation in extremely premature newborns with respiratory distress syndrome. Intensive Care Med 1999;25(1):68–75.

19. Ogawa Y, Miyasaka K, Kawano T, et al. A multicenter randomized trial of high frequency oscillatory ventilation as compared with conventional mechanical ventilation in preterm infants with respiratory failure. Early Hum Dev 1993;32(1):1–10.
20. Clark RH, Gerstmann DR, Null DM, et al. Prospective randomized comparison of high-frequency oscillatory and conventional ventilation in respiratory distress syndrome. Pediatrics 1992;89(1):5–12.
21. Clark RH, Yoder BA, Sell MS. Prospective, randomized comparison of high-frequency oscillation and conventional ventilation in candidates for extracorporeal membrane oxygenation. J Pediatr 1994;124(3):447–54.
22. Courtney SE, Durand DJ, Asselin JM, et al. High-frequency oscillatory ventilation versus conventional mechanical ventilation for very-low-birth-weight infants. N Engl J Med 2002;347(9):643–52.
23. Bollen CW, Uiterwaal CS, Van Vught AJ. Cumulative meta-analysis of high-frequency versus conventional ventilation in premature neonates. Am J Respir Crit Care Med 2003;168(10):1150–5.
24. Fort P, Farmer C, Westerman J, et al. High-frequency oscillatory ventilation for adult respiratory distress syndrome–a pilot study. Crit Care Med 1997;25(6): 937–47.
25. Mehta S, Granton J, MacDonald RJ, et al. High-frequency oscillatory ventilation in adults: the Toronto experience. Chest 2004;126(2):518–27.
26. Derdak S. High-frequency oscillatory ventilation for acute respiratory distress syndrome in adults: a randomized, controlled trial. Am J Respir Crit Care Med 2002;166(6):801–8.
27. Sud S, Sud M, Friedrich JO, et al. High frequency oscillation in patients with acute lung injury and acute respiratory distress syndrome (ARDS): systematic review and meta-analysis. BMJ 2010;340:c2327.
28. Suzuki H, Papazoglou K, Bryan AC. Relationship between PaO2 and lung volume during high frequency oscillatory ventilation. Acta Paediatrica Japonica 1992; 34(5):494–500.
29. Chang HK. Mechanisms of gas transport during ventilation by high-frequency oscillation. respiratory, environmental and exercise physiology. J Appl Physiol 1984;56(3):553–63.
30. Slutsky AS, Drazen JM. Ventilation with small tidal volumes. N Engl J Med 2002; 347(9):630–1.
31. Van Genderingen HR, Van Vught AJ, Duval EL, et al. Attenuation of pressure swings along the endotracheal tube is indicative of optimal distending pressure during high-frequency oscillatory ventilation in a model of acute lung injury. Pediatr Pulmonol 2002;33(6):429–36.
32. Sakai T, Kakizawa H, Aiba S, et al. Effects of mean and swing pressures on piston-type high-frequency oscillatory ventilation in rabbits with and without acute lung injury. Pediatr Pulmonol 1999;27(5):328–35.
33. Pillow JJ, Sly PD, Hantos ZN. Monitoring of lung volume recruitment and derecruitment using oscillatory mechanics during high-frequency oscillatory ventilation in the preterm lamb. Pediatr Crit Care Med 2004;5(2):172–80.
34. Mentzelopoulos SD, Malachias S, Kokkoris S, et al. Comparison of high-frequency oscillation and tracheal gas insufflation versus standard high-frequency oscillation at two levels of tracheal pressure. Intensive Care Med 2010;36(5):810–6.
35. Dreyfuss D, Saumon G. Ventilator-induced lung injury: lessons from experimental studies. Am J Respir Crit Care Med 1998;157:294–323.
36. Santos Dos CC, Slutsky AS. Invited review: mechanisms of ventilator-induced lung injury: a perspective. J Appl Physiol 2000;89:1645–55.

37. Dreyfuss D, Soler P, Basset G, et al. High inflation pressure pulmonary edema. Respective effects of high airway pressure, high tidal volume, and positive end-expiratory pressure. Am Rev Respir Dis 1988;137(5):1159–64.
38. Dreyfuss D, Basset G, Soler P, et al. Intermittent positive-pressure hyperventilation with high inflation pressures produces pulmonary microvascular injury in rats. Am Rev Respir Dis 1985;132(4):880–4.
39. Tremblay L, Valenza F, Ribeiro SP, et al. Injurious ventilatory strategies increase cytokines and c-fos m-RNA expression in an isolated rat lung model. J Clin Invest 1997;99(5):944–52.
40. Webb HH, Tierney DF. Experimental pulmonary edema due to intermittent positive pressure ventilation with high inflation pressures. Protection by positive end-expiratory pressure. Am Rev Respir Dis 1974;110(5):556–65.
41. Tremblay LN, Slutsky AS. Ventilation-induced lung injury: from barotrauma to biotrauma. Proc Assoc Am Physicians 1998;110:482–8.
42. Santos Dos CC, Slutsky AS. Cellular responses to mechanical stress: invited review: mechanisms of ventilator-induced lung injury: a perspective. J Appl Physiol 2000;89(4):1645–55.
43. Terragni PP, Rosboch G, Tealdi A, et al. Tidal hyperinflation during low tidal volume ventilation in acute respiratory distress syndrome. Am J Respir Crit Care Med 2006;175(2):160–6.
44. Muscedere JG, Mullen JB, Gan K, et al. Tidal ventilation at low airway pressures can augment lung injury. Am J Respir Crit Care Med 1994;149(5):1327–34.
45. Gattinoni L, Pesenti A. The concept of "baby lung". Intensive Care Med 2005; 31(6):776–84.
46. Rotta AT, Gunnarsson B, Fuhrman BP, et al. Comparison of lung protective ventilation strategies in a rabbit model of acute lung injury. Crit Care Med 2001;29(11): 2176–84.
47. Imai Y, Nakagawa S, Ito Y, et al. Comparison of lung protection strategies using conventional and high-frequency oscillatory ventilation. J Appl Physiol 2001; 91(4):1836–44.
48. der von HK, Kandler MA, Fink L, et al. High frequency oscillatory ventilation suppresses inflammatory response in lung tissue and microdissected alveolar macrophages in surfactant depleted piglets. Pediatr Res 2004;55(2):339–46.
49. Sedeek KA, Takeuchi M, Suchodolski K, et al. Open-lung protective ventilation with pressure control ventilation, high-frequency oscillation, and intratracheal pulmonary ventilation results in similar gas exchange, hemodynamics, and lung mechanics. Anesthesiology 2003;99(5):1102–11.
50. Bryan CL, Jenkinson SG. Oxygen toxicity. Clin Chest Med 1988;9(1):141–52.
51. Bryan AC, Froese AB. Reflections on the HIFI trial. Pediatrics 1991;87:565–7.
52. Henderson-Smart DJ, Cools F, Bhuta T. Elective high frequency oscillatory ventilation versus conventional ventilation for acute pulmonary dysfunction in preterm infants. Cochrane Database Syst Rev 2007;3:CD000104.
53. Mehta S, Lapinsky SE, Hallett DC, et al. A prospective trial of high frequency oscillatory ventilation in adults with acute respiratory distress syndrome. Crit Care Med 2001;29:1360–9.
54. Derdak S, Mehta S, Stewart TE, et al. High frequency oscillatory ventilation for acute respiratory distress syndrome: a randomized controlled trial. Am J Respir Crit Care Med 2002;166:801–8.
55. Fessler HE, Derdak S, Ferguson ND, et al. A protocol for high-frequency oscillatory ventilation in adults: results from a roundtable discussion. Crit Care Med 2007;35:1649–54.

56. Sedeek KA, Takeuchi M, Suchodolski K, et al. Determinants of tidal volume during high-frequency oscillation. Crit Care Med 2003;31(1):227–31.
57. Hager DN, Fuld M, Kaczka DW, et al. Four methods of measuring tidal volume during high-frequency oscillatory ventilation. Crit Care Med 2006;34(3):751–7.
58. Hager DN, Fessler HE, Kaczka DW, et al. Tidal volume delivery during high-frequency oscillatory ventilation in adults with acute respiratory distress syndrome*. Crit Care Med 2007;35(6):1522–9.
59. Fessler HE, Hager DN, Brower RG. Feasibility of very high-frequency ventilation in adults with acute respiratory distress syndrome*. Crit Care Med 2008;36(4): 1043–8.
60. David M, Weiler N, Heinrichs W, et al. High-frequency oscillatory ventilation in adult acute respiratory distress syndrome. Intensive Care Med 2003;29(10):1656–65.
61. Bollen C, Uiterwaal C, Van Vught A. HFO Outcome determinants. Crit Care 2006; 10(1):R34.
62. Froese AB, Kinsella JP. High-frequency oscillatory ventilation: lessons from the neonatal/pediatric experience. Crit Care Med 2005;33(Suppl 3):S115–21.
63. Ferguson ND, Chiche J, Kacmarek RM, et al. Combining high-frequency oscillatory ventilation and recruitment maneuvers in adults with early acute respiratory distress syndrome: the Treatment with Oscillation and an Open Lung Strategy (TOOLS) Trial pilot study*. Crit Care Med 2005;33(3):479–86.
64. Gattinoni L, Caironi P, Cressoni M, et al. Lung recruitment in patients with the acute respiratory distress syndrome. N Engl J Med 2006;354(17):1775–86.
65. Papazian L, Forel J, Gacouin A, et al. Neuromuscular blockers in early acute respiratory distress syndrome. N Engl J Med 2010;363(12):1107–16.

Airway Pressure Release Ventilation in Acute Respiratory Distress Syndrome

Adrian A. Maung, MD, Lewis J. Kaplan, MD, FCCM, FCCP*

KEYWORDS

- APRV • Airway pressure release ventilation • ARDS • ALI
- PEEP • Alveolar derecruitment

Patients with acute lung injury (ALI) and acute respiratory distress syndrome (ARDS) exhibit multiple areas of lung collapse, often in the dependent regions. The ensuing decrease in gas-exchanging alveoli leads to pulmonary shunting and hypoxemia. Conventional mechanical ventilation strategies can exacerbate this pulmonary pathology through ventilator-induced lung injury (VILI) by both overdistention as well as mechanical shear during repeat openings of the normal, more compliant alveoli. The current accepted lung protective ventilation strategy uses low tidal volume ventilation with moderate positive-end expiratory pressure (PEEP) (ARDSnet).

However, airway pressure release ventilation (APRV) is also increasingly used as an alternative mode of ventilation for both salvage therapy in hypoxemic respiratory failure as well as an alternate means of lung protection in patients with ALI/ARDS. In this article, the authors review the basic principles of APRV, discuss the theoretical and published experimental benefits of APRV, as compared with conventional modes of ventilation, and review the available human clinical data.

WHAT IS APRV?

Stock and Downs first described APRV in 1987 as a modified form of continuous positive airway pressure (CPAP) to enhance oxygenation by augmenting alveolar recruitment.[1] Because fairly high CPAP levels are used, CO_2 clearance must be supported by intermittently releasing the airway pressure and allowing ventilation, hence, the appellation airway pressure release ventilation. The APRV respiratory cycle is, therefore, divided into 2 time periods: a longer T_{high} period at the higher airway

---

The authors have nothing to disclose.
Department of Surgery, Section of Trauma, Surgical Critical Care and Surgical Emergencies, Yale University School of Medicine, 330 Cedar Street, BB310, PO Box 208062, New Haven, CT 06520-8062, USA
* Corresponding author.
E-mail address: lewis.kaplan@yale.edu

Crit Care Clin 27 (2011) 501–509
doi:10.1016/j.ccc.2011.05.003 criticalcare.theclinics.com
0749-0704/11/$ – see front matter

pressure (P_{high}) and a much shorter (typically 0.4–0.8 seconds) T_{low} period during which pressure is released to P_{low} to allow for CO_2 clearance (**Fig. 1**). Because most of the respiratory cycle (80%–95%) is spent at P_{high}, the generated mean airway pressure is higher than in conventional ventilation modes without a corresponding increase in peak airway pressure.[2] The short release times retain a residual volume of air, thus, creating intentional auto-PEEP. Both the higher mean airway pressure and the auto-PEEP prevent collapse of alveoli and progressively recruit additional lung units to participate in gas exchange by matching the regional time constant variations in injured segments of lung.

It is essential to note that patients may breathe at any point in the phase cycle because of the unique valve construction of ventilators capable of providing APRV. In this way, APRV is fundamentally different from traditional cyclic ventilation where patients are constrained to either inspiration or exhalation occurring only during predefined periods. A full discussion of managing ventilator settings in APRV is beyond the scope of this article, but several reviews are available.[2–4]

Mechanics and Hemodynamic Effects of APRV

Oxygenation in APRV occurs by a combination of several mechanisms: (1) alveolar recruitment, (2) intrinsic PEEP, and (3) increased pulmonary and systemic blood flow.[5–8] CO_2 clearance occurs as a result of the combined effects of P_{high}, T_{high}, and T_{low} on recruiting alveoli and maintaining the lung at volumes approaching total lung capacity (TLC). At P_{high}, the chest wall resistance, compliance and elastance in concert with elastic recoil of the lung are balanced against the applied airway pressure. When that airway pressure is released, forces tending to expel gas are unopposed, generating gas flow rates that routinely approach negative 80 L/min (see **Fig. 1**). Thus, ventilation may occur over a short period of time, allowing a short T_{low} to be employed.

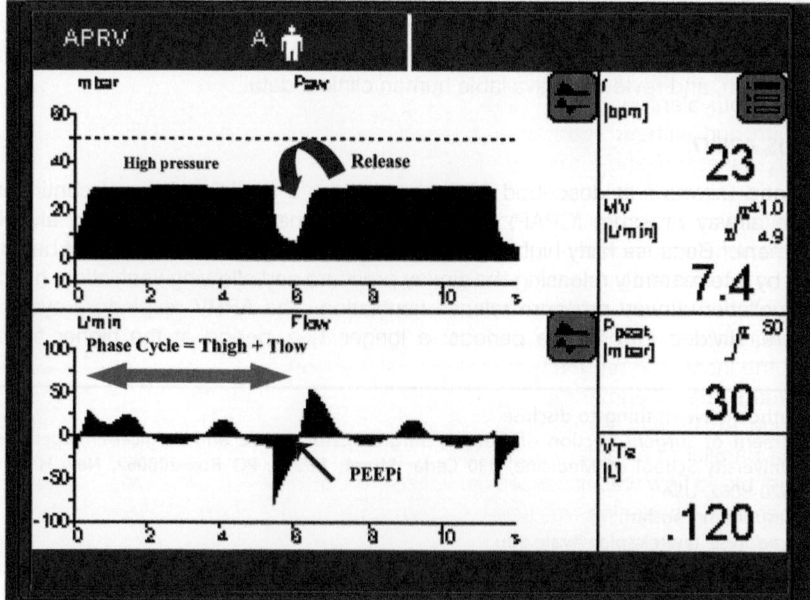

Fig. 1. Airway pressure release ventilation.

Moreover, the tremendous alveolar recruitment also affects pulmonary and systemic blood flow in a salutary fashion.[5,6,8] One byproduct of the vast alveolar recruitment achieved with APRV is reduction and even near elimination of hypoxic pulmonary vasoconstriction.[5,8,9] Reduction of pulmonary hypoxic vasoconstriction ultimately depends on the degree of recruitment achieved; the advantage of APRV is that it achieves much greater recruitment than other conventional modes of mechanical ventilation. By ameliorating hypoxic pulmonary vasoconstriction, one increases the effective cross-sectional area of the pulmonary vascular bed, reduces pulmonary vascular resistance, and, in turn, decreases the effective pressure against which the right ventricle ejects. The increase in right ventricle ejection fraction leads to decreased end-systolic volume and, thus, decreased end-systolic pressure. The decreased right ventricle pressure augments right atrial emptying and increases venous return. Increased venous return generates increased cardiac output by an increase in stroke volume, a low oxygen cost method of augmenting cardiac performance.

Note that the increase in cardiac performance is akin to the volume of recruitable cardiac performance targeted during resuscitation from septic shock. Moreover, with increased myofibrillar stretch, increased contractility is also observed as measured by left ventricle stroke work index.[8] Such benefits also allow reduction in vasopressor agents required for maintenance of mean arterial pressure in the setting of sepsis or injury.[8,9] Importantly, increased cardiac performance as a result of increased pulmonary flow is an important and perhaps overlooked element in critical care management schemes, and occurs at a time that oxygenation is being maximized when using APRV. Patients being managed on APRV realize the full benefits of the mode when they are allowed to engage in spontaneous ventilation.[10,11]

The Role of Spontaneous Breathing

During the last 2 decades, assisted forms of spontaneous breathing have risen to the forefront of critical care medicine as a desirable tool in the intensivist's armamentarium.[12] Wrigge and colleagues[6] investigated the effect of spontaneous ventilation on lung volume using both computed tomographic (CT) scanning and nitrogen-washout techniques in a porcine model of oleic acid acute lung injury. Pigs sustained equivalent lung injury and were then divided into 2 groups managed on APRV with and without spontaneous breathing. Spontaneous breathing increased paO_2, CT-assessed end-expiratory lung volume, and a CT-guided aeration index. Importantly, nitrogen-washout characteristics indicated that recruitment was not static, but steadily improved over the course of the 4-hour experiment, demonstrating a dynamic benefit to spontaneous breathing with APRV (**Fig. 2**). Importantly, the investigators noted that the increased aeration and lung volume was derived from dependent region recruitment rather than overdistention of compliant regions, supporting a lung protective role for APRV. The question unanswered by this experiment was whether the increased recruitment was matched by increased perfusion.

Two years later, Neumann and colleagues[5] investigated whether alveolar recruitment using APRV with spontaneous breathing augmented pulmonary blood flow in a fashion parallel to alveolar recruitment. In an identical model of lung injury to that of Wrigge, blood flow was assessed using positron emission tomographic (PET) scanning, whereas CT scanning was used to interrogate lung recruitment. Recruitment and blood flow was assessed, progressing from the sternum to the spine, to determine regionalization of changes in alveolar volume and corresponding blood flow. Similar recruitment was identified as in the 2003 Wrigge and colleagues study when using APRV with spontaneous breathing (**Fig. 3**). Perhaps most importantly, regional blood

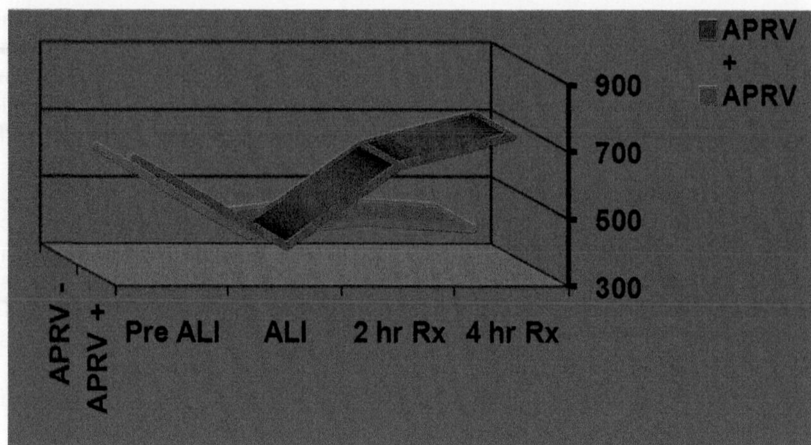

Fig. 2. End-expiratory lung volumes with (+) and without (-) spontaneous breathing during airway pressure release ventilation. Nitrogen washout-derived end-expiratory lung volumes (mL) in a porcine model of oleic acid injury demonstrating the benefit of spontaneous breathing with APRV (*green*) as measured by steadily increased lung volumes compared with ARPV without spontaneous breathing. APRV +, APRV with spontaneous breathing; ARPV -, APRV without spontaneous breathing; Pre ALI, before instillation of oleic acid; Rx, treatment. (*Adapted from* Wrigge H, Zinserling J, Neumann P, et al. Spontaneous breathing improves lung aeration in oleic acid-induced lung injury. Anesthesiology 2003;99(2):376–84; with permission.)

flow increased in a parallel fashion, with the greatest benefit noted in the group with spontaneous breathing. Therefore, this group established that APRV with spontaneous breathing decreased pulmonary shunt with the maximal decrease being observed in dependent regions that were previously derecruited and underperfused. Increased pulmonary blood flow with ventilation and perfusion redistribution should allow for efficient gas exchange and may allow the clinician to use a lower minute ventilation to achieve similar ventilator goals.

End-Organ Blood Flow

Although ventilator management augments systemic oxygenation for patients suffering from a variety of maladies, APRV has been demonstrated to increase cardiac performance as well as pulmonary blood flow. Whether these flow changes may be observed in other end-organ systems, such as the kidney, may be logically predicted. Decreased intrathoracic pressure and right-sided pressures may lead to a lower venous pressure for in-line organs, such as the liver, kidney, and brain. Decreased venous pressure should augment the net flux of blood across these systems at a given mean arterial pressure (MAP) using the straightforward mathematics used to calculate organ blood flow (MAP–mean organ venous outflow pressure = organ perfusion pressure). Recognizing that cerebral perfusion pressure (CPP) depends on intracranial pressure (ICP), and that ICP is tied to brain parenchymal volume, cerebrospinal fluid, and intracranial blood volume, one may reason that reduced venous pressure will allow for enhanced cerebral venous drainage, lower ICP, and improved CPP. Clearly, such benefits, if realizable, would be desirable as part of an end-organ blood flow management scheme to support O_2 delivery and use.

To investigate whether these notions were accurate, 12 patients with ALI were managed with APRV with or without spontaneous breathing.[10] As a means of

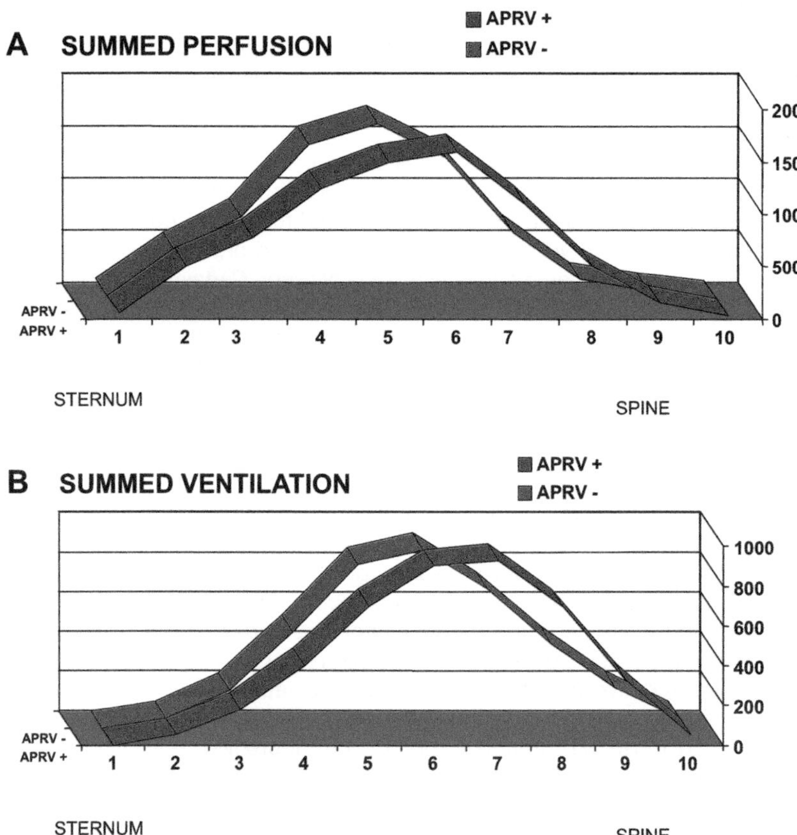

Fig. 3. Regional changes in alveolar ventilation and perfusion with (+) and without (-) spontaneous breathing during APRV. (*A*) Summed perfusion, (*B*) summed ventilation. (*Adapted from* Neumann P, Wrigge H, Zinserling J, et al. Spontaneous breathing affects the spatial ventilation and perfusion distribution during mechanical ventilatory support. Crit Care Med 2005;33(5):1090–5; with permission.)

supplemental investigation, patients managed with APRV without spontaneous breathing were managed to establish either no change in minute ventilation (V_E) or no change in airway pressure (P_{aw}) compared with those with spontaneous breathing. Cardiac index, glomerular filtration rate (GFR), and effective renal blood flow (eRBF) were assessed. Although cardiac index was maximized using APRV without spontaneous breathing and constant P_{aw} (similar to the Kaplan study), GFR and eRBF were optimized with spontaneous breathing. This observation was important because it supported the concept that the intensivist's target of optimized end-organ perfusion may not correlate with gross measures of systemic blood flow. More subtly, and perhaps more importantly, this study demonstrated that a ventilator strategy can modify end-organ perfusion independent of plasma volume expander-based changes in effective circulating volume or the use of vasopressor agents.

It is perhaps noteworthy that this observation, coupled with the physiology previously outlined, fit together nicely with the concept of stressed volume as advanced by Magder.[13] It is intuitively attractive that APRV manifests its' observed changes in effective circulating volume by manipulating and recruiting volume from capacitance vessels, thereby augmenting patients' stressed volume. Further investigation, however, is required before accepting this theory as fact. However, Hering's[11] group also noted similar results with intestinal blood flow in an identical model. It is similarly attractive that patients at risk for intestinal ischemia during resuscitation would be patients targeted for management with APRV and spontaneous breathing. Such patients are those with rising intra-abdominal pressures who are at risk of developing intra-abdominal hypertension and then the abdominal compartment syndrome. APRV with spontaneous breathing may ameliorate the need for as vigorous volume expansion by recruiting stressed volume, and reducing the end-organ venous pressure as a means of augmenting organ blood flow and O_2 delivery. Certainly, such a management strategy would be predicted to modify the abdominal perfusion pressure and, thus, intestinal perfusion pressure (small and large bowel). It is unclear whether such a strategy would decrease the incidence of unanticipated abdominal compartment syndrome and the rate of unintended relaparotomy for decompression, but this strategy is conceptually attractive.

Patient and Family Comfort

APRV has been documented to increase patient comfort compared with ventilator modes that deliver gas in abnormal fashions, such as inverse ratio pressure control ventilation.[8,9] Reductions in sedative needs as guided by stimulated Bispectral Index criteria as well as more traditional sedative protocols surface as additional benefits in the current literature.[9] The singular importance of these observations is not in reductions in direct financial costs by reduced medication use but in the underlying implications. Reduced sedative needs indicate increased patient comfort. Less sedated patients are better able to participate in their care (physically, emotionally, and cognitively), excluding those with traumatic brain injury. Moreover, remaining uncertain about the depth of sedation and analgesia for patients receiving neuromuscular blockers is curtailed by enabling the use of interactive sedation and analgesia assessment scales in awake patients. Patients may participate in turning as well as self-repositioning, a critically essential element in avoiding both pressure ulceration and nursing injury with the steadily growing severely obese patient population. Current studies are underway to track these elements.

Family comfort is enhanced when patients are able to interact with their family. Certainly, heavy sedation or neuromuscular blockade abolishes communication between patients and their family or support individuals. Two studies demonstrate reductions or elimination of neuromuscular blockade and heavy sedation using APRV instead of conventional ventilation for managing ALI or ARDS.[8,9] Eliminating the use of neuromuscular blocking agents in the intensive care unit (ICU) will eliminate the prolonged neuromuscular blockade syndrome in those patients. Although APRV may be combined with prone positioning for ALI/ARDS management, prone-positioning protocols often use neuromuscular blockade. Seemingly paradoxically, neuromuscular blockade may reduce the effectiveness of the prone position by failing to maximally redistribute both gas and blood flow.[14] Thus, using APRV may simplify and optimize the use of adjunctive measures supporting pulmonary recruitment.

APRV in the Operating Room

Therapeutic interventions for critically ill patients with ALI/ARDS may require transport to the operating room (OR). In addition, it is not infrequent that patients who are optimized with regard to ventilator settings undergo a moderate-length operative procedure and return to the ICU hypoxemic and hypercarbic, yet, at no time in the OR was hypoxia or hypercarbia an issue. In this discrete patient population with evolving or recovering ALI or ARDS, alveolar derecruitment is the common thread uniting the clinical observations. The reader should note that modern OR practice uses ventilator tidal volumes that are commonly set at less than what are employed in the ICU, as is the rate of mechanical ventilation. Thus, there is commonly an absolute decrease in inspiratory time and a concomitant increase in expiratory time. These practices are further enabled by anesthesia machines that are incapable of delivering PEEP (rare), or the lack of applied PEEP (more common), rendering recruitment maintenance in the OR problematic. Indeed, a recent review of intraoperative management techniques to avoid postoperative pulmonary complications advocated for limited use of PEEP.[15] This issue is complex, spanning anesthesia technique, ventilator mode, patient position, and procedure that ultimately affect gas distribution.

Multiple controllable factors promote derecruitment and atelectasis. Indeed, recruitment strategies employed after returning to the ICU typically resolve the issues accrued during the period of OR ventilation. Not all of the derecruitment occurs in the OR because significant derecruitment may occur if patients are disconnected from an appropriately adjusted ventilator and are hand ventilated using an bag valve mask bag for transport to and from the ICU. This situation can be corrected by employing transportation on a standard ventilator as opposed to a transport ventilator with reduced capabilities. Other etiologies of derecruitment separate from intraoperative ventilator strategy include closure of an open anterior abdominal wall with cephalad displacement of the diaphragms, or a thoracic procedure that requires single-lung ventilation.

One strategy to ameliorate swings in paO_2, $paCO_2$, and alveolar shear forces is to use APRV in the OR, especially for patients already being managed with APRV in the ICU or those with prolonged inspiratory times on modes, such as inverse ratio pressure control or inspiratory time–governed volume-cycled ventilation. Such a strategy was created and employed by Bratzke and colleagues[16] in 1998 and used quite successfully during operative undertakings.[16] Notably, the investigators described a reduced minute ventilation need as well as lower peak airway pressures compared with volume-cycled ventilation.

The authors apply APRV in the OR for major surgery, and have done so for the past 14 years. Of course, ICU-based procedures may also proceed unimpeded on APRV. Similar to the OR, deep sedation using fentanyl and propofol may be used instead of neuromuscular blockade. One disadvantage of using APRV in the OR is that it requires careful communication between the ICU service, the surgeon, and the anesthesiologist regarding the management of patients on a nonstandard mode of ventilation, because noncritical care–trained anesthesiologists may not have experience or comfort managing APRV settings, because the "user interface" of the device is rather different from many anesthesia machines. This aspect of care represents a patient safety issue regarding device manipulation, because the conceptual framework required to safely and effectively use APRV is readily taught and understood by clinicians of diverse backgrounds.

HUMAN STUDIES OF APRV

The clinical evidence evaluating the use of APRV is currently limited to retrospective studies and small, randomized trials. Small studies have demonstrated that compared with conventional ventilation, patients ventilated with APRV have lower peak airway pressures but higher mean airway pressures with comparable oxygenation and ventilation parameters.[17–19] Putensen and colleagues[9] randomized 30 trauma patients to either APRV with spontaneous breathing or pressure-controlled ventilation. The

APRV group had improved lung compliance and oxygenation with shorter duration of ventilator support, ICU length of stay, and decreased need for sedation and vasopressors.

Varpula and colleagues[20] randomized 58 patients with ALI to either APRV or pressure-controlled synchronized intermittent mandatory ventilation (SIMV) with pressure support. Although the inspiratory pressure was lower in the APRV group, other physiologic variables of oxygenation, ventilation, and hemodynamic variables were comparable between the 2 groups. The investigators concluded that the 2 modes of ventilation were equivalent. The same investigators also examined the effects of prone positioning in 33 patients with ALI who were ventilated with APRV versus pressure-controlled SIMV.[14] Patients ventilated with APRV had a significantly increased improvement in oxygenation following the second pronation episode. Dart and colleagues[21] performed a retrospective analysis of 46 trauma patients with and without ALI/ARDS. Patients who were converted to APRV had improved PaO_2/FiO_2 ratio as well as lower peak airway pressures.

Currently, there is only 1 prospective study, albeit a small one, comparing APRV directly to low tidal volume ventilation (LOVT).[22] Maxwell and colleagues randomized 63 trauma patients to APRV or LOVT using volume-control SIMV with pressure support. Their results suggested that APRV had a similar safety profile to LOVT, although there was a trend for increased ventilator days, ICU length of stay, and ventilator-associated pneumonia in the APRV group. This study has been criticized for both using SIMV with pressure support instead of volume assist-control ventilation used in the ARDSnet trials, and that many of the patients did not meet criteria for ARDS. It is clear that further study is required to evaluate for superiority of APRV compared with other ventilator modes. However, it is unlikely to occur because this would require a large, randomized prospective controlled trial. Instead, the available data suggests equivalence to conventional modes of ventilation, establishing APRV as one effective mode of lung protective ventilation in the intensivist's armamentarium for patients with ALI/ARDS.

SUMMARY

APRV is an alternative mode of ventilation that is increasingly used in patients with acute respiratory failure, ALI, and ARDS. Animal and clinical studies have demonstrated that, compared with conventional ventilation, APRV has beneficial effects on lung recruitment, oxygenation, end-organ blood flow, pulmonary vasoconstriction, and sedation requirements. Further studies, however, are required to directly compare APRV to ARDSnet protocol ventilation, specifically in patients with ALI/ARDS, and to determine whether managing ALI/ARDS with APRV will also achieve mortality reduction. For now, APRV may be used as a safe, effective alternative to conventional ventilation in patients with ALI and ARDS that may have its best role in providing optimal alveolar recruitment and hypoxemic salvage.

REFERENCES

1. Downs JB, Stock MC. Airway pressure release ventilation: a new concept in ventilatory support. Crit Care Med 1987;15(5):459–61.
2. Modrykamien A, Chatburn RL, Ashton RW. Airway pressure release ventilation: an alternative mode of mechanical ventilation in acute respiratory distress syndrome. Cleve Clin J Med 2011;78(2):101–10.
3. Frawley P, Habashi N. Airway pressure release ventilation and pediatrics: theory and practice. Crit Care Nurs Clin North Am 2004;16(3):337–48, viii.

4. Frawley P, Habashi N. Airway pressure release ventilation: theory and practice. AACN Clin Issues 2001;12(2):234–46 [quiz: 328–9].
5. Neumann P, Wrigge H, Zinserling J, et al. Spontaneous breathing affects the spatial ventilation and perfusion distribution during mechanical ventilatory support. Crit Care Med 2005;33(5):1090–5.
6. Wrigge H, Zinserling J, Neumann P, et al. Spontaneous breathing improves lung aeration in oleic acid-induced lung injury. Anesthesiology 2003;99(2):376–84.
7. Habashi NM. Other approaches to open-lung ventilation: airway pressure release ventilation. Crit Care Med 2005;33(3 Suppl):S228–40.
8. Kaplan LJ, Bailey H, Formosa V. Airway pressure release ventilation increases cardiac performance in patients with acute lung injury/adult respiratory distress syndrome. Crit Care 2001;5(4):221–6.
9. Putensen C, Zech S, Wrigge H, et al. Long-term effects of spontaneous breathing during ventilatory support in patients with acute lung injury. Am J Respir Crit Care Med 2001;164(1):43–9.
10. Hering R, Peters D, Zinserling J, et al. Effects of spontaneous breathing during airway pressure release ventilation on renal perfusion and function in patients with acute lung injury. Intensive Care Med 2002;28(10):1426–33.
11. Hering R, Viehöfer A, Zinserling J, et al. Effects of spontaneous breathing during airway pressure release ventilation on intestinal blood flow in experimental lung injury. Anesthesiology 2003;99(5):1137–44.
12. Burchardi H. New strategies in mechanical ventilation for acute lung injury. Eur Respir J 1996;9(5):1063–72.
13. Magder S, De Varennes B. Clinical death and the measurement of stressed vascular volume. Crit Care Med 1998;26(6):1061–4.
14. Varpula T, Jousela I, Niemi R, et al. Combined effects of prone positioning and airway pressure release ventilation on gas exchange in patients with acute lung injury. Acta Anaesthesiol Scand 2003;47(5):516–24.
15. Weingarten TN, Whalen FX, Warner DO, et al. Comparison of two ventilatory strategies in elderly patients undergoing major abdominal surgery. Br J Anaesth 2010;104(1):16–22.
16. Bratzke E, Downs JB, Smith RA. Intermittent CPAP: a new mode of ventilation during general anesthesia. Anesthesiology 1998;89(2):334–40.
17. Garner W, Downs JB, Stock MC, et al. Airway pressure release ventilation (APRV). A human trial. Chest 1988;94(4):779–81.
18. Davis K, Johnson DJ, Branson RD, et al. Airway pressure release ventilation. Arch Surg 1993;128(12):1348–52.
19. Räsänen J, Cane RD, Downs JB, et al. Airway pressure release ventilation during acute lung injury: a prospective multicenter trial. Crit Care Med 1991;19(10):1234–41.
20. Varpula T, Valta P, Niemi R, et al. Airway pressure release ventilation as a primary ventilatory mode in acute respiratory distress syndrome. Acta Anaesthesiol Scand 2004;48(6):722–31.
21. Dart BW, Maxwell RA, Richart CM, et al. Preliminary experience with airway pressure release ventilation in a trauma/surgical intensive care unit. J Trauma 2005;59(1):71–6.
22. Maxwell RA, Green JM, Waldrop J, et al. A randomized prospective trial of airway pressure release ventilation and low tidal volume ventilation in adult trauma patients with acute respiratory failure. J Trauma 2010;69(3):501–10 [discussion: 511].

Prone-Positioning Therapy in ARDS

Sharon Dickinson, RN, MSN, CNS-BC, ANP, CCRN,
Pauline K. Park, MD, FCCM, Lena M. Napolitano, MD*

KEYWORDS

- Acute respiratory distress syndrome
- Prone-positioning therapy • Hypoxemia • Acute lung injury
- Prone • Prone position

The prone position has been used to improve oxygenation in patients with severe hypoxemia and acute respiratory failure since 1974.[1] The prone position has been documented to induce an increase in both end-expiratory lung volume and alveolar recruitment. All studies with the prone position document an improvement in systemic oxygenation in 70% to 80% of patients with acute respiratory distress syndrome (ARDS), and the maximal improvements are seen in the most hypoxemic patients.

This article reviews the data regarding efficacy for use of the prone position in patients with ARDS. The authors also describe the simple, safe, quick, and inexpensive procedure that they use to prone a patient with severe ARDS on a standard bed in the intensive care unit (ICU) at the University of Michigan.[2]

PHYSIOLOGIC EFFECTS OF PRONE POSITION IN ARDS

When the ARDS patient is prone, the mass of the dorsal lung, which reinflates (ie, dorsal becomes the nondependent lung regions), is greater than the potential mass of the ventral (now dependent) lung regions, which may collapse (**Fig. 1**).[3] When lung perfusion is substantially unmodified, the overall ventilation/perfusion (V/Q) matching improves as new pulmonary units are recruited for more effective gas exchange.

This mechanism is probably the primary one for the improvement in oxygenation in the prone ARDS patient, although other mechanisms (including a different shape of the diaphragm, changes of hypoxic pulmonary vasoconstriction, and a differential production of nitric oxide in different lung regions) may play a role.[4] Both prone and semirecumbent positions facilitate the reaeration of dependent and caudal lung regions by partially relieving cardiac and abdominal compression, with resultant improvement in gas exchange.

Conflicts of Interest: None.
Division of Acute Care Surgery, Department of Surgery, University of Michigan Health System, 1500 East Medical Center Drive, 1C340A-UH, SPC 5033, Ann Arbor, MI 48109-5033, USA
* Corresponding author.
E-mail address: lenan@med.umich.edu

Crit Care Clin 27 (2011) 511–523
doi:10.1016/j.ccc.2011.05.010 criticalcare.theclinics.com
0749-0704/11/$ – see front matter

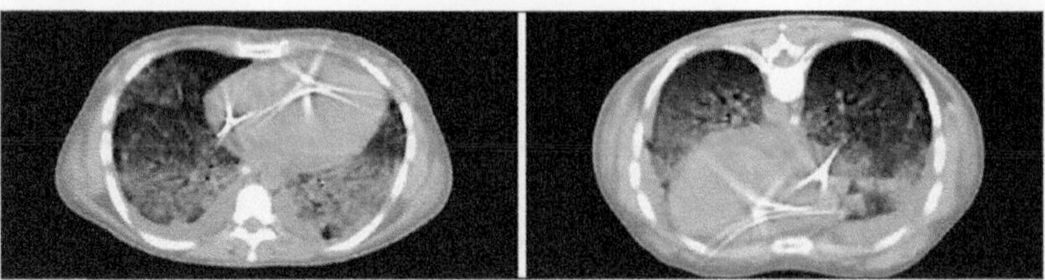

Fig. 1. Computed tomography scan of the lungs showing ARDS when the patient is lying supine (*left*) and prone (*right*). Note the density redistribution in the prone compared with the supine position. (*From* Gattinoni L, Protti A. Ventilation in the prone position: for some but not for all? CMAJ 2008;178(9):1174–6; with permission.)

Additional data confirm that the prone position may also limit ventilator-induced lung injury.[5] It has been postulated that the prone position leads to more homogeneous lung inflation and more homogeneous alveolar ventilation, suggesting that the strain applied to the lung parenchyma and its associated stress are more homogeneously distributed than in the supine position; this may decrease ventilator-induced lung injury.[6]

PRONE POSITION IN ARDS: EVIDENCE FOR EFFICACY

Changes in patient positioning can have a dramatic effect on oxygenation and ventilation in severe ARDS. Changing the patient position to prone or a steep lateral decubitus position can improve the distribution of perfusion to ventilated lung regions, decreasing intrapulmonary shunt and improving oxygenation.[7] The use of intermittent prone positioning has been documented to significantly improve oxygenation in 60% to 70% of acute lung injury (ALI) and ARDS patients.[1,8]

The Prone-Supine I Study[9] was a multicenter, randomized trial, in patients aged 16 years or older with ALI or ARDS, of conventional treatment compared with placing patients (n = 295) in a prone position for 6 or more hours daily for 10 days. No differences in mortality or complications were identified for the prone versus conventional positioning group at any time point during the study, with up to 6 months of follow-up. The mean increase in the partial pressure of oxygen/fraction of inspired oxygen (PaO_2/FiO_2) ratio was greater in the prone than in the supine group (63 $\pm$ 67 vs 45 $\pm$ 68, P = .02). Of note is that the mean PaO_2 of 85 to 88 mm Hg and mean PaO_2/FiO_2 ratio of 125 to 129 are quite high, that is, these patients did not have severe hypoxemia or severe ARDS (PaO_2/FiO_2 ratio <100) and therefore these patients may not have been likely to benefit from the prone intervention as regards mortality. A retrospective analysis of patients in the prone-position arm of this study revealed that ALI/ARDS patients who responded to prone positioning with a reduction in their partial pressure of carbon dioxide ($PaCO_2$) of 1 mm Hg or more showed an increase in survival at 28 days with a decrease in the mortality rate from 52% to 35%.[10]

A multicenter, randomized, controlled clinical trial[11] of supine versus prone positioning in 102 pediatric patients failed to demonstrate a significant difference in the main outcome measure, which was ventilator-free days to day 28. There were also no differences in the secondary end points study that included proportion alive and ventilator-free on day 28, mortality, time to recovery from lung injury, organ-failure free days, and functional health.

The Prone-Supine II Study[12] is the largest clinical trial (N = 342) in adult ARDS patients, conducted in 23 centers in Italy and 2 in Spain. Patients underwent supine or prone (20 hours per day) positioning during mechanical ventilation. Prone and supine patients from the entire study population had similar 28-day (31.0% vs 32.8%; relative risk [RR], 0.97; 95% confidence interval [CI], 0.84–1.13; P = .72) and 6-month (47.0% vs 52.3%; RR, 0.90; 95% CI, 0.73–1.11; P = .33) mortality rates, despite significantly higher complication rates in the prone group. Outcomes were also similar for patients with moderate hypoxemia in the prone and supine groups at 28 days (25.5% vs 22.5%; RR, 1.04; 95% CI, 0.89–1.22; P = .62) and at 6 months (42.6% vs 43.9%; RR, 0.98; 95% CI, 0.76–1.25; P = .85). Of importance, the 28-day mortality of patients with severe hypoxemia was decreased in the prone group (37.8% in the prone group and 46.1% in the supine group [RR, 0.87; 95% CI, 0.66–1.14; P = .31]), while their 6-month mortality was 52.7% and 63.2%, respectively (RR, 0.78; 95% CI, 0.53–1.14; P = .19).

A recent systematic review of the effect of mechanical ventilation in the prone position on clinical outcomes in patients with acute hypoxemic respiratory failure reported that it does not reduce mortality or duration of ventilation despite improved oxygenation and a decreased risk of pneumonia (**Figs. 2** and **3**).[13] However, despite there being no significant effect on mortality reduction, these data do confirm a significant improvement in oxygenation, and support the use of prone-position ventilation as a rescue strategy in patients with severe hypoxemia. Additional systematic reviews

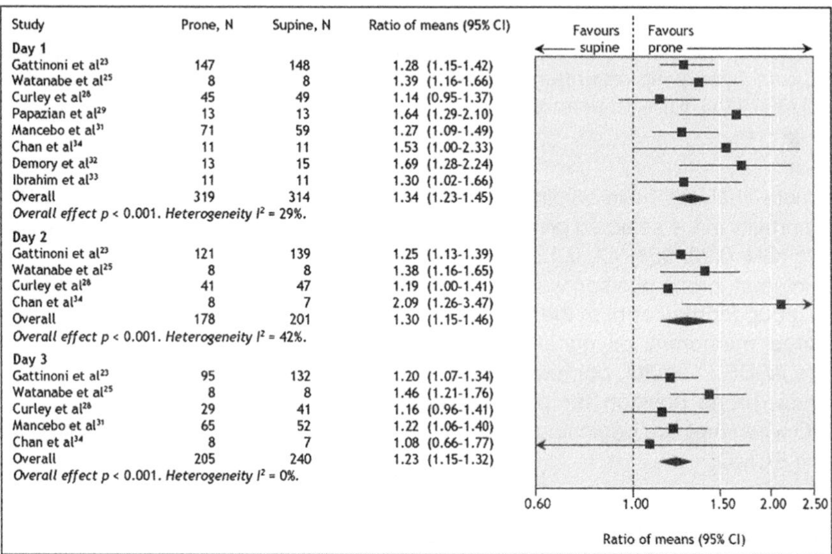

Fig. 2. Effect of prone position ventilation on oxygenation. Effect of ventilation in the prone position on daily ratio of partial pressure of oxygen to inspired fraction of oxygen. A random-effects model was used in the analysis. Values were recorded at the end of the period of prone positioning (prone group) and simultaneously in the supine group. Ratio of means = mean ratio of partial pressure of oxygen to inspired fraction of oxygen in the prone group divided by that in the supine group. I^2 = percentage of total variation across studies owing to between-study heterogeneity rather than chance. CI, confidence interval. Reference citations apply to references as listed in the source article. (*From* Sud S, Sud M, Friedrich JO, et al. Effect of mechanical ventilation in the prone position on clinical outcomes in patients with acute hypoxemic respiratory failure: a systematic review and meta-analysis. CMAJ 2008;178(8):1153–61; with permission.)

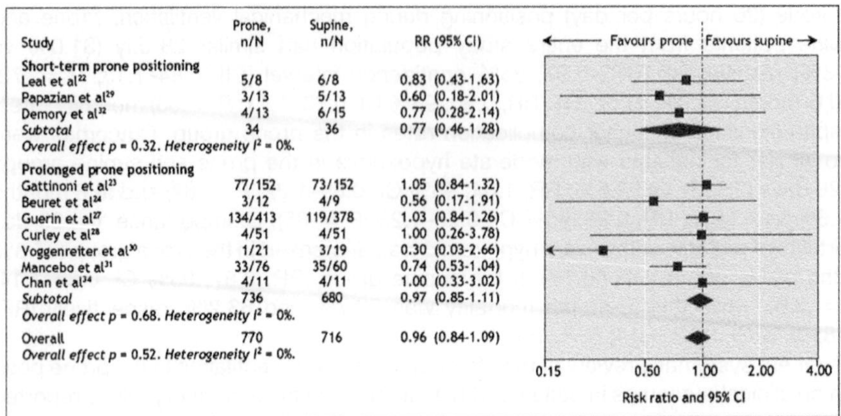

Fig. 3. Effect of prone position ventilation on mortality. A random-effects model was used for analysis. The duration of prone positioning was up to 24 hours for 1 to 2 days in the short-term trials and up to 24 hours daily for more than 2 days in the prolonged-duration trials. The trial by Gattinoni and colleagues[9] included data only for patients with acute hypoxemic respiratory failure. Including all patients from this trial (7/25 deaths in the prone group and 14/28 deaths in the supine group) did not change the result (RR 0.95, 95% CI 0.83–1.08; *P* = .41). I^2 = percentage of total variation across studies owing to between-study heterogeneity rather than chance. CI, confidence interval; RR, relative risk. Reference citations apply to references as listed in the source article. (*From* Sud S, Sud M, Friedrich JO, et al. Effect of mechanical ventilation in the prone position on clinical outcomes in patients with acute hypoxemic respiratory failure: a systematic review and meta-analysis. CMAJ 2008;178(8):1153–61; with permission.)

and meta-analyses have confirmed similar findings. Furthermore, the pooled OR for ICU mortality in the selected group of the more severely ill patients favored prone positioning (OR, 0.29; 95% CI, 0.12–0.70).[14–18]

Of interest, prone position was used in 42% of patients in the conventional management group (control arm) of the CESAR trial, the multicenter randomized trial of extracorporeal membrane oxygenation (ECMO) versus conventional therapy for treating severe ARDS in adults, compared with only 4% in the ECMO group.[19] The authors also use prone position for posterior dependent lung recruitment in patients on ECMO when they are beginning to recruit the native lung and progressing toward trialing off ECMO.

UPDATED META-ANALYSES OF RANDOMIZED TRIALS IN SEVERE ARDS

In patients with ALI or ARDS, more recent randomized controlled trials (RCTs) showed a consistent trend of mortality reduction with prone ventilation. An updated meta-analysis included 2 subgroups of studies: those that included all ALI or hypoxemic patients, and those that restricted inclusion to only ARDS patients. In the overall meta-analysis that included 7 RCTs with 1675 adult patients (862 in prone position), prone position was not associated with a mortality reduction (OR 0.91, 95% CI 0.75–1.2, *P* = .39). However, in the 4 most recent RCTs that enrolled only patients with ARDS, and that also applied the longest prone position durations and used lung-protective ventilation, prone position was associated with significantly reduced mortality (OR 0.71, 95% CI 0.5–0.99, *P* = .048; number needed to treat = 11)

(**Fig. 4**). Prone position was not associated with any increase in major airway complications in this meta-analysis.[20]

Gattinoni and colleagues[21] performed an individual patient meta-analysis of the 4 major clinical trials,[9,12,22,23] which documented that with prone positioning, the absolute mortality of severely hypoxemic ARDS patients may be reduced by approximately 10% (**Fig. 5**). This study also suggested that long-term prone positioning may expose patients with less severe ARDS to unnecessary complications. A recent review of all published meta-analyses on the efficacy of prone position in ALI and ARDS concluded that prone ventilation was associated with reduced mortality in patients with severe hypoxemic respiratory failure.[24]

EXTENDED PRONE POSITION VENTILATION

Extended prone position ventilation (extended PPV) in severe ARDS has been confirmed in a recent pilot feasibility study. Extended PPV was defined as PPV for 48 hours or until the oxygenation index was 10 or less. A prospective interventional study[25] in 15 patients confirmed that there was a statistically significant improvement in oxygenation (PaO_2/FiO_2 92 $\pm$ 12 vs 227 $\pm$ 43, $P<.0001$) and oxygenation index (22 $\pm$ 5 vs 8 $\pm$ 2, $P<.0001$), reduction of $PaCO_2$ (54 $\pm$ 9 vs 39 $\pm$ 4, $P<.0001$) and plateau pressure (32 $\pm$ 2 vs 27 $\pm$ 3, $P<.0001$), and improved static compliance (21 $\pm$ 3 vs 37 $\pm$ 6, $P<.0001$) with extended PPV. All the parameters continued to improve significantly while the patients remained in prone position and did not change on the patients' return to the supine position. The results obtained suggest that extended PPV is safe and effective in patients with severe ARDS when it is performed by trained staff and within an established protocol. Extended PPV is emerging as an effective rescue therapy for patients with severe ARDS and severe hypoxemia.

A prospective randomized study (n = 136),[23] with guidelines established for ventilator settings and weaning, examined the efficacy of the prolonged prone position

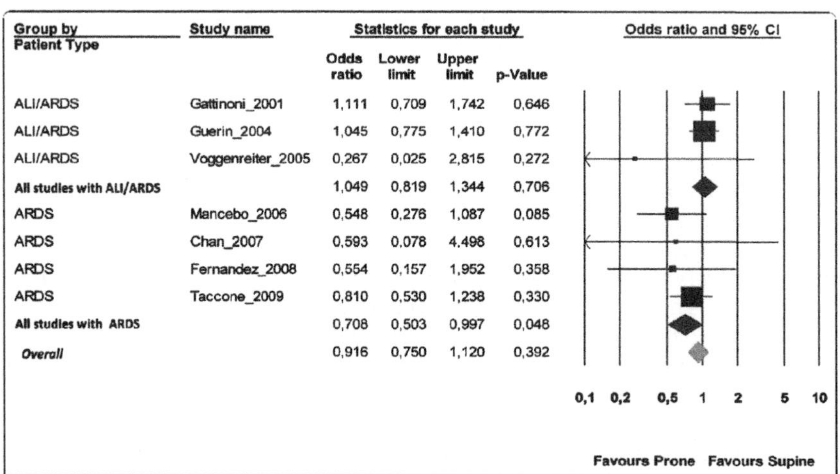

Fig. 4. Effect of prone position on ICU mortality. Point estimates (by random-effects model) are reported separately for the groups of studies that included both ALI and ARDS, those that included only ARDS patients, and the pooled overall effects of all patients included in the meta-analysis. (*From* Abroug F, Ouanes-Besbes L, Dachraoui F, et al. An updated study-level meta-analysis of randomised controlled trials on proning in ARDS and acute lung injury. Crit Care 2011;15(1):R6; with permission.)

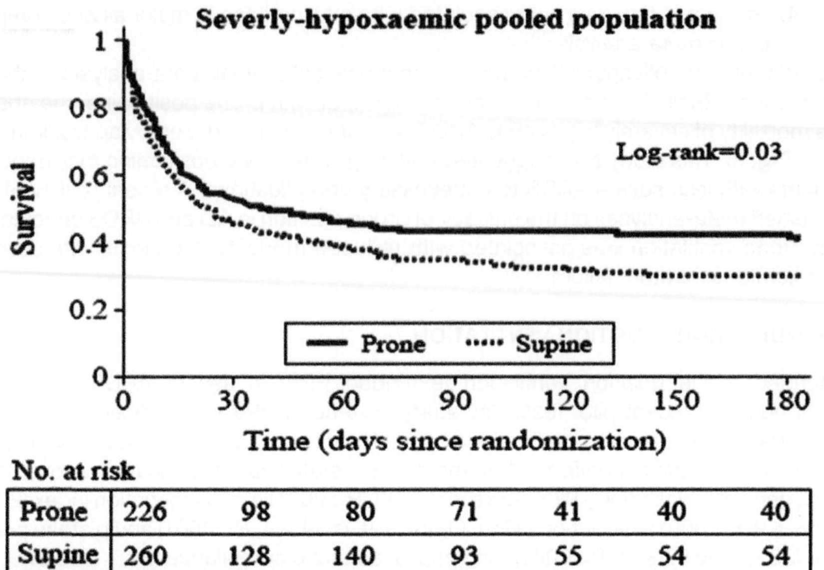

No. at risk

Prone	226	98	80	71	41	40	40
Supine	260	128	140	93	55	54	54

Fig. 5. Survival in ARDS patients with severe hypoxemia. Kaplan-Meier estimates of survival rates at the latest follow-up of the prone and supine patients from the studies included in the pooled analysis of the 4 largest existing trials investigating the effects of prone positioning in patients with severe hypoxemia (defined as PaO_2/FiO_2 ratio <100 mm Hg). (*From* Gattinoni L, Carlesso E, Taccone P, et al. Prone positioning improves survival in severe ARDS: a pathophysiologic review and individual patient meta-analysis. Minerva Anestesiol 2010;76(6):448–54; with permission.)

(continuous prone position for 20 hours daily) in severe ARDS patients with 48 hours of tracheal intubation. Multivariate analysis documented that randomization to the supine position was an independent risk factor for mortality (OR 2.53, $P = .03$). These investigators concluded that prone ventilation is feasible and safe, and may reduce mortality in patients with severe ARDS when it is initiated early and applied for most of the day.

An open randomized controlled trial[26] in 17 medical-surgical ICUs enrolled 40 mechanically ventilated patients with early and refractory ARDS despite protective ventilation in the supine position. Patients were randomized to remain supine or be moved to early (within 48 hours) and continuous (≥20 hours per day) prone position until recovery or death. The trial was prematurely stopped, due to a low patient recruitment rate. PaO_2/FiO_2 tended to be higher in prone than in supine patients after 6 hours (202 ± 78 vs 165 ± 70 mm Hg); this difference reached statistical significance on day 3 (234 ± 85 vs 159 ± 78). Prone-related side effects were minimal and reversible. Sixty-day survival reached the targeted 15% absolute increase in prone patients (62% vs 47%), but failed to reach significance because of the small sample. This study adds data to reinforce the potential beneficial effect of early continuous prone positioning on survival in ARDS patients.

COMPLICATIONS ASSOCIATED WITH PRONE POSITION

Prone positioning has associated risks to both the patient and the health care worker. One hindrance to use of the prone position in ARDS patients has been the difficulty of safely moving a patient with severe hypoxemia due to ARDS. Complications can arise in the process and include unplanned extubation, lines being pulled, and tubes becoming kinked. In addition, proning obese patients can be labor intensive and can result in staff injuries. However, the technique can be performed safely by trained and dedicated critical care staff who are aware of its potential benefits in critically ill patients with ARDS and severe hypoxemia.

Complications that have been reported with prone positioning include inadvertent extubation, airway complications, pressure sores, and brachial plexus injuries.[27] Some of these complications are fully preventable with proper technique and careful attention to detail. Avoidance of pressure ulceration requires the use of appropriate cushioning of the dependent portions of the body.

In the Prone-Supine I Study, Gattinoni and colleagues[9] reported complications related to pressure in 36% of patients and cannula loss in 1.2% of patients. In a comprehensive review conducted by Curley and colleagues,[11] displacement of venous lines and indwelling catheters was found to be the most common complication, occurring in 0.6% of turning cycles (supine to prone and back to supine). In the more recent Prone-Supine II Study,[12] a significantly greater proportion of patients in the prone group experienced at least one complication (94.6% vs 76.4%) and the incidence of most of the complications was significantly higher in the prone group (**Table 1**). However, other reports have confirmed the safety of prone positioning with open abdomen[28] and with high-flow venous access.[29]

Table 1
Incidence of complications during the 28-day Prone-Supine II Study

	Patients, %[a]				Events/100 Days of Study[b]				Events During Positional
Complication	All	Prone	Supine	*P* Value[c]	All	Prone	Supine	*P* Value[c]	Changes, %[d]
Entire Population									
Need for increased sedation/muscle relaxants	68.1	80.4	56.3	<.001	15.2	17.9	12.5	<.001	26.9
Airway obstruction	42.1	50.6	33.9	.002	8.4	10.3	6.6	<.001	20.4
Transient desaturation	57.0	63.7	50.6	.01	13.4	15.4	11.3	<.001	21.3
Vomiting	20.8	29.1	12.6	<.001	3.0	4.4	1.7	<.001	35.1
Hypotension, arrhythmias, increased vasopressors	63.2	72.0	54.6	<.001	15.2	18.0	12.4	<.001	22.0
Loss of venous access	9.9	16.1	4.0	<.001	0.7	1.23	0.25	<.001	36.6
Displacement of endotracheal tube	7.6	10.7	4.6	.03	0.6	0.87	0.40	.02	40.0
Displacement of thoracotomy tube	2.9	4.2	1.7	.21	0.2	0.25	0.11	.23	30.0

[a] Percentage of patients who experienced at least 1 episode of the complication considered during the 28-day study period.
[b] Number of days with at least 1 event, divided by 100 patient-days (2760 patient-days for the prone group and 2764 patient-days for the supine group).
[c] For comparison between prone and supine groups.
[d] Percentage of events in the prone group that occurred during the positional changes.

Data from Taccone P, Pesenti A, Latini R, et al. Prone positioning in patients with moderate and severe acute respiratory distress syndrome: a randomized controlled trial. JAMA 2009;302:1977–84.

METHODS FOR PRONE POSITIONING

Several methods for prone positioning have been developed. The authors use a simple, manual 3-step procedure (**Figs. 6** and **7**) that takes 4 staff members (2 on each side of the bed) to manage all lines and tubes. First, patients are moved to the edge of the bed with a full sheet. This sheet is then wrapped around the patient's

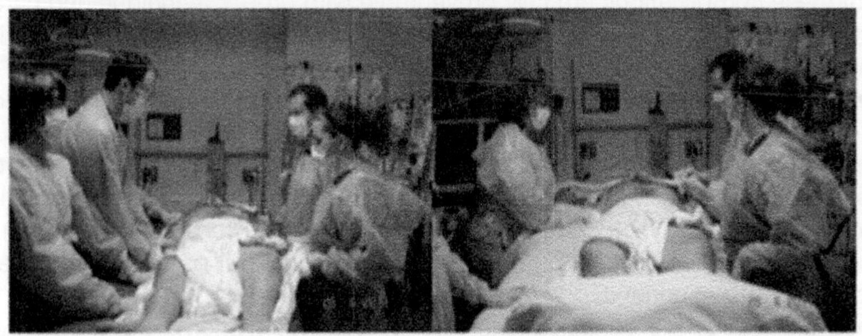

With flat sheet, pull patient to one side of the bed.

Tuck flat sheet around patient arm in order to protect it and move patient.

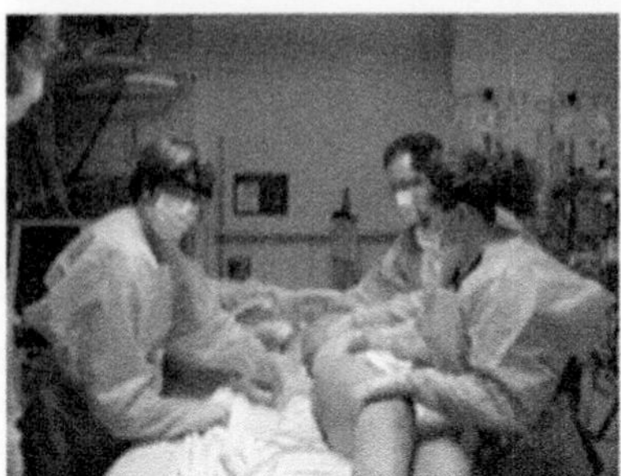

Place a second flat sheet on the bed, tuck under patient. Everything will pull through when you turn the patient.

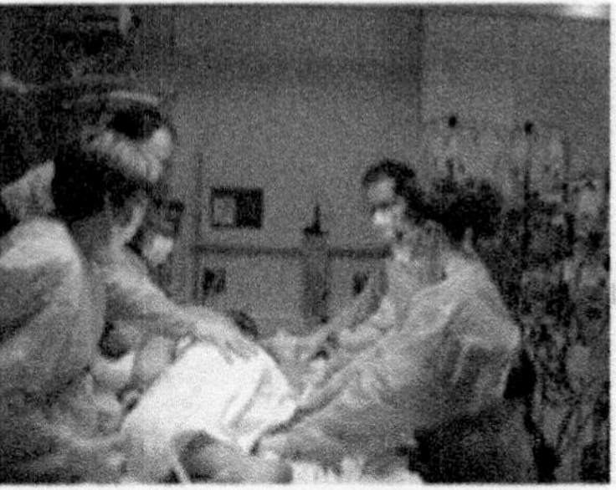

Carefully turn the patient over and position prone by pulling the sheet. This will allow the arm and sheet to pulled across the bed.

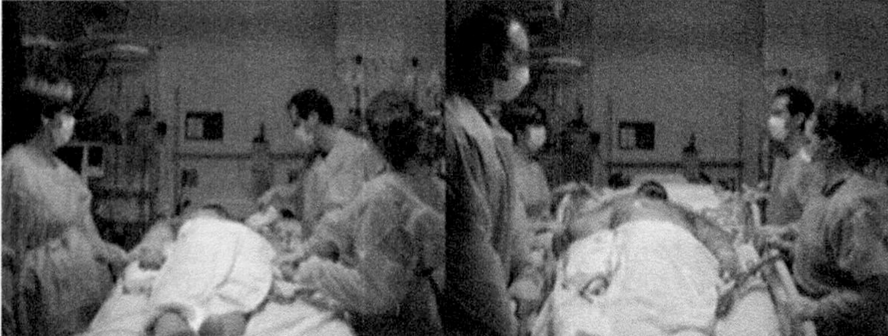

Discard the sheet that was pulled through, position lines and tubes.

Patient now prone. Place arms in swimmers position (one positioned up toward head, one at side. Place in Reverse Trendelenberg.

Fig. 6. Simple steps to placing an ARDS patient in the prone position: University of Michigan method.

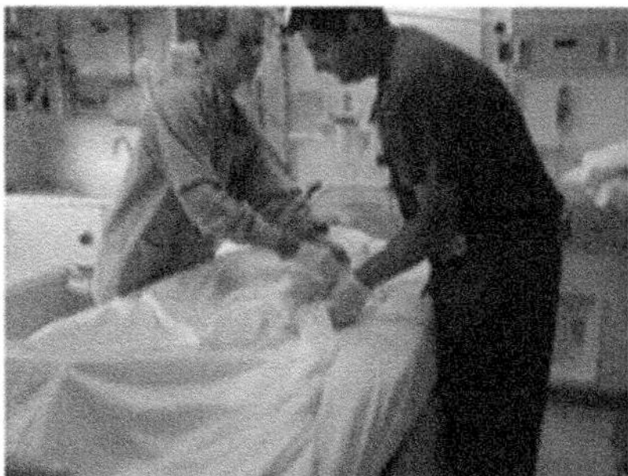

To place supine reverse the process, place flat sheet over patient, tucking in one side under arm.

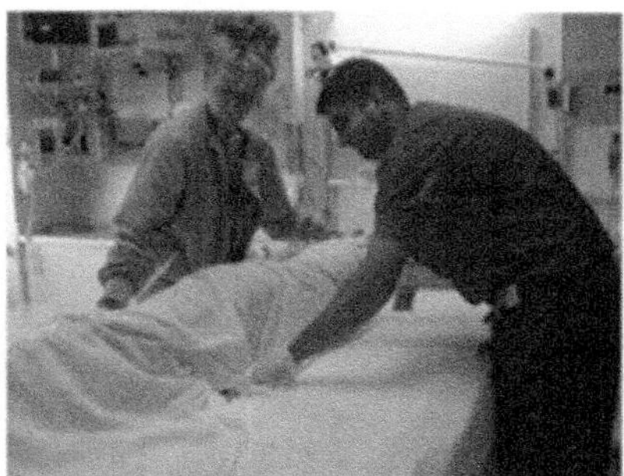

Place a second flat sheet on the bed, tuck under patient. Everything will pull through when you turn the patient.

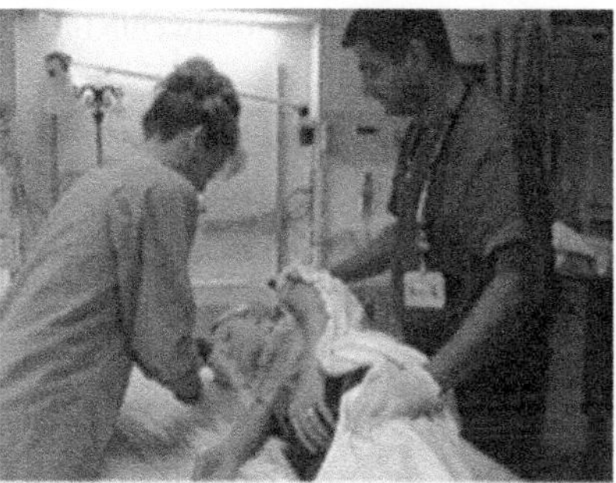

Carefully turn the patient over and position prone by pulling the sheet. This will allow the arm and sheet to pulled across the bed.

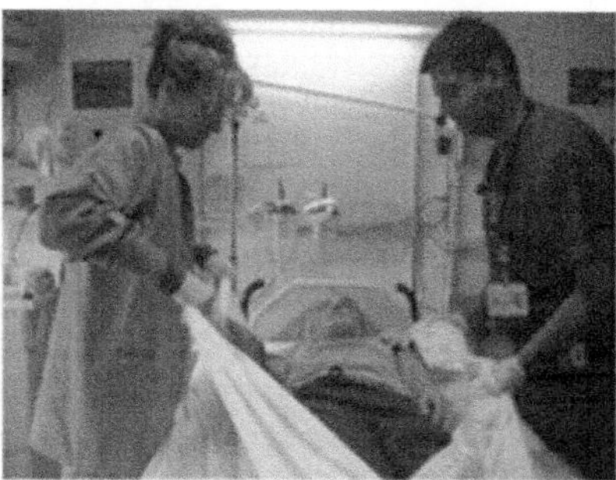

Discard the sheet that was pulled through, position lines and tubes, center patient in the bed.

Fig. 7. Simple steps to return the patient to the supine position after proning: University of Michigan method.

arm that is located toward the middle of the bed. A second flat sheet is tucked under the covered arm and then the patient is rolled further as far as possible to the side of the bed. Finally, the patient is carefully turned back over by pulling the first sheet from the side of the bed back toward the middle of the bed. The wrapped arm is gently pulled from under the patient while pulling the second sheet fully under the patient.

Box 1
Requirements for safe prone positioning in ALI/ARDS patients

- Preoxygenate the patient with FiO_2 1.0
- Secure the endotracheal tube and arterial and central venous catheters
- Adequate number of staff to assist in the turn and to monitor the turn
- Supplies to turn (pads for bed, sheet, protection for the patient, or specialty bed)
- Knowledge of how to perform the turn or use the specialty bed
- Knowledge of how to supine the patient in the event of an emergency

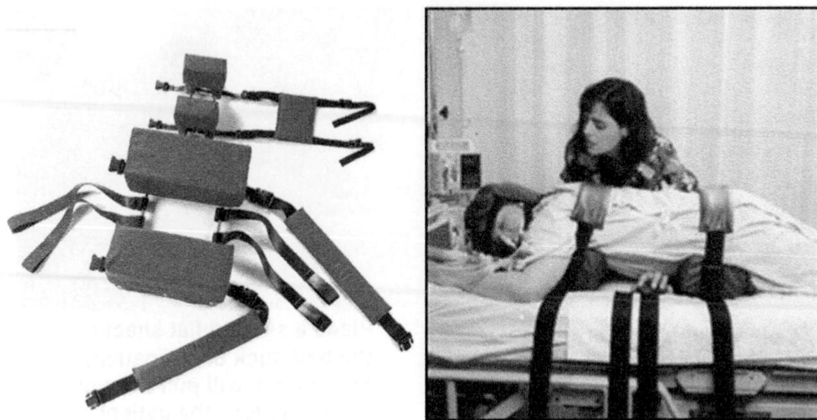

Fig. 8. Use of the Vollman Prone Positioner. (© 2007 Hill-Rom Services, Inc. REPRINTED WITH PERMISSION-ALL RIGHTS RESERVED.)

This maneuver releases the first sheet that can be thrown away, and leaves the second sheet under the patient to reverse the patient to a supine position later. This technique is simple and easy to perform, but most importantly allows the ICU staff full access to the patient, particularly to provide posterior skin care.

In their ICU, the authors have standardized this process and prone patients frequently. This prone-position procedure is routinely completed in less than 5 minutes by the ICU staff with the patient on a standard ICU bed. After the patient is prone, appropriate padding of the chest, extremities, and face and neck is necessary. The bed is then placed in a slight reverse Trendelenburg position to minimize pressure in the head and neck area.

In response to perceived difficulties in placing ALI/ARDS patients in the prone position, several manufacturers have developed devices, frames, or complete bed systems to help staff efficiently and safely prone patients. These methods may require extensive staff training and are often quite expensive, limiting their availability at some hospitals; the authors do not use these methods in their ICU (**Box 1**).

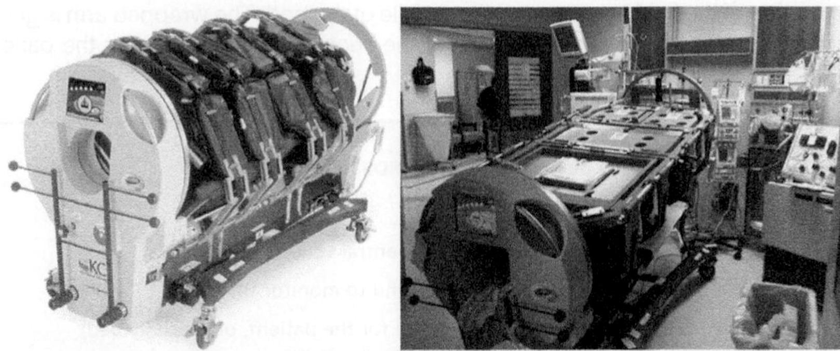

Fig. 9. The use of the Rotoprone Therapy System (KCI USA, Inc, San Antonio, TX). This is an automated system that allows multiple intervals of prone therapy over an extended time. (*Courtesy of* Rotoprone Therapy System, KCI USA, Inc, San Antonio, TX; with permission.)

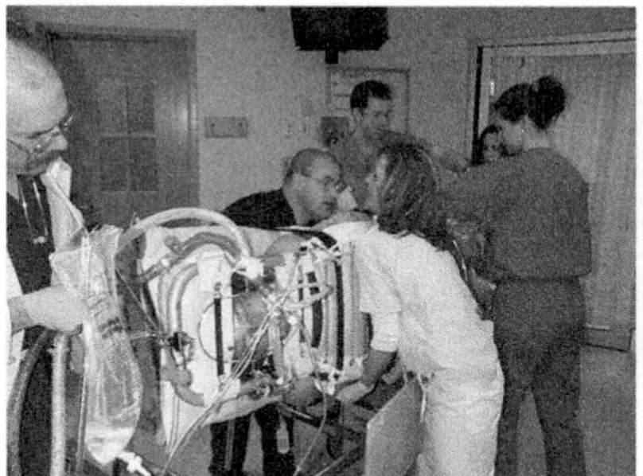
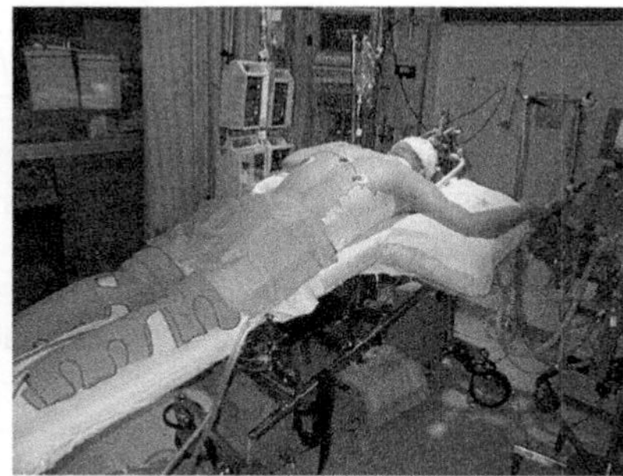

Fig. 10. Another method used for prone positioning is the Stryker frame (Stryker, Kalamazoo, MI).

One method used to establish the prone position is via the use of the Vollman Prone Positioner (Hill-Rom Services Inc, Batesville, IN, USA) (**Fig. 8**). Others use the Rotoprone Therapy System (KCI USA Inc, San Antonio, TX, USA) (**Fig. 9**), which is an automated system that allows multiple intervals of prone therapy over an extended time. This technique has some advantages due to its automated use, but is somewhat limited because of the daily expense of bed rental. In the Prone-Supine II Study, prone positioning was applied using this rotational bed in 20 participating centers and applied manually in the remaining 5 centers.[12] There is some concern, however, that easy access to the patient in the Rotoprone bed is limited. Others implement prone positioning with the use of a Stryker frame (Stryker, Kalamazoo, MI, USA) (**Fig. 10**); however, care must be taken to appropriately pad all exposed areas to prevent ulcerations, because there is a metal frame.

SUMMARY

In the authors' experience, the use of the prone position is an effective strategy for the treatment of severe hypoxemia in patient with ARDS. To establish the prone position, the authors favor a simple technique that uses 4 staff members and a regular ICU bed with no specialized equipment. More recent studies document the benefit of extended prone position therapy (>20 hours per day) in ARDS. A recent review of all published meta-analyses on the efficacy of prone position in ALI and ARDS concluded that prone ventilation was associated with reduced mortality in the cohort of patients with severe hypoxemia, defined as PaO_2/FiO_2 ratio less than 100 mm Hg. In addition, prone positioning serves a role as rescue therapy for patients with ARDS and refractory life-threatening hypoxemia.

REFERENCES

1. Piehl MA, Brown RS. Use of extreme position changes in acute respiratory failure. Crit Care Med 1976;4:13–4.
2. Dirkes S, Dickinson S. Common questions about prone positioning for ARDS. Am J Nurs 1998;98(6):16JJ, 16NN, 16PP.
3. Gattinoni L, Pelosi P, Vitale G, et al. Body position changes redistribute lung computed-tomographic density in patients with acute respiratory failure. Anesthesiology 1991;74:15–23.
4. Gattinoni L, Caironi P. Prone positioning: beyond physiology. Anesthesiology 2010;113(6):1262–4.

5. Broccard AF, Shapiro RS, Schmitz LL, et al. Influence of prone position on the extent and distribution of lung injury in a high tidal volume oleic acid model of acute respiratory distress syndrome. Crit Care Med 1997;25:16–27.
6. Valenza F, Guglielmi M, Maffioletti M, et al. Prone position delays the progression of ventilator-induced lung injury in rats: does lung strain distribution play a role? Crit Care Med 2005;33:361–7.
7. Richter T, Bellani G, Scott Harris R, et al. Effect of prone position on regional shunt, aeration, and perfusion in experimental acute lung injury. Am J Respir Crit Care Med 2005;172(4):480–7.
8. Douglas WW, Rehder K, Beynen FM, et al. Improved oxygenation in patients with acute respiratory failure: the prone position. Am Rev Respir Dis 1977;115:559–66.
9. Gattinoni L, Tognoni G, Pesenti A, et al. Effect of prone positioning on the survival of patients with acute respiratory failure. N Engl J Med 2001;345:568–73.
10. Gattinoni L, Vagginelli F, Carlesso E, et al. Decrease in PaCO with prone position is predictive of improved outcome in acute respiratory distress syndrome. Crit Care Med 2003;31(12):2727–33.
11. Curley MA, Hibberd PL, Fineman LD, et al. Effect of prone positioning on clinical outcomes in children with acute lung injury: a randomized controlled trial. JAMA 2005;294(2):229–37.
12. Taccone P, Pesenti A, Latini R, et al. Prone positioning in patients with moderate and severe acute respiratory distress syndrome: a randomized controlled trial. JAMA 2009;302:1977–84.
13. Sud S, Sud M, Friedrich JO, et al. Effect of mechanical ventilation in the prone position on clinical outcomes in patients with acute hypoxemic respiratory failure: a systematic review and meta-analysis. CMAJ 2008;178(8):1153–61.
14. Kopterides P, Siempos II, Armaganidis A. Prone positioning in hypoxemic respiratory failure: meta-analysis of randomized controlled trials. J Crit Care 2009; 24(1):89–100.
15. Abroug F, Ouanes-Besbes L, Elatrous S, et al. The effect of prone positioning in acute respiratory distress syndrome or acute lung injury: a meta-analysis. Areas of uncertainty and recommendations for research. Intensive Care Med 2008; 34(6):1002–11.
16. Alsaghir AH, Martin CM. Effect of prone positioning in patients with acute respiratory distress syndrome: a meta-analysis. Crit Care Med 2008;36(2):603–9.
17. Tiruvoipati R, Bangash M, Manktelow B, et al. Efficacy of prone ventilation in adult patients with acute respiratory failure: a meta-analysis. J Crit Care 2008;23(1): 101–10.
18. Wells DA, Gillies D, Fitzgerald DA. Positioning for acute respiratory distress in hospitalised infants and children. Cochrane Database Syst Rev 2005;(2):CD003645.
19. Peek GJ, Mugford M, Tiruvoipati R, et al, CESAR trial collaboration. Efficacy and economic assessment of conventional ventilatory support versus extracorporeal membrane oxygenation for severe adult respiratory failure (CESAR): a multicentre randomised controlled trial [Erratum in: Lancet 2009;374(9698):1330]. Lancet 2009;374(9698):1351–63.
20. Abroug F, Ouanes-Besbes L, Dachraoui F, et al. An updated study-level meta-analysis of randomised controlled trials on proning in ARDS and acute lung injury. Crit Care 2011;15(1):R6.
21. Gattinoni L, Carlesso E, Taccone P, et al. Prone positioning improves survival in severe ARDS: a pathophysiologic review and individual patient meta-analysis. Minerva Anestesiol 2010;76(6):448–54.

22. Guerin C, Gaillard S, Lemasson S, et al. Effects of systematic prone positioning in hypoxemic acute respiratory failure: a randomized controlled trial. JAMA 2004; 292:2379–87.
23. Mancebo J, Fernandez R, Blanch L, et al. A multicenter trial of prolonged prone ventilation in severe acute respiratory distress syndrome. Am J Respir Crit Care Med 2006;173(11):1233–9.
24. Cesana BM, Antonelli P, Chiumello D, et al. Positive end-expiratory pressure, prone positioning, and activated protein C: a critical review of meta-analyses. Minerva Anestesiol 2010;76(11):929–36.
25. Romero CM, Cornejo RA, Galvez LR, et al. Extended prone position ventilation in severe acute respiratory distress syndrome: a pilot feasibility study. J Crit Care 2009;24(1):81–8.
26. Fernandez R, Trenchs X, Klamburg J, et al. Prone positioning in acute respiratory distress syndrome: a multicenter randomized clinical trial. Intensive Care Med 2008;34(8):1487–91.
27. Goettler CE, Pryor JP, Reilly PM. Brachial plexopathy after prone positioning. Crit Care 2002;6(6):540–2.
28. Schiller HJ, Reilly PM, Anderson HL, et al. The 'open abdomen' is not a contraindication to prone positioning for severe ARDS. Chest 1996;110:142S.
29. Goettler CE, Pryor JP, Hoey BA, et al. Prone positioning does not affect cannula function during extra-corporeal membrane oxygenation or continuous renal replacement therapy. Crit Care Med 2001;29(Suppl):173A.

Surfactant Therapy for Acute Lung Injury and Acute Respiratory Distress Syndrome

Krishnan Raghavendran, MD[a,*], D. Willson, MD[b], R.H. Notter, MD, PhD[c]

KEYWORDS

• ALI • ARDS • Surfactant • Lungs

The extensive pulmonary alveolar and capillary networks make the lungs highly susceptible to cell and tissue injury from pathogens or toxic environmental agents present either in the circulation or in the external environment. The medical consequences of acute pulmonary injury are frequently defined as the syndromes of acute lung injury (ALI) and acute respiratory distress syndrome (ARDS). The American-European Consensus Conference (AECC) in 1994 defined ARDS as respiratory failure of acute onset with a arterial partial pressure of oxygen (Pao_2)/fraction of inspired oxygen (Fio_2) ratio less than 200 mm Hg (regardless of the level of positive end-expiratory pressure [PEEP]), bilateral infiltrates on frontal chest radiograph, and a pulmonary capillary wedge pressure less than 18 mm Hg (if measured) or no evidence of left atrial hypertension.[1] ALI is defined identically except for a higher Pao_2/Fio_2 limit of less than 300 mm Hg.[1] The AECC definitions of ALI/ARDS are widely used clinically, although they have nontrivial deficiencies in discrimination. The AECC definitions are often supplemented by lung injury or critical care scores such as the Murray[2] or Acute Physiology and Chronic Health Evaluation (APACHE) II[3] scores in adults, or the Pediatric Risk of Mortality (PRISM),[4,5] Pediatric Index Of Mortality (PIM),[6] or oxygenation index (OI)[7] in children. Expanded definitions of ALI/ARDS have also been developed using the Delphi technique.[8]

The support of NIH grants HL-1020113 (K.R.) and HL094641 (R.H.N.) is gratefully acknowledged.
[a] Division of Acute Care Surgery, Department of Surgery, University of Michigan Health System, 1500 East Medical Center Drive, 1C340A-UH, SPC 5033, Ann Arbor, MI 48109-5033, USA
[b] Departments of Pediatrics and Anesthesia, University of Virginia Childrens Hospital, University of Virginia Health Services System, PO Box 800-386, Charlottesville, VA 22908-0386, USA
[c] Departments of Pediatrics and Environmental Medicine, University of Rochester School of Medicine, 601 Elm Wood Avenue, Box 850, Rochester, NY 14642, USA
* Corresponding author.
E-mail address: kraghave@umich.edu

Crit Care Clin 27 (2011) 525–559
doi:10.1016/j.ccc.2011.04.005 **criticalcare.theclinics.com**
0749-0704/11/$ – see front matter

The incidence of ALI/ARDS has been variably reported to be 50,000 to 190,000 cases per year in the United States.[1,9–15] Comprehensive studies by Rubenfeld and colleagues[14] and Goss and colleagues[15] have placed the incidence of ALI at 22 to 86 cases per 100,000 persons per year,[14,15] with 40% to 43% of these patients having ARDS.[14] The incidence of ALI/ARDS is lower in pediatric age groups, but still equates to thousands of affected children per year.[16–20] Overall mortality in adult and pediatric patients with these lung injury syndromes still remain high at 25% to 50%.[1,9–15,17–20] Rubenfeld and colleagues[14] reported mortalities of 38.5% for ALI and 41% for ARDS, with an estimated 74,500 deaths per year and an aggregate 3.6 million hospital days of care in the United States. Further details on the incidence and mortality of ALI/ARDS are given elsewhere in this issue.

There is clearly a significant need for improved therapy for ALI/ARDS, and this article focuses primarily on the potential benefits of exogenous surfactant replacement. In targeting this and other therapeutic interventions to the most applicable subgroups of patients, it is helpful to distinguish between ALI/ARDS associated with direct pulmonary causes compared with systemic (indirect, extrapulmonary) causes (**Table 1**). Direct pulmonary causes of ALI/ARDS include pulmonary viral or bacterial infections; aspiration (eg, gastric aspiration, meconium aspiration in infants); blunt thoracic trauma with lung contusion; near drowning; thoracic radiation; and the inhalation of oxygen, smoke, or other toxicants. Indirect (systemic) causes of ALI/ARDS include sepsis, closed-space burn injury, hypovolemic shock, generalized trauma with long bone fracture, multiple transfusions, pancreatitis, and other primary extrapulmonary insults. Indirect forms of ALI/ARDS have substantial multiorgan symptoms that significantly affect long-term patient outcomes, reducing the impact and effectiveness of pulmonary-based therapies like exogenous surfactant

Table 1
Causes of neonatal respiratory distress syndrome (NRDS), clinical ALI, and ARDS

Syndrome	Primary	Patient	Associated	Predisposing
NRDS	Surfactant deficiency caused by immature alveolar type II epithelial cells	Premature infants	Complications of prematurity	Premature birth
ARDS/ALI (direct injury)	Direct injury to the lungs	Any age	Added pathology from the specific lung injury insult can also occur	Aspiration Pulmonary infection Lung contusion Near drowning Hyperoxia Smoke inhalation Other inhaled toxins Lung radiation
ARDS/ALI (indirect injury)	Lung injury results from an extrapulmonary insult and inflammation	Any age	SIRS, MODS, MOF, and less-severe forms of multiorgan pathology	Sepsis Hypovolemic shock Nonthoracic trauma Burn injury Pancreatitis

Abbreviations: MODS, multiple organ dysfunction syndrome; MOF, multiple organ failure; SIRS, systemic inflammatory response syndrome.

Data from Notter RH. Lung surfactants: basic science and clinical applications. New York: Marcel Dekker; 2000.

administration. As detailed later, post-hoc analyses in 2 clinical trials of surfactant therapy in ALI/ARDS suggest greater efficacy in direct, as opposed to indirect, forms of pulmonary injury.[21,22]

SURFACTANT DYSFUNCTION IN ALI/ARDS

There are several pathways by which lung surfactant activity can be compromised during acute pulmonary injury, as summarized in **Figs. 1** and **2**. Impairments in lung surfactant activity, and reductions in the content or composition of active large surfactant aggregates, have been reported in bronchoalveolar lavage (BAL), edema fluid, or tracheal aspirates from patients with ALI/ARDS or other diseases involving lung injury.[23–35] Research in the last 2 decades has clarified many pathways and mechanisms contributing to surfactant dysfunction in acute pulmonary injury (for detailed review see Refs.[36–38]). One important mechanism of surfactant dysfunction in ALI/ARDS involves detrimental physicochemical interactions with substances in the alveoli as a result of permeability edema or inflammation (**Box 1**). Extensive biophysical studies have documented that the surface activity of lung surfactant is significantly impaired by injury-related inhibitors such as plasma and blood proteins,[39–46] meconium,[47] cell membrane lipids,[41,46,48] fluid free fatty acids,[46,49–51] reactive oxidants,[49,52–54] and lytic enzymes including proteases[55] and phospholipases.[56,57] Mechanistically, albumin and other blood proteins impair surface activity primarily by competitive adsorption that reduces the entry of active surfactant components into the alveolar air-water interface.[43,58] In contrast, cell membrane lipids, lysophospholipids, or fatty acids act in part by mixing into the surface film and compromising its ability to reach low surface tension during dynamic compression.[41,46,50,58] Phospholipases, proteases, and reactive oxygen-nitrogen species act to chemically alter functionally essential surfactant lipids or proteins.[55,57,59] It is well documented that surface activity deficits from all these mechanisms can be mitigated in vitro by increasing the concentration of active surfactant even if inhibitor substances remain present,[36–38] supporting the conceptual usefulness of exogenous surfactant supplementation strategies.

Another type of surfactant dysfunction that occurs in many forms of lung injury is the depletion or alteration of active large surfactant aggregates. Surfactant exists in the alveolar hypophase in a size-distributed microstructure of aggregates, the largest of which typically have the greatest surface activity and the highest apoprotein content.[51,60–66] Total lavaged surfactant phospholipid is unchanged or even increased in amount in many animal models of ALI/ARDS, but the percentage of large surfactant aggregates is frequently reduced and the activity of remaining aggregates impaired.[51,67–70] The percentage of large aggregates and their content of surfactant protein (SP)–A and SP-B have also been shown to be reduced in BAL from patients with ARDS.[28–30] Large surfactant aggregates can, in principle, be affected by several pathways in ALI/ARDS, including physical interactions with injury-induced substances in the alveoli, alterations in intra-alveolar aggregate processing, or changes in surfactant reuptake, metabolism, or recycling in type II cells.[51,67–70] Again, depleted large aggregates can theoretically be replenished by delivering supplemental exogenous surfactant.

Surfactant dysfunction, including both inhibitor-induced activity reductions and large aggregate depletion, has been widely shown in animal models of acute inflammatory lung injury in vivo.[36,37,70–79] The ability of exogenous surfactant therapy to improve acute respiratory symptoms in animal models of ALI/ARDS in vivo is similarly well documented (**Box 2**). Examples of animal models found to display acute improvements in arterial

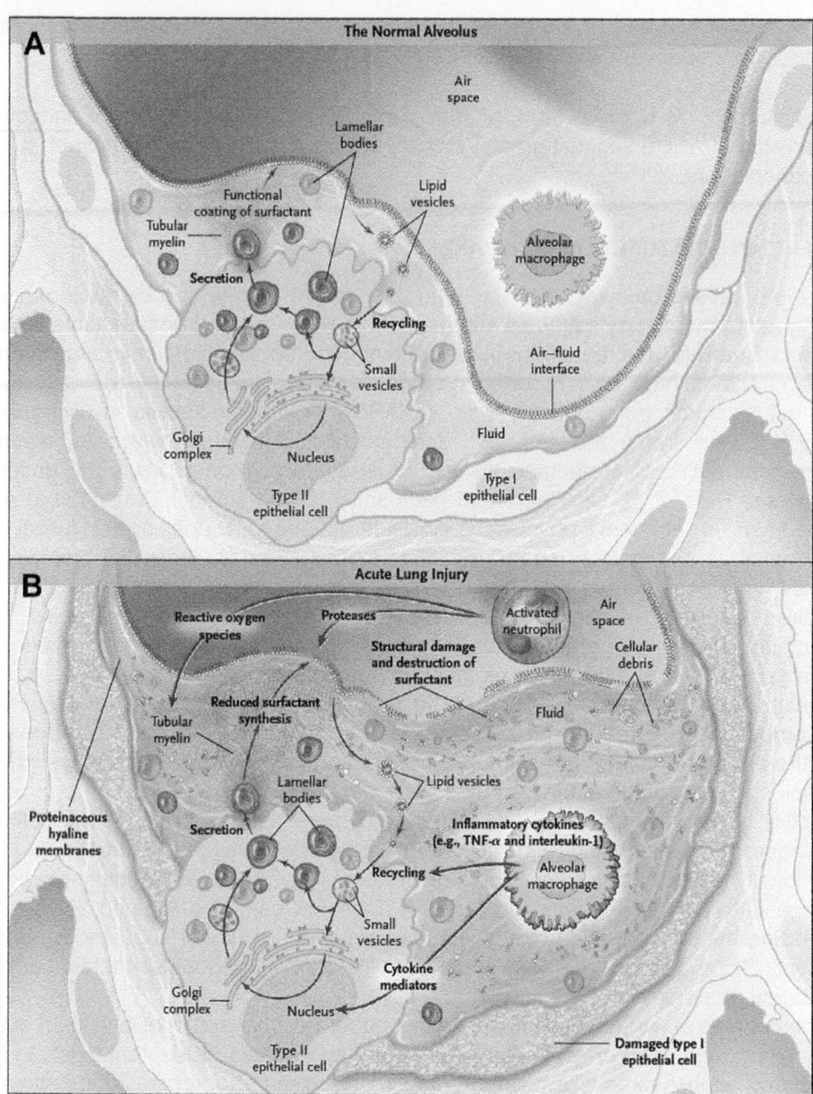

Fig. 1. Surfactant production and recycling in the normal alveolus (*A*) and changes in surfactant metabolism in acute pulmonary injury (*B*). In the normal alveolus (*A*), surfactant is synthesized and packaged into lamellar bodies in the cytoplasm of type II epithelial cells. The exocytotic lamellar body organelles secrete surfactant into the alveolar hypophase, where it forms tubular myelin and other active large lipid-protein aggregates. Surfactant lipids and proteins adsorb to the alveolar air-liquid interface as a highly active film that lowers and varies surface tension during breathing. Surfactant activity is physiologically essential in reducing the work of breathing, stabilizing alveoli against collapse and overdistension, and lowering the hydrostatic driving force for pulmonary edema. In injured lungs (*B*), multiple inflammatory cytokines and chemokines can influence the metabolism of alveolar surfactant (synthesis, secretion, reuptake, recycling) by altering type II pneumocyte function and responses. Surfactant metabolism in type II cells can also be altered as a result of type I cell injury, because they are stem cells for the alveolar epithelium. In addition, inflammation and permeability injury can lead to the presence of reactive species and other substances in the interstitium and alveoli that can interact chemically or physically with lung surfactant lipids and proteins. Examples of specific pathways by which the surface-active function of alveolar surfactant can be impaired during acute pulmonary injury are described further in Fig. 2. TNF, tumor necrosis factor. (*From* Baudouin SV. Exogenous surfactant replacement in ARDS–one day, someday, or never? N Engl J Med 2004;351:854; with permission. Copyright (c) 2004 Massachusetts Medical Society.)

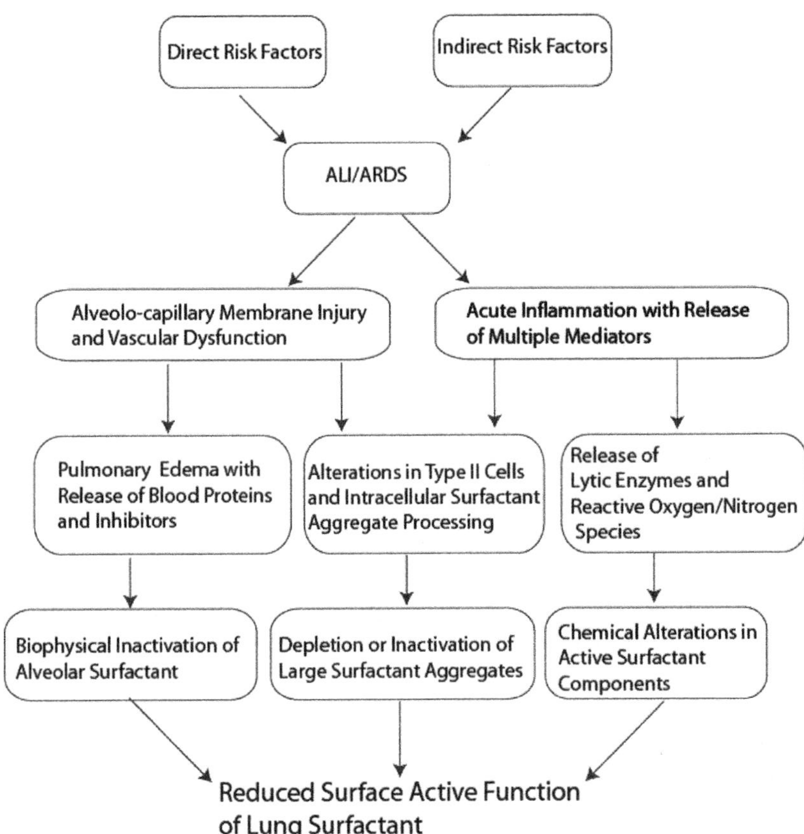

Fig. 2. Causes of decreases in lung surfactant surface-active function during acute pulmonary injury (ALI/ARDS). Although available amounts of surfactant may be decreased as a result of type II cell injury in some forms of ALI/ARDS, surfactant deficiency is typically much less prominent than surfactant dysfunction (reduced surface activity). Dysfunction of alveolar surfactant can result from several pathways in injured lungs, with one prominent mechanism being inactivation from biophysical interactions with inhibitor compounds like plasma/blood proteins or cellular lipids that enter the alveoli in edema fluid. Alveolar surfactant can also be chemically degraded or modified by substances present in the innate inflammatory response such as lytic enzymes (proteases, phospholipases) or reactive oxygen/nitrogen species. In addition, injury-induced depletion or compositional changes in large alveolar surfactant aggregates may lead to a decrease in overall surface-active function because such aggregates normally have the highest apoprotein content and surface activity. (*Data from* Wang Z, Holm BA, Matalon S, et al. Surfactant activity and dysfunction in lung injury. In: Notter RH, Finkelstein JN, Holm BA, editors. Lung injury: mechanisms, pathophysiology, and therapy. Boca Raton (FL): Taylor & Francis; 2005. p. 297–352; and Notter RH. Lung surfactants: basic science and clinical applications. New York: Marcel Dekker; 2000.)

oxygenation and/or lung mechanics following surfactant therapy are acid aspiration,[80–82] meconium aspiration,[83–86] antilung serum,[87] bacterial or endotoxin injury,[88–93] pulmonary contusion,[78] bilateral vagotomy,[94] hyperoxia,[95–99] in vivo lavage,[100–105] *N*-nitroso-*N*-methylurethane injury,[106–108] and viral pneumonia.[109,110] Animals studies of acute injury are typically not designed to assess efficacy based on long-term outcomes. However, improvements in acute respiratory function should ultimately be associated with

Box 1
Examples of injury-induced endogenous compounds that inhibit lung surfactant activity through physical or chemical interactions

Biophysical inhibitors

- Plasma and blood proteins (eg, albumin, hemoglobin, fibrinogen, fibrin monomer)
- Cell membrane lipids
- Lysophospholipids
- Fluid free fatty acids
- Glycolipids and sphingolipids
- Meconium in term infants

Chemically acting inhibitors

- Lytic enzymes (proteases, phospholipases)
- Reactive oxygen species and reactive nitrogen species
- Antibodies to surfactant proteins

See text for literature citations and discussion.

improved long-term outcomes if they are not outweighed by other untreated and continuing aspects of lung injury disorders in patients with ALI/ARDS.

FACTORS AFFECTING THE EFFICACY OF EXOGENOUS SURFACTANT THERAPY IN ALI/ARDS

Several factors make developing exogenous surfactant therapy for ALI/ARDS more difficult compared with the case of surfactant-deficient premature infants with the

Box 2
Animal models of acute pulmonary injury shown to respond to exogenous surfactant therapy in vivo.

Acid aspiration[80–82]
Meconium aspiration[83–86]
Antilung serum infusion[87]
Bacterial or endotoxin injury[88–93]
Pulmonary contusion[78]
Bilateral vagotomy[94]
Hyperoxic lung injury[95–99]
In vivo lung lavage with mechanical ventilation[100–105]
N-Nitroso-*N*-methylurethane lung injury[106–108]
Viral pneumonia[109,110]
See text for discussion

Data from Notter RH. Lung surfactants: basic science and clinical applications. New York: Marcel Dekker; 2000; and Chess P, Finkelstein JN, Holm BA, et al. Surfactant replacement therapy in lung injury. In: Notter RH, Finkelstein JN, Holm BA, editors. Lung injury: mechanisms, pathophysiology, and therapy. Boca Raton (FL): Taylor & Francis; 2005. p. 617–63.

neonatal respiratory distress syndrome (NRDS). Premature infants with NRDS have a primary deficiency of surfactant caused by a lack of mature alveolar type II epithelial cells at birth. The delivery of exogenous surfactant at or near parturition thus provides a direct and specific treatment of the disease, normalizing respiration until sufficient numbers of functional type II cells are available to synthesize/secrete active endogenous surfactant. Type II cell maturation commonly occurs during a matter of days even in premature infants if the lungs are not significantly injured by mechanical ventilation and oxygen therapy during intensive care. Exogenous surfactant is also typically given to premature infants in the immediate postnatal period when pulmonary edema and inflammation are minimal, and drug delivery and distribution following intratracheal instillation is facilitated further by the absorption of fetal lung liquid that occurs at this time. This combination of specificity in terms of therapeutic target (surfactant deficiency) plus drug deliverability makes surfactant therapy in NRDS effective and life saving in premature infants.

In ALI/ARDS, the major rationale for surfactant therapy is the presence of surfactant dysfunction in the injured lungs, although the therapy also treats surfactant deficiency if present. Surfactant dysfunction in ALI/ARDS is most prominent in the acute exudative phase of disease, and it is here that surfactant therapy has the greatest theoretic benefits. However, several complexities not present in the case of NRDS exist. Although all forms of ALI/ARDS share aspects of lung injury, these conditions are clinical syndromes encompassing diverse causes with individual features and varying levels of lung injury and systemic disorders. Combining this pathophysiologic heterogeneity in the single rubric of ALI/ARDS significantly reduces the resolving power of clinical trials. The use of subclassifications such as direct pulmonary and indirect systemic forms of ALI/ARDS as in **Table 1** helps to address some of this heterogeneity, but broad groups of individuals with multiple causes are still combined. Moreover, even for patients with a single lung injury cause, the pathology present is much more complicated than simple surfactant deficiency of prematurity. Acute pulmonary injury is complex and multifaceted, and includes not only surfactant dysfunction but also prominent aspects of inflammation, vascular dysfunction, oxidant injury, cellular injury, and edema. Edema and inflammation in patients with ALI/ARDS make it more difficult to deliver and distribute exogenous surfactant to the alveoli. Also, the presence of significant aspects of pathology not targeted by surfactant therapy may substantially affect patient outcomes, making it more difficult to discern the intrinsic efficacy of this intervention per se. The complex pathophysiology of acute pulmonary injury is a major factor in the rationale for combination therapy approaches in ALI/ARDS, as described later. However, whether dealing with single-agent or combination interventions, evaluating clinical therapies in ALI/ARDS for outcomes such as survival requires multicenter controlled studies of substantial size, with patient populations and outcome variables chosen as rigorously as possible.[111]

CLINICAL EXOGENOUS SURFACTANT DRUGS

To be effective in ALI/ARDS, exogenous surfactants must have high intrinsic surface activity plus the ability to resist inactivation. Clinical exogenous surfactants used to treat surfactant-related lung disease are listed in **Box 3**. The table classifies clinical surfactants into 3 groups: (1) organic solvent extracts of lavaged endogenous lung surfactant from animals; (2) organic solvent extracts of processed animal lung tissue with or without additional synthetic additives; and (3) synthetic preparations not containing animal-derived material. Meaningful evaluations of surfactant therapy in ALI/ARDS must account for differences in surfactant drug activity and inhibition resistance

Box 3
Clinical exogenous surfactant drugs for treating diseases that involve lung surfactant deficiency or dysfunction

1. Organic solvent extracts of lavaged animal lung surfactant
   a. Infasurf (calf lung surfactant extract [CLSE])
   b. Bovine lipid extract surfactant (bLES)
   c. Alveofact
2. Supplemented or unsupplemented organic solvent extracts of processed animal lung tissue
   a. Survanta
   b. Surfactant-TA
   c. Curosurf
3. Synthetic exogenous lung surfactants
   a. Exosurf
   b. Artificial lung-expanding compound (ALEC)
   c. Surfaxin (KL4)
   d. Venticute (recombinant SP-C surfactant)
   e. Novel lipid/peptide synthetic surfactants (eg, Super Mini-B surfactants)

Curosurf (Chesi Farmaceutici; Dey Laboratories), Infasurf (ONY, Inc; Forest Laboratories), and Survanta (Abbott/Ross Labs) are approved by the Food and Drug Administration (FDA) in the United States. Exosurf (Glaxo-Wellcome) is also FDA-approved, but is no longer used clinically. Surfaxin (KL4, Discovery Labs) is undergoing clinical evaluation. Specifically bioengineered synthetic lipid/peptide surfactants having the potential for even greater activity in ALI/ARDS are currently being developed, including preparations containing novel phospholipase-resistant lipids plus highly active peptides incorporating the most active sequences in human SP-B (eg, Super Mini-B peptide[121]). Further details on the composition, activity, and inhibition resistance of clinical exogenous surfactants are reviewed elsewhere (eg, Refs.[37,201,280,281]).

Data from Notter RH. Lung surfactants: basic science and clinical applications. New York: Marcel Dekker; 2000; and Chess P, Finkelstein JN, Holm BA, et al. Surfactant replacement therapy in lung injury. In: Notter RH, Finkelstein JN, Holm BA, editors. Lung injury: mechanisms, pathophysiology, and therapy. Boca Raton (FL): Taylor & Francis; 2005. p. 617–63.

that can significantly affect therapeutic efficacy, and many such differences stem from composition-based differences, as noted later.

Organic solvent extracts of lavaged alveolar surfactant (category 1 in **Box 3**) in principle contain all the lipids and hydrophobic proteins in endogenous surfactant, although composition can still vary in among preparations because of differences in extraction and processing methods. Surfactant preparations extracted from minced or homogenized lungs (category 2) contain some nonsurfactant tissue-derived components, and also require more elaborate processing that can alter composition relative to native surfactant. For example, the content of functionally important SP-B is reduced to a low level in Survanta during processing from bovine lungs.[42,112–114] Synthetic lung surfactants (category 3) have significant conceptual advantages compared with animal-derived surfactants in purity, reproducibility, manufacturing quality control efficiency, and scale-up economy. They are also free from the risk of pathogens such as prions, and are not subject to cultural/religious considerations affecting bovine or porcine surfactants. However, it has proved to be challenging to bioengineer fully synthetic surfactants having high activity equivalent to native surfactant.

Two early synthetic surfactants (Exosurf and ALEC) are no longer used clinically because of their lower activities relative to animal-derived surfactants. The synthetic preparation KL4 (Surfaxin) contains a peptide of 21 amino acids that approximates the ratio of positive and uncharged amino acid residues in SP-B,[115,116] but does not incorporate active regions of molecular structure of the human protein, whereas recombinant SP-C surfactant (Venticute) contains no SP-B peptide. Recent advances in molecular bioengineering and peptide chemistry have increased the potential to design and produce new, highly active, synthetic lung surfactants, and several approaches are currently being studied (see Refs.[117–120] for review). These approaches include fully synthetic lipid/peptide surfactants bioengineered to contain peptides incorporating the most active amino acid sequences in human SP-B, such as Super Mini-B peptide.[121] Synthetic exogenous surfactants containing Super Mini-B or related peptides that mimic active human SP-B can also incorporate novel lipids with beneficial molecular properties such as phospholipid resistance. One particularly active synthetic lipid analogue of dipalmitoyl phosphatidylcholine (DPPC), the most prevalent phospholipid in native surfactant, is the phospholipase-resistant diether compound designated DEPN-8.[117,122–125] Synthetic surfactants containing DEPN-8 or other phospholipase-resistant lipids plus active SP-B peptides may have particular potential usefulness in treating ALI/ARDS,[59,117,124–127] where these lytic enzymes can be elaborated in high concentrations in the interstitium and alveoli of injured lungs.[128–134] New synthetic surfactants can also potentially be bioengineered to include novel peptide components incorporating the most active regions of other human surfactant apoproteins in combination with SP-B peptides and lipids [117]

CLINICAL EXPERIENCE WITH EXOGENOUS SURFACTANT THERAPY IN ALI/ARDS

Several clinical studies have reported pulmonary benefits following the instillation of exogenous surfactants to term infants, children, or adults with lung injury-related acute respiratory failure or ALI/ARDS (**Table 2**).[21,135–150] However, many of these positive clinical studies are small case studies or treatment trials that documented improvements only in acute lung function (oxygenation). Randomized controlled trials of surfactant therapy in patients with ALI/ARDS have had limited success in improving long-term outcomes including survival, particularly in adults.[151,152] Nonetheless, there are several populations of patients with lung injury–related respiratory failure in which therapy with active exogenous surfactant drugs has been documented to be effective in improving clinically significant outcomes, particularly in pediatric patients, encompassing full-term infants to older children and including young adults up to 21 years of age. No studies on surfactant use in infants, children, or adults have shown any significant adverse long-term effects from the therapy, although transient hypoxia and some hemodynamic instability surrounding intratracheal or bronchoscopic instillation are common. More detailed review of specific studies of surfactant therapy in various age groups with lung injury is given later.

Surfactant Therapy in Preterm Infants with Established NRDS

Multiple studies confirm the efficacy of surfactant therapy in preventing and treating NRDS in preterm infants (eg, see the meta-analyses in Refs.[153,154]). The use of surfactant for treatment of NRDS is associated with a decreased risk of pneumothorax, pulmonary interstitial emphysema, bronchopulmonary dysplasia, and a decreased risk of mortality (**Fig. 3**).[153] Furthermore, multiple doses resulted in greater improvements in

Table 2
Selected controlled and uncontrolled clinical studies reporting benefits of exogenous surfactant therapy in acute respiratory failure (ALI/ARDS)

Study	Patients (N)	Disease	Surfactant	Outcomes
Günther et al (B)[135]	Adults (27)	ARDS	Alveofact	Improved surfactant function
Walmrath et al (B)[196]	Adults (10)	ARDS, sepsis	Alveofact	Improved oxygenation
Spragg et al (B)[137]	Adults (6)	ARDS, multiple causes	Curosurf	Improved oxygenation and biophysical function
Wiswell et al (B)[138]	Adults (12)	ARDS, multiple causes	Surfaxin	Improved oxygenation
Amital et al (A)[282]	Adults (42)	Lung transplant	Infasurf	Improved oxygenation, better graft function
Spragg et al[22]	Adults (40)	ARDS, multiple causes	Venticute	Improved oxygenation, decreased IL-6 in BAL
Willson et al (A)[139,140]	Children (29 and 42)	ARDS, multiple causes	Infasurf	Improved oxygenation
Willson et al (A)[21]	Children (152)	ARDS, multiple causes	Infasurf	Improved survival and improved ventilation
Lopez-Herce et al (B)[141]	Children (20)	ARDS + postoperative cardiac	Curosurf	Improved oxygenation
Hermon et al (B)[142]	Children (19)	ARDS + postoperative cardiac	Curosurf or Alveofact	Improved oxygenation
Herting et al (B)[143]	Children (8)	Pneumonia	Curosurf	Improved oxygenation
Moller et al (A)[159]	Children (35)	ARDS, multiple causes	Alveofact	Improved oxygenation
Auten et al (B)[144]	Infants (14)	MAS or pneumonia	Infasurf (CLSE)	Improved oxygenation
Lotze et al (A)[145,146]	Infants (28 & 328)	ECMO, multiple indications	Survanta	Improved oxygenation, decreased ECMO
Khammash et al (B)[147]	Infants (20)	MAS	bLES	Improved oxygenation
Findlay et al (A)[148]	Infants (40)	MAS	Survanta	Improved oxygenation, decreased pneumothorax and mechanical ventilation
Luchetti (A) et al[149,150]	Infants (20 and 40)	RSV bronchiolitis	Curosurf	Improved oxygenation

The tabulated studies of Willson and colleagues,[21,140] Findlay and colleagues,[148] Moller and colleagues,[159] Lotze and colleagues,[145,146] Luchetti and colleagues,[149,150] and Amital and colleagues[282] were controlled trials (A), whereas/although the remaining studies were uncontrolled treatment trials (B) as detailed in the text.

Abbreviations: BAL, bronchoalveolar lavage; MAS, meconium aspiration syndrome; RSV, respiratory syncytial virus.

Data from Willson DF, Chess PR, Notter RH. Surfactant for pediatric acute lung injury. Pediatr Clin N Am 2008;55:545–5; and Chess P, Finkelstein JN, Holm BA, et al. Surfactant replacement therapy in lung injury. In: Notter RH, Finkelstein JN, Holm BA, editors. Lung injury: mechanisms, pathophysiology, and therapy. Boca Raton (FL): Taylor & Francis; 2005. p. 617–63.

Analysis 1.11. Comparison 1 Animal derived surfactant extract treatment of RDS (all infants), Outcome 11 Effect on Neonatal Mortality.

Review: Animal derived surfactant extract for treatment of respiratory distress syndrome

Comparison: 1 Animal derived surfactant extract treatment of RDS (all infants)

Outcome: 11 Effect on Neonatal Mortality

Study or subgroup	Treatment n/N	Control n/N	Risk Ratio M-H,Fixed,95% CI	Risk Ratio M-H,Fixed,95% CI
1 Bovine surfactant extract				
Subtotal (95% CI)	**0**	**0**		**0.0 [0.0, 0.0]**
Total events: 0 (Treatment), 0 (Control)				
Heterogeneity: not applicable				
Test for overall effect: not applicable				
2 Modified bovine surfactant extract				
Chen 1990	0/9	0/9		0.0 [0.0, 0.0]
Fujiwara 1990	8/54	10/46		0.68 [0.29, 1.58]
Gitlin 1987	3/18	6/23		0.64 [0.18, 2.21]
Horbar 1989	13/78	14/81		0.96 [0.48, 1.92]
Horbar 1990	12/50	16/52		0.78 [0.41, 1.48]
Liechty 1991	74/402	108/395		0.67 [0.52, 0.87]
Raju 1987	2/17	6/13		0.25 [0.06, 1.06]
Soll 1988	6/17	5/14		0.99 [0.38, 2.56]
Subtotal (95% CI)	**645**	**633**		**0.70 [0.57, 0.86]**
Total events: 118 (Treatment), 165 (Control)				
Heterogeneity: $Chi^2 = 3.48$, df = 6 (P = 0.75); I^2 =0.0%				
Test for overall effect: Z = 3.36 (P = 0.00079)				
3 Porcine surfactant extract				
European 1988	24/77	35/69		0.61 [0.41, 0.92]
Subtotal (95% CI)	**77**	**69**		**0.61 [0.41, 0.92]**
Total events: 24 (Treatment), 35 (Control)				
Heterogeneity: not applicable				
Test for overall effect: Z = 2.36 (P = 0.019)				
4 Human amniotic fluid surfactant extract				
Hallman 1985	3/22	6/23		0.52 [0.15, 1.84]
Subtotal (95% CI)	**22**	**23**		**0.52 [0.15, 1.84]**
Total events: 3 (Treatment), 6 (Control)				
Heterogeneity: not applicable				
Test for overall effect: Z = 1.01 (P = 0.31)				
Total (95% CI)	**744**	**725**		**0.68 [0.57, 0.82]**
Total events: 145 (Treatment), 206 (Control)				
Heterogeneity: $Chi^2 = 4.00$, df = 8 (P = 0.86); I^2 =0.0%				
Test for overall effect: Z = 4.11 (P = 0.000040)				

0.1 0.2 0.5 1 2 5 10

Fig. 3. The effect of exogenous surfactant on mortality in infants with NRDS, showing the results of meta-analyses of data on infant mortality from clinical trials of surfactant replacement therapy with modified bovine surfactant, porcine surfactant extract, and human amniotic fluid surfactant extract. Overall, treatment with animal-derived surfactant extracts significantly decreased the risk of neonatal mortality (typical relative risk 0.68; 95% CI 0.57, 0.82; typical risk difference −0.09, 95% CI −0.13, −0.05). The number of patients needed to be treated to prevent 1 neonatal death was 11 (95% CI 8, 20). Significant heterogeneity was not noted between the trials analyzed. Meta analysis also indicated that the subgroup of trials using modified bovine surfactant extract also had a significant decrease in the risk of neonatal mortality (typical relative risk 0.70; 95% CI 0.57, 0.86; typical risk difference −0.08; 95% CI −0.12, −0.03). In addition, the trial of porcine surfactant extract (European 1988) individually showed a decrease in the risk of mortality (relative risk 0.61; 95% CI 0.41, 0.92). (*Adapted from* Seger N, Soll R. Animal derived surfactant extract for treatment of respiratory distress syndrome. Cochrane Database Syst Rev 2009;2:CD007836; with permission.)

oxygenation and ventilator requirements, a decreased risk of pneumothorax, and a trend toward improved survival.[154]

Surfactant Therapy in Term Infants with Acute Respiratory Failure

The best-studied use of surfactant therapy in term infants with acute pulmonary injury is in meconium aspiration syndrome.[144–148] When aspirated during delivery, usually in association with fetal distress, meconium obstructs the airways and causes severe inflammatory lung injury. Meconium also acts biophysically to directly inhibit lung surfactant activity.[47,155] Initial uncontrolled studies by Auten and colleagues[144] and Khammash and colleagues[147] reported significant improvements in lung function following exogenous surfactant administration to term infants with meconium aspiration. Subsequently, Findlay and colleagues[148] studied 40 term infants randomized to surfactant-treated and placebo groups, and showed that this therapy not only improved oxygenation but also led to a reduced incidence of pneumothorax, a decreased duration of mechanical ventilation and oxygen therapy, a reduced time of hospitalization, and fewer infants meeting criteria for extracorporeal membrane oxygenation (ECMO). Beneficial results from exogenous surfactant administration have also been found in 2 controlled studies by Lotze and colleagues[145,146] in term infants referred for ECMO with severe acute respiratory failure (meconium aspiration was a prevalent diagnosis in these patients). In an initial study, 28 infants treated with 4 doses of Survanta (150 mg/kg) had improved pulmonary mechanics, decreased duration of ECMO treatment, and a lower incidence of complications after ECMO compared with control infants.[145] A larger multicenter controlled trial in 328 term infants also reported significant improvements in respiratory status and a reduction in the need for ECMO following surfactant treatment.[146]

In addition to having efficacy in treating meconium aspiration, surfactant therapy also has clinical benefits in term infants with acute respiratory failure from respiratory syncytial virus (RSV) infection.[149,150,156] Luchetti and colleagues[149] reported that 10 infants with severe RSV bronchiolitis treated with tracheally instilled porcine-derived surfactant (Curosurf, 50 mg/kg body weight) had improved gas exchange, a reduced duration of mechanical ventilation, and a reduced length of stay in the pediatric intensive care unit compared with an equal number of control infants not receiving exogenous surfactant. A subsequent multicenter controlled trial in 40 infants with RSV-associated respiratory failure showed that instillation of Curosurf improved gas exchange and respiratory mechanics, and shortened the duration of mechanical ventilation and hospitalization.[150] Tibby and colleagues[156] also reported that 9 infants with severe RSV bronchiolitis who received 2 doses of Survanta (100 mg/kg) had a more rapid improvement in oxygenation and ventilation indices in the first 60 hours compared with 10 control infants receiving air placebo. Exogenous surfactant administration is now used in many neonatal intensive care units as a standard treatment of respiratory failure in term infants with meconium aspiration or pulmonary viral/bacterial infection. Surfactant therapy has also been studied in infants with congenital diaphragmatic hernia, but its use remains controversial in this context.[157,158]

Surfactant Therapy in Children with ALI/ARDS

Exogenous surfactant therapy has also been found to be beneficial in improving lung function in children with ARDS-related respiratory failure.[21,139,140] In an initial treatment study in 29 children (0.1–16 years of age) with acute respiratory failure at 6 centers, Willson and colleagues[139] showed that instillation of Infasurf (70 mg/kg) improved lung function defined prospectively as a 25% decrease in OI (OI $=100 \times$ mean airway pressure [MAP] $\times$ Fio_2/Pao_2). A subsequent randomized controlled trial in 42 children (aged 1 day to 18 years) at 8 centers showed that patients receiving 1 or 2 doses of Infasurf (70 mg/kg instilled intratracheally in 4 aliquots) had significantly better OI values during the 50 hours after treatment (**Fig. 4**).[140] Statistically significant differences in survival were not found in this small study, but several prospectively chosen outcome variables, including days of mechanical ventilation and days in the intensive care unit, were significantly improved by Infasurf. Patients treated with surfactant also had a significant increase in ventilator-free days during the first 14 days of hospitalization and a higher incidence of extubation by 72 hours.[140] Moller and colleagues[159] also reported that children with ARDS showed an immediate improvement in oxygenation and less need for rescue therapy following treatment with Survanta, although this study was underpowered for more definitive outcomes. Most recently, a large, blinded, randomized, controlled study by Willson and colleagues[21] in 152 pediatric patients with ALI/ARDS (77 surfactant treated and 75 placebo) yielded positive results, showing both immediate improvements in oxygenation as well as a significant survival advantage for patients receiving calfactant (Infasurf) relative to placebo (**Table 3**). Patients aged 1 week to 21 years in this 21-center study were enrolled within 48 hours of endotracheal intubation with radiographic evidence of bilateral lung disease and an OI greater than 7. Patients with preexisting lung, cardiac, or central nervous system disorders were excluded. Ventilator-free days and mortality were primary outcomes. Surfactant treatment resulted in decreased OI, decreased mortality, and a higher percentage of response to conventional mechanical ventilation compared with air placebo (see **Table 3**). A post-hoc analysis indicated that most of these beneficial effects were confined to patients with direct-injury forms of ALI/ARDS (**Table 4**).

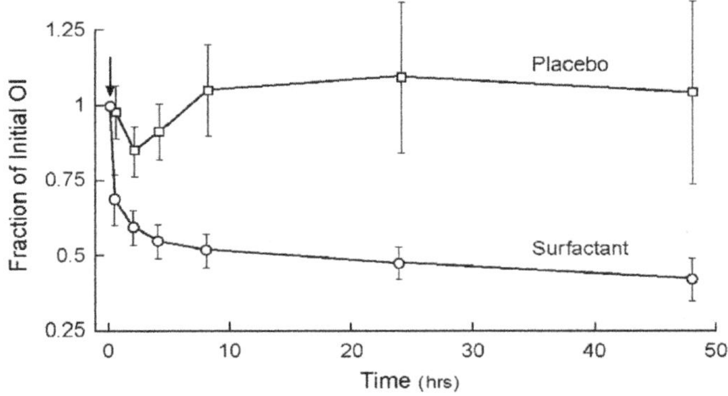

Fig. 4. Improvements in OI after instillation of exogenous surfactant in children with ALI/ARDS.[140] Patients ranging in age from 1 day to 18 years in 8 pediatric intensive care units were randomized to surfactant or control groups in the 1999 study of Willson and colleagues.[140] Patients treated with surfactant received a dose of Infasurf of 80 mL/m^2 body surface (70 mg/kg body weight) by tracheal instillation during hand ventilation with 100% oxygen (*arrow*). Control patients received hand ventilation and 100% oxygen alone. Ten of 21 patients treated with surfactant received a second dose 12 or more hours after the first. Significant improvements were found in lung function in patients receiving exogenous surfactant therapy. OI is defined as 100 × MAP × Fio_2/Pao_2, where MAP is mean airway pressure, Fio_2 is fraction of inspired oxygen, and Pao_2 is arterial partial pressure of oxygen. Data are mean ± standard deviation. (*Data from* Willson DF, Bauman LA, Zaritsky A, et al. Instillation of calf lung surfactant extract (calfactant) is beneficial in pediatric acute hypoxemic respiratory failure. Crit Care Med 1999;27:188–95.)

Table 3
Clinical outcomes from the controlled 2005 study of Willson and colleagues[21] on surfactant therapy in pediatric patients up to age 21 years with ALI/ARDS

	Infasurf (n = 77)	Placebo (n = 75)	*P* Value
Mortality			
Died (in hospital)	15 (19%)	27 (36%)	0.03
Died without extubation	12 (16%)	24 (32%)	0.02
Failed CMV[a]	13 (21%)	26 (42%)	0.02
ECMO	3	3	—
Use of nitric oxide	9	10	0.80
HFOV after entry	7	15	0.07
Secondary Outcomes			
PICU LOS	15.2 ± 13.3	13.6 ± 11.6	0.85
Hospital LOS	26.8 ± 26	25.3 ± 32.2	0.91
Days O_2 therapy	17.3 ± 16	18.5 ± 31	0.93
Hospital charges[b]	$205 ± 220	$213 ± 226	0.83
Hospital Charges/d[b]	$7.5 ± 7.6	$7.9 ± 7.5	0.74

In addition to improving mortality and reducing the percentage of patients who failed CMV, instilled Infasurf (70 mg/kg) also significantly improved OI compared with placebo (*P* = .01 see the findings from an earlier trial by the same group shown in **Fig. 1**).

Abbreviations: CMV, conventional mechanical ventilation; ECMO, extracorporeal membrane oxygenation; HFOV, high-frequency oscillatory ventilation; LOS, length of stay.

[a] Some patients who failed CMV had more than 1 nonconventional therapy (ECMO, inhaled nitric oxide [INO], or HFOV).

[b] Costs are given in thousands of dollars.

Data from Willson DF, Thomas NJ, Markovitz BP, et al. Effect of exogenous surfactant (calfactant) in pediatric acute lung injury: a randomized controlled trial. JAMA 2005;293:470–6.

Table 4
Efficacy of exogenous surfactant therapy in direct and indirect lung injury in the controlled 2005 study of Willson and colleagues[21] in children up to age 21 years with ALI/ARDS

	Placebo	Calfactant	*P* value
Direct lung injury (n)	48	50	—
OI ↓ 25% or more	31%	66%	0.0006
Ventilator days	17 ± 10	13 ± 9	0.05
Died	38%	8%	0.0005
Indirect lung injury (n)	27	27	—
OI ↓ 25% or more	41%	37%	0.79
Ventilator days	17 ± 10	18 ± 10	0.75
Died	33%	41%	0.65

Treatment was with Infasurf (Calfactant) at a dose of 70 mg/kg body weight.[21] Percentages of patients with an OI decrease of greater than 25%, days on mechanical ventilation, and percentage mortality were calculated in a post-hoc analysis. The efficacy of exogenous surfactant therapy is confined to patients with direct pulmonary forms of ALI/ARDS. See text for details.

Data from Willson DF, Thomas NJ, Markovitz BP, et al. Effect of exogenous surfactant (calfactant) in pediatric acute lung injury: a randomized controlled trial. JAMA 2005;293:470–6.

Surfactant Therapy in Adults with ALI/ARDS

In adults with ALI/ARDS, uncontrolled treatment studies have documented improved respiratory function (oxygenation) with surfactant administration,[135,136] but results from controlled clinical trials have been less successful. An initial large and highly visible prospective controlled study of surfactant therapy in adults with ARDS in 1996 was definitively negative.[151] Anzueto and colleagues[151] administered nebulized Exosurf versus placebo to 725 adults with ARDS secondary to sepsis and found no improvement in any measure of oxygenation and no effect on morbidity or mortality. However, interpretation of these negative results is confounded because sepsis is an indirect cause of ALI/ARDS that has substantial systemic consequences. Detailed laboratory and clinical studies have documented that Exosurf has low activity compared with animal-derived surfactants,[42,160–168] and the drug is no longer used in the United States for this reason. In addition, the aerosol method of surfactant administration used by Anzueto and colleagues[151] has not been shown to be as effective as direct airway instillation in delivering and distributing surfactant to the alveoli. A second disappointing controlled clinical trial of surfactant therapy in adults with ALI/ARDS was that of Gregory and colleagues[152] in 1997, who reported small benefits in oxygenation in the subgroup of 43 patients who received 4 doses of 100 mg/kg of Survanta, but no advantage in survival. However, this trial again focused on sepsis-induced lung injury in which significant systemic symptoms are present. In addition, Survanta contains only small amounts of SP-B,[42,112–114] which is the most biophysically active apoprotein in native surfactant.[169–177]

In 2003, Spragg and colleagues[22] performed a controlled trial of recombinant SP-C (rSP-C) surfactant (Venticute) in adults with ARDS and reported immediate improvements in oxygenation, but no improvement in duration of mechanical ventilation, lengths of stay, or mortality. However, post-hoc analysis did suggest that the response in the subgroup of patients with ARDS caused by direct lung injury was positive.[22] A recent large follow-up trial randomized adults with ARDS in association with direct lung injury from pneumonia or aspiration to receive Venticute (up to 8 doses administered in 96 hours, n = 419) or usual care (n = 424).[178] However, there was no improvement in oxygenation from Venticute in this large study.[178] In examining this lack of efficacy, the study investigators reported that a partial inactivation of rSP-C surfactant occurred in the clinical trial because of a step in the resuspension process (shear-induced loss of drug activity).[178] Also, as noted earlier, Venticute contains rSP-C but not highly active SP-B. There is thus a continuing need for further evaluations of surfactant therapy in adults with ARDS using the most active and inhibition-resistant drugs. In addition, effective delivery of exogenous surfactants to the alveoli must also be accomplished in trials of surfactant therapy in ARDS, as discussed later.

DELIVERY AND DOSAGE OF EXOGENOUS SURFACTANTS IN ALI/ARDS

Delivery of Exogenous Surfactant

To effectively treat surfactant dysfunction in injured lungs, exogenous surfactants of high activity must be delivered in adequate concentrations to the alveoli (the site of surfactant action). The primary method used to administer exogenous surfactants to patients in ALI/ARDS is intratracheal instillation through an endotracheal tube, as is done in the case of premature infants. Airway instillation of surfactant via a bronchoscope is also sometimes used in older patients as an alternative. Exogenous surfactant material instilled into the larger airways has the capacity to spread and distribute to the periphery of the lung.[179–181] Spreading from central airways toward the alveoli is promoted by surface tension gradients (ie, surface tension is reduced in the initial region where surfactant is instilled, and transport is then driven toward peripheral regions where surface tension is higher and surfactant concentration is lower).

The delivery and distribution of instilled exogenous surfactants in injured lungs can potentially be facilitated by the use of specific modes or strategies of mechanical ventilation. For example, studies have suggested that the distribution and/or efficacy of instilled exogenous surfactant can be improved by jet ventilation[182,183] and partial liquid ventilation.[184–186] Additional mechanism-based research on the impact of specific ventilation methods and strategies on the delivery, distribution, and efficacy of exogenous surfactants may be important for optimizing this therapy in ALI/ARDS. The delivery and distribution of surfactant drugs in injured lungs could also potentially be improved by the use of low-viscosity formulations to reduce transport resistance after tracheal or bronchoscopic instillation. Whole surfactant and animal-derived exogenous surfactants have complex, non-Newtonian, concentration-dependent viscosities that vary significantly among preparations.[187,188] For a given surfactant preparation at fixed shear rate, viscosity can be significantly reduced by modifying the physical formulation by changes in dispersion methodology, ionic environment, or temperature.[187,188]

An alternative to administering exogenous surfactants by instillation is to deliver them in aerosol form. In theory, aerosolization can reduce required surfactant doses if efficient alveolar delivery can be achieved by controlling particle size. Phospholipid aerosols with stable particle sizes appropriate for alveolar deposition in normal lungs can be formed by ultrasonic or jet nebulization,[189–191] and exogenous surfactants have been aerosolized to animals and patients with surfactant deficiency or dysfunction.[89,103,108,151,192–194] However, the theoretic potential of aerosols to improve alveolar deposition and lower required surfactant doses has not yet been replicated in practice. Aerosol methods to date have not been shown to deliver and distribute exogenous surfactants as effectively as instillation in clinical studies, although this may change in the future as technology for aerosol formation and delivery advances. A recent report, using dry-powder aerosolization of SP-C in animal models of ALI, showed that a lot of surfactant with intact biophysical properties could be delivered.[195]

Dosage of Exogenous Surfactants

Typical doses of surfactant drugs instilled intratracheally in premature infants with NRDS are 100 mg/kg body weight. This dose is significantly more than the amount needed to cover the surface of the alveolar network with a tightly packed surfactant film (only about 3 mg/kg of phospholipid-rich surfactant at an average molecular weight of 750 Da are needed to form a monomolecular film at a limiting area of 40 $Å^2$/molecule over an alveolar surface of 1 m^2/kg body weight[37,190]). Excess exogenous surfactant that reaches the alveoli following instillation provides a reservoir of material in the hypophase that can adsorb into the air-water interface when needed, and excess surfactant is also available for incorporation into endogenous surfactant pools via type II cell uptake and recycling pathways.

For ALI/ARDS, surfactant dosage amounts are typically increased on a body weight (or body surface area) basis. For older children and adults, this represents a substantial increase in the total amount of surfactant that needs to be administered. To achieve a dose comparable with the 100 mg/kg level used in premature infants weighing 1 kg, the typical 70-kg adult requires 7 g of exogenous surfactant. Clinical studies instilling exogenous surfactants in patients with ALI/ARDS have used a range of doses as high as 300 mg/kg[196] and as low as 25 mg/kg.[22] An instilled dose of 100 mg/kg in an adult with ALI/ARDS requires an instilled fluid volume of about 90 to 280 mL at the phospholipid concentrations of current clinical surfactant drugs in saline (~25–80 mg/mL). Although it is important to minimize instilled surfactant volumes in patients with edema and severe respiratory failure, this has disadvantages as well as advantages. In particular, instilled surfactant volume can affect intrapulmonary distribution, which is already compromised by edema and inflammation in patients with ALI/ARDS. Several studies in animal models of ALI/ARDS have indicated that the distribution of exogenous surfactant can be improved by instilling larger fluid volumes or using associated BAL.[197–200]

POTENTIAL FOR COMBINING EXOGENOUS SURFACTANT WITH OTHER THERAPIES IN ALI/ARDS

The earlier discussion has focused on exogenous surfactant therapy as an individual intervention. However, even if extrapulmonary symptoms are absent or minimal in patients with ALI/ARDS, the multifaceted pathophysiology of lung injury itself is still present. Individual pharmacologic agents such as exogenous surfactant may mitigate their intended target of pathology, but a benefit to survival and other long-term clinical outcomes in patients may be obscured by remaining aspects of the lung injury. A large body of scientific research elucidating many of the mechanisms of pulmonary injury and inflammation now exists and is continuing to expand rapidly. Such research has already identified multiple biologic processes and pharmacologic agents that could potentially be used concurrently with exogenous surfactant to treat complementary targets in the pathophysiology of ALI/ARDS. When studied individually in cell or animal research on lung injury, many agents have shown measurable benefits, but have not been found to improve survival and other significant outcomes in patients with ALI/ARDS. Rational mechanism-based combination therapies that concurrently target different aspects of lung injury pathology may have more success in improving long-term patient outcomes, as reviewed in detail elsewhere.[111,201] Combination therapies for ALI/ARDS could include not only pharmacologic agents but also multimodal strategies incorporating nonpharmacologic interventions such as different protocols or modes of mechanical ventilation or patient positioning.

Potential biologic targets in addition to surfactant dysfunction in the acute exudative phase of ALI/ARDS include hypoperfusion and ventilation/perfusion mismatching, arterial hypoxemia, edema, inflammation, oxidant injury, and injury to alveolar epithelial and capillary endothelial cells (**Table 5**). Agents and interventions targeting many of these abnormalities are discussed elsewhere in this issue, and many may have potential usefulness in combination therapy approaches with exogenous surfactant. Examples of pharmacologic agents in addition to exogenous surfactant that have been tested individually in patients with ALI/ARDS or sepsis include vasoactive agents such as inhaled nitric oxide (INO), almitrine, or prostacyclin[202–218]; β-2 agonists such as salbutamol to reduce edema,[219–221] anticoagulants like tissue factor pathway inhibitor (TFPI) and antithrombotic protein C (APC)[222–224]; antiinflammatory antibodies or receptor antagonists such as anti–tumor necrosis factor (TNF) α[225–228] and interleukin (IL)-1 receptor antagonist (IL-1Ra)[229,230]; antiinflammatory agents like pentoxifylline and corticosteroids[231–241]; and antioxidants like *N*-acetylcysteine[242–244] and superoxide dismutase.[245,246] Nonpharmacologic interventions that could be used in combination therapies include modes or strategies of mechanical ventilation that enhance alveolar recruitment and minimize ventilator-induced lung injury.[247–259] Prone positioning can also be used to enhance alveolar recruitment and ventilation in patients with ALI/ARDS (eg, see Ward.[260]). These agents and interventions, and their

Table 5
Selected biologic targets for pharmacotherapy that can be used in addition to surfactant therapy in ALI/ARDS

Target	Contributing Abnormalities/ Processes	Selected Desired Outcomes
Hypoperfusion and ventilation/perfusion mismatching	Hypoxic vasoconstriction Inappropriate vasodilation Microvascular occlusion	Treat with agents to vasodilate ventilated lung regions, vasoconstrict nonventilated lung regions, and reduce microvascular thrombosis
Surfactant dysfunction or deficiency	Physicochemical inhibitors of surfactant in edema or inflammation, or injury to type II pneumocytes	Deliver exogenous surfactant to reverse surfactant dysfunction/deficiency to improve alveolar stability, reduce edema, and normalize P-V mechanics
Overexuberant inflammation	Activation/recruitment of inflammatory leukocytes and overexuberant production of inflammatory mediators	Deliver agents to remove or deplete activated neutrophils, macrophages, or other leukocytes, or to block the effects of specific inflammatory mediators
Arterial hypoxemia, alveolar and interstitial edema	Decreased gas exchange, increased permeability, and decreased resorptive capacity of the alveolocapillary membrane	Delivery of agents to reduce edema coupled with mechanical ventilation strategies to raise arterial oxygenation without increasing permeability injury
Death/injury of cells in airways and alveolocapillary membrane	Loss of normal ciliated airway epithelium alveolar type I cells, and microvascular endothelial cells	Reduce cell death and the severity of cellular injury by delivering antioxidants or other cell-protective agents

Examples of pharmacologic targets that could potentially be targeted in combination therapies with exogenous surfactant (also listed) in the acute exudative phase of ALI/ARDS are summarized. A variety of additional targets in the later fibroproliferative/fibrotic phase of ALI/ARDS also exist.

Data from Pryhuber GS, D'Angio CT, Finkelstein JN, et al. Combined-modality therapies for lung injury. In: Notter RH, Finkelstein JN, Holm BA, editors. Lung injury: mechanisms, pathophysiology, and therapy. Boca Raton (FL): Taylor & Francis; 2005. p. 779–838.

potential usefulness in combination therapies for acute exudative ALI/ARDS, are detailed more fully elsewhere.[111,201] As a representative example, the possible benefit of concurrent use of exogenous surfactant therapy with INO is discussed briefly later.

Clinical studies have shown that INO alone improves arterial oxygenation and reduces pulmonary artery pressure in adults with ARDS[202–210] and in infants or children with acute respiratory failure.[261–266] The rationale for combination therapy with INO and exogenous surfactant is based on their complementary mechanisms of action in improving ventilation/perfusion matching and gas exchange. INO dilates the vasculature in ventilated lung units, whereas surfactant improves ventilation by decreasing surface tension and enhancing alveolar stability and recruitment. Exogenous surfactant therapy would theoretically increase the ventilated lung area accessible to INO, whereas the latter would increase the perfusion of these ventilated areas. Additive improvements in lung function from the simultaneous use of INO and exogenous surfactant have been shown in premature surfactant-deficient lambs with congenital diaphragmatic hernia,[267] as well as in animal models of ALI/ARDS.[268–273] A stepwise, multiple regression analysis of neonates with hypoxic respiratory failure being weaned from INO has shown that therapeutic surfactant significantly enhanced oxygenation reserve.[274] Clinical benefits have been reported from exogenous surfactant therapy and INO in a small case series in full-term infants with severe acute respiratory failure.[275] These findings support more extensive study of combination therapy with surfactant and INO in ALI/ARDS. This recommendation is also the conclusion of a review of newborns less than 5 days old and at 35 weeks' gestation or more diagnosed with hypoxemic respiratory failure (OI>15) from meconium aspiration, sepsis/pneumonia, or persistent pulmonary hypertension in the eras preceding (1993–1994) and following (1996–1997) the simultaneous availability of high-frequency oscillatory ventilation, INO, and exogenous surfactant.[276] The simultaneous availability of these therapies was associated with a reduced percentage of infants requiring rescue therapy with ECMO (42.8% vs 27.7%) that was not fully attributable to the reported efficacy of the individual agents alone.[276] The efficacy of INO has also been reported to be additive with those of PEEP[277] and patient prone positioning.[278]

Developing and testing combination interventions for ALI/ARDS is challenging no matter what agents or specific treatments are involved. Controlled clinical trials are essential for defining the efficacy of any specific combination therapies in ALI/ARDS. However, the complexity, time, and cost associated with such clinical trials make it particularly important also to make maximum use of laboratory studies in animal and cell models to evaluate a broader range of potential combination regimens so that clinical testing can be focused on the most promising interventions. Because of the rapid pace of progress in understanding inflammation and lung injury at the molecular and cellular level, there is reason for optimism about the potential for eventually developing combination therapies able to effect substantial improvements in survival and other long-term outcomes for patients (or targeted patient subgroups) with ALI/ARDS.

SUMMARY AND FUTURE PROSPECTS FOR SURFACTANT THERAPY IN ALI/ARDS

Exogenous surfactant therapy is a standard life-saving intervention for the prevention and treatment of NRDS in premature infants, and basic science and clinical evidence strongly support its use in at least some patients with lung injury–associated respiratory failure, as described in this article. The efficacy of surfactant therapy in term infants with meconium aspiration is sufficiently well documented to have become a standard intervention in many neonatal intensive care units. Surfactant therapy is also used routinely in infants and children with lung injury–related acute respiratory failure from pulmonary viral or bacterial infections (pneumonia). Controlled trials of exogenous surfactant therapy in children up to 21 years of age with ALI/ARDS have also shown significant benefits, with significant survival advantages in direct pulmonary forms of ALI/ARDS documented in the randomized controlled trial of Willson and colleagues.[21]

Current clinical evidence supporting the use of surfactant in adults with ALI/ARDS is less compelling than in infants and children. However, the surfactants that have been most extensively studied in adults with ARDS (Exosurf and Survanta) have known limitations in composition and activity compared with several other available preparations. Adult studies to date have also not focused on direct pulmonary forms of ALI/ARDS, in which surfactant therapy is most likely to be effective as a targeted intervention. In addition, neonatal data suggest that early surfactant administration generates improved responses compared with delayed administration (eg, Kendig and colleagues[279]), possibly as a result of better intrapulmonary drug distribution coupled with minimized ventilator-induced lung injury. Similar advantages might accompany early, as opposed to later, surfactant administration in patients with ALI/ARDS, if individuals who are at greater risk for progression to respiratory failure can be accurately identified nearer the start of their clinical course. Although it is challenging and expensive to examine surfactant therapy in controlled clinical trials, further studies of direct pulmonary forms of ALI/ARDS with the most active available exogenous surfactants delivered effectively to the alveoli are warranted based on current pathophysiologic understanding and extensive biophysical and animal research.

An additional consideration for surfactant therapy in ALI/ARDS involves its use in combination with agents or interventions targeting other aspects of the complex pathophysiology of acute pulmonary injury. A combination therapy approach seems particularly relevant for adults with ALI/ARDS, for which responses to exogenous surfactant have so far been disappointing. The use of multiple therapeutic agents or interventions based on a mechanistic rationale for synergy may significantly enhance outcomes in patients with complex inflammatory lung injury disorders. This article gives examples of specific biologic targets, pharmacologic agents, and other interventions that might be synergistic with exogenous surfactant in ALI/ARDS. Given the known contributions of surfactant dysfunction in inflammatory lung injury, it seems likely that surfactant therapy alone or in combination with other agents will ultimately be applicable for at least some adult as well as pediatric patients with ALI/ARDS caused by direct forms of pulmonary injury.

REFERENCES

1. Bernard GR, Artigas A, Brigham KL, et al. The American-European Consensus Conference on ARDS: definitions, mechanisms, relevant outcomes, and clinical trial coordination. Am J Respir Crit Care Med 1994;149:818–24.
2. Murray JF, Matthay MA, Luce JM, et al. An expanded definition of the adult respiratory distress syndrome. Am Rev Respir Dis 1988;138:720–3.
3. American College of Chest Physicians Society of Critical Care Medicine Consensus Conference Committee. Definitions for sepsis and organ failure and guidelines for the use of innovative therapies for sepsis. Crit Care Med 1992;20:864–74.
4. Pollack MM, Patel KM, Ruttimann UE. PRISM III: an updated pediatric risk of mortality score. Crit Care Med 1996;24:743–52.
5. Slater A, Shann F, ANZICS Paediatric Study Group. The suitability of the Pediatric Index of Mortality (PIM), PIM2, the Pediatric Risk of Mortality (PRISM), and PRISM III for monitoring the quality of pediatric intensive care in Australia and New Zealand. Pediatr Crit Care Med 2004;5:447–54.
6. Shann F, Pearson G, Slater A, et al. Paediatric index of mortality (PIM): a mortality prediction model for children in intensive care. Intensive Care Med 1997;23:201–7.
7. Trachsel D, McCrindle BW, Nakagawa S, et al. Oxygenation index predicts outcome in children with acute hypoxemic respiratory failure. Am J Respir Crit Care Med 2005;172:206–11.
8. Ferguson ND, Davis AM, Slutsky AS, et al. Development of a clinical definition for acute respiratory distress syndrome using the Delphi technique. J Crit Care 2005;20:147–54.

9. Hudson LD, Milberg JA, Anardi D, et al. Clinical risks for development of the acute respiratory distress syndrome. Am J Respir Crit Care Med 1995;151: 293–301.
10. Krafft P, Fridrich P, Pernerstorfer T, et al. The acute respiratory distress syndrome; definitions, severity, and clinical outcome. An analysis of 101 clinical investigations. Intensive Care Med 1996;22:519–29.
11. Doyle RL, Szaflarski N, Modin GW, et al. Identification of patients with acute lung injury: predictors of mortality. Am J Respir Crit Care Med 1995;152:1818–24.
12. Ware LB, Matthay MA. The acute respiratory distress syndrome. N Engl J Med 2000;342:1334–48.
13. Rubenfeld GD. Epidemiology of acute lung injury. Crit Care Med 2003; 31(Suppl):S276–84.
14. Rubenfeld GD, Caldwell E, Peabody E, et al. Incidence and outcomes of acute lung injury. N Engl J Med 2005;353:1685–93.
15. Goss CH, Brower RG, Hudson LD, et al. ARDS Network. Incidence of acute lung injury in the United States. Crit Care Med 2003;31:1607–11.
16. Pfenninger J, Gerber A, Tschappeler H, et al. Adult respiratory distress syndrome in children. J Pediatr 1982;101:352–7.
17. Bindl L, Dresbach K, Lentze M. Incidence of acute respiratory distress syndrome in German children and adolescents: a population based study. Crit Care Med 2005;33:209–12.
18. Manzano F, Yuste E, Colmenero M, et al. Incidence of acute respiratory distress syndrome and its relation to age. J Crit Care 2005;20:274–80.
19. Randolph AG, Wypij D, Venkataraman ST, et al. Effect of mechanical ventilator weaning protocols on respiratory outcomes in infants and children. A randomized controlled trial. JAMA 2002;288:2561–8.
20. Flori HR, Glidden DV, Rutherford GW, et al. Pediatric acute lung injury. Prospective evaluation of risk factors associated with mortality. Am J Respir Crit Care Med 2005;171:995–1001.
21. Willson DF, Thomas NJ, Markovitz BP, et al. Effect of exogenous surfactant (calfactant) in pediatric acute lung injury: a randomized controlled trial. JAMA 2005;293:470–6.
22. Spragg RG, Lewis JF, Wurst W, et al. Treatment of acute respiratory distress syndrome with recombinant surfactant protein C surfactant. Am J Respir Crit Care Med 2003;167:1562–6.
23. Petty T, Reiss O, Paul G, et al. Characteristics of pulmonary surfactant in adult respiratory distress syndrome associated with trauma and shock. Am Rev Respir Dis 1977;115:531–6.
24. Hallman M, Spragg R, Harrell JH, et al. Evidence of lung surfactant abnormality in respiratory failure. J Clin Invest 1982;70:673–83.
25. Seeger W, Pison U, Buchhorn R, et al. Surfactant abnormalities and adult respiratory failure. Lung 1990;168(Suppl):891–902.
26. Pison U, Seeger W, Buchhorn R, et al. Surfactant abnormalities in patients with respiratory failure after multiple trauma. Am Rev Respir Dis 1989;140: 1033–9.
27. Gregory TJ, Longmore WJ, Moxley MA, et al. Surfactant chemical composition and biophysical activity in acute respiratory distress syndrome. J Clin Invest 1991;88:1976–81.
28. Günther A, Siebert C, Schmidt R, et al. Surfactant alterations in severe pneumonia, acute respiratory distress syndrome, and cardiogenic lung edema. Am J Respir Crit Care Med 1996;153:176–84.

29. Veldhuizen RAW, McCaig LA, Akino T, et al. Pulmonary surfactant subfractions in patients with the acute respiratory distress syndrome. Am J Respir Crit Care Med 1995;152:1867–71.
30. Griese M. Pulmonary surfactant in health and human lung diseases: state of the art. Eur Respir J 1999;13:1455–76.
31. Mander A, Langton-Hewer S, Bernhard W, et al. Altered phospholipid composition and aggregate structure of lung surfactant is associated with impaired lung function in young children with respiratory infections. Am J Respir Cell Mol Biol 2002;27:714–21.
32. Schmidt R, Meier U, Markart P, et al. Altered fatty acid composition of lung surfactant phospholipids in interstitial lung disease. Am J Physiol Lung Cell Mol Physiol 2002;283:L1079–85.
33. Skelton R, Holland P, Darowski M, et al. Abnormal surfactant composition and activity in severe bronchiolitis. Acta Paediatr 1999;88:942–6.
34. LeVine AM, Lotze A, Stanley S, et al. Surfactant content in children with inflammatory lung disease. Crit Care Med 1996;24:1062–7.
35. Dargaville PA, South M, McDougall PN. Surfactant abnormalities in infants with severe viral bronchiolitis. Arch Dis Child 1996;75:133–6.
36. Wang Z, Holm BA, Matalon S, et al. Surfactant activity and dysfunction in lung injury. In: Notter RH, Finkelstein JN, Holm BA, editors. Lung injury: mechanisms, pathophysiology, and therapy. Boca Raton (FL): Taylor & Francis; 2005. p. 297–352.
37. Notter RH. Lung surfactants: basic science and clinical applications. New York: Marcel Dekker; 2000.
38. Notter RH, Wang Z. Pulmonary surfactant: physical chemistry, physiology and replacement. Rev Chem Eng 1997;13:1–118.
39. Holm BA, Notter RH, Finkelstein JH. Surface property changes from interactions of albumin with natural lung surfactant and extracted lung lipids. Chem Phys Lipids 1985;38:287–98.
40. Seeger W, Stohr G, Wolf HRD, et al. Alteration of surfactant function due to protein leakage: special interaction with fibrin monomer. J Appl Physiol 1985;58:326–38.
41. Holm BA, Notter RH. Effects of hemoglobin and cell membrane lipids on pulmonary surfactant activity. J Appl Physiol 1987;63:1434–42.
42. Seeger W, Grube C, Günther A, et al. Surfactant inhibition by plasma proteins: differential sensitivity of various surfactant preparations. Eur Respir J 1993;6:971–7.
43. Holm BA, Enhorning G, Notter RH. A biophysical mechanism by which plasma proteins inhibit lung surfactant activity. Chem Phys Lipids 1988;49:49–55.
44. Fuchimukai T, Fujiwara T, Takahashi A, et al. Artificial pulmonary surfactant inhibited by proteins. J Appl Physiol 1987;62:429–37.
45. Keough KWM, Parsons CS, Tweeddale MG. Interactions between plasma proteins and pulmonary surfactant: pulsating bubble studies. Can J Physiol Pharmacol 1989;67:663–8.
46. Wang Z, Notter RH. Additivity of protein and non-protein inhibitors of lung surfactant activity. Am J Respir Crit Care Med 1998;158:28–35.
47. Moses D, Holm BA, Spitale P, et al. Inhibition of pulmonary surfactant function by meconium. Am J Obstet Gynecol 1991;164:477–81.
48. Cockshutt A, Possmayer F. Lysophosphatidylcholine sensitizes lipid extracts of pulmonary surfactant to inhibition by plasma proteins. Biochim Biophys Acta 1991;1086:63–71.

49. Seeger W, Lepper H, Hellmut RD, et al. Alteration of alveolar surfactant function after exposure to oxidant stress and to oxygenated and native arachidonic acid in vitro. Biochim Biophys Acta 1985;835:58–67.
50. Hall SB, Lu ZR, Venkitaraman AR, et al. Inhibition of pulmonary surfactant by oleic acid: mechanisms and characteristics. J Appl Physiol 1992;72:1708–16.
51. Hall SB, Hyde RW, Notter RH. Changes in subphase surfactant aggregates in rabbits injured by free fatty acid. Am J Respir Crit Care Med 1994;149: 1099–106.
52. Hickman-Davis JM, Fang FC, Nathan C, et al. Lung surfactant and reactive oxygen-nitrogen species: antimicrobial activity and host-pathogen interactions. Am J Physiol Lung Cell Mol Physiol 2001;281:L517–23.
53. Haddad IY, Ischiropoulos H, Holm BA, et al. Mechanisms of peroxynitrite-induced injury to pulmonary surfactants. Am J Physiol 1993;265:L555–64.
54. Amirkhanian JD, Merritt TA. Inhibitory effects of oxyradicals on surfactant function: utilizing in vitro Fenton reaction. Lung 1998;176:63–72.
55. Pison U, Tam EK, Caughey GH, et al. Proteolytic inactivation of dog lung surfactant-associated proteins by neutrophil elastase. Biochim Biophys Acta 1989;992:251–7.
56. Holm BA, Kelcher L, Liu M, et al. Inhibition of pulmonary surfactant by phospholipases. J Appl Physiol 1991;71:317–21.
57. Enhorning G, Shumel B, Keicher L, et al. Phospholipases introduced into the hypophase affect the surfactant film outlining a bubble. J Appl Physiol 1992; 73:941–5.
58. Holm BA, Wang Z, Notter RH. Multiple mechanisms of lung surfactant inhibition. Pediatr Res 1999;46:85–93.
59. Wang Z, Schwan AL, Lairson LL, et al. Surface activity of a synthetic lung surfactant containing a phospholipase-resistant phosphonolipid analog of dipalmitoyl phosphatidylcholine. Am J Physiol Lung Cell Mol Physiol 2003;285:L550–9.
60. Magoon MW, Wright JR, Baritussio A, et al. Subfractionation of lung surfactant: implications for metabolism and surface activity. Biochim Biophys Acta 1983; 750:18–31.
61. Wright JR, Benson BJ, Williams MC, et al. Protein composition of rabbit alveolar surfactant subfractions. Biochim Biophys Acta 1984;791:320–32.
62. Gross NJ, Narine KR. Surfactant subtypes in mice: characterization and quantitation. J Appl Physiol 1989;66:342–9.
63. Putz G, Goerke J, Clements JA. Surface activity of rabbit pulmonary surfactant subfractions at different concentrations in a captive bubble. J Appl Physiol 1994;77:597–605.
64. Putman E, Creuwels LAJM, Van Golde LMG, et al. Surface properties, morphology and protein composition of pulmonary surfactant subtypes. Biochem J 1996;320:599–605.
65. Veldhuizen RAW, Hearn SA, Lewis JF, et al. Surface-area cycling of different surfactant preparations: SP-A and SP-B are essential for large aggregate integrity. Biochem J 1994;300:519–24.
66. Gross NJ. Extracellular metabolism of pulmonary surfactant: the role of a new serine protease. Annu Rev Physiol 1995;57:135–50.
67. Lewis JF, Ikegami M, Jobe AH. Altered surfactant function and metabolism in rabbits with acute lung injury. J Appl Physiol 1990;69:2303–10.
68. Putman E, Boere AJ, van Bree L, et al. Pulmonary surfactant subtype metabolism is altered after short-term ozone exposure. Toxicol Appl Pharmacol 1995; 134:132–8.

69. Atochina EN, Beers MF, Scanlon ST, et al. *P. carinii* induces selective alterations in component expression and biophysical activity of lung surfactant. Am J Physiol Lung Cell Mol Physiol 2000;278:L599–609.
70. Davidson BA, Knight PR, Wang Z, et al. Surfactant alterations in acute inflammatory lung injury from aspiration of acid and gastric particulates. Am J Physiol Lung Cell Mol Physiol 2005;288:L699–708.
71. Lewis JF, Jobe AH. Surfactant and the adult respiratory distress syndrome. Am Rev Respir Dis 1993;147:218–33.
72. Seeger W, Günther A, Walmrath HD, et al. Alveolar surfactant and adult respiratory distress syndrome. Pathogenic role and therapeutic prospects. Clin Investig 1993;71:177–90.
73. Lachmann B, van Daal G-J. Adult respiratory distress syndrome: animal models. In: Robertson B, van Golde LM, Batenburg JJ, editors. Pulmonary surfactant: from molecular biology to clinical practice. Amsterdam: Elsevier Science Publishers; 1992. p. 635–63.
74. Russo TA, Bartholomew LA, Davidson BA, et al. Total extracellular surfactant is increased but abnormal in a rat model of Gram-negative bacterial pneumonitis. Am J Physiol Lung Cell Mol Physiol 2002;283:L655–63.
75. Russo TA, Wang Z, Davidson BA, et al. Surfactant dysfunction and lung injury due to the *E. coli* virulence factor hemolysin in a rat pneumonia model. Am J Physiol Lung Cell Mol Physiol 2007;292:L632–43.
76. Wright TW, Notter RH, Wang Z, et al. Pulmonary inflammation disrupts surfactant function during *P. carinii* pneumonia. Infect Immun 2001;69:758–64.
77. Bruckner L, Gigliotti F, Wright TW, et al. *Pneumocystis carinii* infection sensitizes the lung to radiation-induced injury after syngeneic marrow transplantation: role of $CD4^+$ T-cells. Am J Physiol Lung Cell Mol Physiol 2006;290:L1087–96.
78. Raghavendran K, Davidson BA, Knight PR, et al. Surfactant dysfunction in lung contusion with and without superimposed gastric aspiration in a rat model. Shock 2008;30:508–17.
79. Wright TW, Pryhuber G, Chess PR, et al. TNF receptor signaling contributes to chemokine secretion, inflammation, and respiratory deficits during *Pneumocystis carinii* pneumonia. J Immunol 2004;172:2511–22.
80. Kobayashi T, Ganzuka M, Taniguchi J, et al. Lung lavage and surfactant replacement for hydrochloric acid aspiration in rabbits. Acta Anaesthesiol Scand 1990;34:216–21.
81. Zucker A, Holm BA, Wood LDH, et al. Exogenous surfactant with PEEP reduces pulmonary edema and improves lung function in canine aspiration pneumonitis. J Appl Physiol 1992;73:679–86.
82. Schlag G, Strohmaier W. Experimental aspiration trauma: comparison of steroid treatment versus exogenous natural surfactant. Exp Lung Res 1993;19:397–405.
83. Al-Mateen KB, Dailey K, Grimes MM, et al. Improved oxygenation with exogenous surfactant administration in experimental meconium aspiration syndrome. Pediatr Pulmonol 1994;17:75–80.
84. Sun B, Curstedt T, Robertson B. Exogenous surfactant improves ventilation efficiency and alveolar expansion in rats with meconium aspiration. Am J Respir Crit Care Med 1996;154:764–70.
85. Cochrane CG, Revak SD, Merritt TA, et al. Bronchoalveolar lavage with KL4-surfactant in models of meconium aspiration syndrome. Pediatr Res 1998;44:705–15.
86. Sun B, Curstedt T, Song GW, et al. Surfactant improves lung function and morphology in newborn rabbits with meconium aspiration. Biol Neonate 1993;63:96–104.

87. Lachmann B, Hallman M, Bergman K-C. Respiratory failure following anti-lung serum: study on mechanisms associated with surfactant system damage. Exp Lung Res 1987;12:163–80.
88. Nieman G, Gatto L, Paskanik A, et al. Surfactant replacement in the treatment of sepsis-induced adult respiratory distress syndrome in pigs. Crit Care Med 1996; 24:1025–33.
89. Lutz C, Carney D, Finck C, et al. Aerosolized surfactant improves pulmonary function in endotoxin-induced lung injury. Am J Respir Crit Care Med 1998; 158:840–5.
90. Lutz CJ, Picone A, Gatto LA, et al. Exogenous surfactant and positive end-expiratory pressure in the treatment of endotoxin-induced lung injury. Crit Care Med 1998;26:1379–89.
91. Tashiro K, Li W-Z, Yamada K, et al. Surfactant replacement reverses respiratory failure induced by intratracheal endotoxin in rats. Crit Care Med 1995;23:149–56.
92. Eijking EP, van Daal GJ, Tenbrinck R, et al. Effect of surfactant replacement on *Pneumocystis carinii* pneumonia in rats. Intensive Care Med 1990;17:475–8.
93. Sherman MP, Campbell LA, Merritt TA, et al. Effect of different surfactants on pulmonary group B streptococcal infection in premature rabbits. J Pediatr 1994;125:939–47.
94. Berry D, Ikegami M, Jobe A. Respiratory distress and surfactant inhibition following vagotomy in rabbits. J Appl Physiol 1986;61:1741–8.
95. Matalon S, Holm BA, Notter RH. Mitigation of pulmonary hyperoxic injury by administration of exogenous surfactant. J Appl Physiol 1987;62:756–61.
96. Loewen GM, Holm BA, Milanowski L, et al. Alveolar hyperoxic injury in rabbits receiving exogenous surfactant. J Appl Physiol 1989;66:1987–92.
97. Engstrom PC, Holm BA, Matalon S. Surfactant replacement attenuates the increase in alveolar permeability in hyperoxia. J Appl Physiol 1989;67:688–93.
98. Matalon S, Holm BA, Loewen GM, et al. Sublethal hyperoxic injury to the alveolar epithelium and the pulmonary surfactant system. Exp Lung Res 1988;14: 1021–33.
99. Novotny WE, Hudak BB, Matalon S, et al. Hyperoxic lung injury reduces exogenous surfactant clearance in vitro. Am J Respir Crit Care Med 1995;151:1843–7.
100. Lachmann B, Fujiwara T, Chida S, et al. Surfactant replacement therapy in experimental adult respiratory distress syndrome (ARDS). In: Cosmi EV, Scarpelli EM, editors. Pulmonary surfactant system. Amsterdam: Elsevier; 1983. p. 221–35.
101. Kobayashi T, Kataoka H, Ueda T, et al. Effect of surfactant supplementation and end expiratory pressure in lung-lavaged rabbits. J Appl Physiol 1984;57: 995–1001.
102. Berggren P, Lachmann B, Curstedt T, et al. Gas exchange and lung morphology after surfactant replacement in experimental adult respiratory distress induced by repeated lung lavage. Acta Anaesthesiol Scand 1986;30:321–8.
103. Lewis JF, Goffin J, Yue P, et al. Evaluation of exogenous surfactant treatment strategies in an adult model of acute lung injury. J Appl Physiol 1996;80: 1156–64.
104. Walther FJ, Hernandez-Juviel J, Bruni R, et al. Spiking Survanta with synthetic surfactant peptides improves oxygenation in surfactant-deficient rats. Am J Respir Crit Care Med 1997;156:855–61.
105. Walther F, Hernandez-Juviel J, Bruni R, et al. Protein composition of synthetic surfactant affects gas exchange in surfactant-deficient rats. Pediatr Res 1998; 43:666–73.

106. Harris JD, Jackson F, Moxley MA, et al. Effect of exogenous surfactant instillation on experimental acute lung injury. J Appl Physiol 1989;66:1846–51.
107. Lewis JF, Ikegami M, Jobe AH. Metabolism of exogenously administered surfactant in the acutely injured lungs of adult rabbits. Am Rev Respir Dis 1992;145:19–23.
108. Lewis J, Ikegami M, Higuchi R, et al. Nebulized vs. instilled exogenous surfactant in an adult lung injury model. J Appl Physiol 1991;71:1270–6.
109. van Daal GJ, So KL, Gommers D, et al. Intratracheal surfactant administration restores gas exchange in experimental adult respiratory distress syndrome associated with viral pneumonia. Anesth Analg 1991;72:589–95.
110. van Daal GJ, Bos JA, Eijking EP, et al. Surfactant replacement therapy improves pulmonary mechanics in end-stage influenza A pneumonia in mice. Am Rev Respir Dis 1992;145:859–63.
111. Pryhuber GS, D'Angio CT, Finkelstein JN, et al. Combined-modality therapies for lung injury. In: Notter RH, Finkelstein JN, Holm BA, editors. Lung injury: mechanisms, pathophysiology, and therapy. Boca Raton (FL): Taylor & Francis; 2005. p. 779–838.
112. Mizuno K, Ikegami M, Chen C-M, et al. Surfactant protein-B supplementation improves *in vivo* function of a modified natural surfactant. Pediatr Res 1995; 37:271–6.
113. Hamvas A, Cole FS, deMello DE, et al. Surfactant protein B deficiency: antenatal diagnosis and prospective treatment with surfactant replacement. J Pediatr 1994;125:356–61.
114. Notter RH, Wang Z, Egan EA, et al. Component-specific surface and physiological activity in bovine-derived lung surfactants. Chem Phys Lipids 2002;114:21–34.
115. Cochrane CG, Revak SD. Pulmonary surfactant protein B (SP-B): structure-function relationships. Science 1991;254:566–8.
116. Cochrane CG, Revak SD, Merritt TA, et al. The efficacy and safety of KL4-surfactant in preterm infants with respiratory distress syndrome. Am J Respir Crit Care Med 1996;153:404–10.
117. Notter RH, Schwan AL, Wang Z, et al. Novel phospholipase-resistant lipid/peptide synthetic lung surfactants. Mini Rev Med Chem 2007;7:932–44.
118. Mingarro I, Lukovic D, Vilar M, et al. Synthetic pulmonary surfactant preparations: new developments and future trends. Curr Med Chem 2008;15:303–403.
119. Walther FJ, Waring AJ, Sherman MA, et al. Hydrophobic surfactant proteins and their analogues. Neonatology 2007;91:303–10.
120. Curstedt T, Johansson J. New synthetic surfactant–how and when? Biol Neonate 2006;89:336–9.
121. Walther FJ, Waring AJ, Hernandez-Juviel JM, et al. Critical structural and functional roles for the N-terminal insertion sequence in surfactant protein B analogs. PLoS ONE 2010;5:e8672.
122. Turcotte JG, Sacco AM, Steim JM, et al. Chemical synthesis and surface properties of an analog of the pulmonary surfactant dipalmitoyl phosphatidylcholine analog. Biochim Biophys Acta 1977;488:235–48.
123. Turcotte JG, Lin WH, Pivarnik PE, et al. Chemical synthesis and surface activity of lung surfactant phospholipid analogs. II. Racemic N-substituted diether phosphonolipids. Biochim Biophys Acta 1991;1084:1–12.
124. Wang Z, Chang Y, Schwan AL, et al. Activity and inhibition resistance of a phospholipase-resistant synthetic exogenous surfactant in excised rat lungs. Am J Respir Cell Mol Biol 2007;37:387–94.
125. Walther FJ, Waring AJ, Hernandez-Juviel JM, et al. Dynamic surface activity of a fully-synthetic phospholipase-resistant lipid/peptide lung surfactant. PLoS ONE 2007;2(10):e1039.

126. Notter RH, Wang Z, Wang Z, et al. Synthesis and surface activity of diether-linked phosphoglycerols: potential applications for exogenous lung surfactants. Bioorg Med Chem Lett 2007;17:113–7.
127. Chang Y, Wang Z, Schwan AL, et al. Surface properties of sulfur- and ether-linked phosphonolipids with and without purified hydrophobic lung surfactant proteins. Chem Phys Lipids 2005;137:77–93.
128. Kim DK, Fukuda T, Thompson BT, et al. Bronchoalveolar lavage fluid phospholipase A_2 activities are increased in human adult respiratory distress syndrome. Am J Physiol 1995;269:L109–18.
129. Touqui L, Arbibe L. A role for phospholipase A_2 in ARDS pathogenesis. Mol Med Today 1999;5:244–9.
130. Vadas P. Elevated plasma phospholipase A_2 levels: correlation with the hemodynamic and pulmonary changes in gram-negative septic shock. J Lab Clin Med 1984;104:873–81.
131. Vadas P, Pruzanski W. Biology of disease: role of secretory phospholipases A_2 in the pathobiology of disease. Lab Invest 1986;55:391–404.
132. Ackerman SJ, Kwatia MA, Doyle CB, et al. Hydrolysis of surfactant phospholipids catalyzed by phospholipase A_2 and eosinophil lysophospholipases causes surfactant dysfunction: a mechanism for small airway closure in asthma. Chest 2003;123:255S.
133. Attalah HL, Wu Y, Alaoui-El-Azher M, et al. Induction of type-IIA secretory phospholipase A_2 in animal models of acute lung injury. Eur Respir J 2003;21:1040–5.
134. Nakos G, Kitsiouli E, Hatzidaki E, et al. Phospholipases A_2 and platelet-activating–factor acetylhydrolase in patients with acute respiratory distress syndrome. Crit Care Med 2003;33:772–9.
135. Gunther A, Schmidt R, Harodt J, et al. Bronchoscopic administration of bovine natural surfactant in ARDS and septic shock: impact on biophysical and biochemical surfactant properties. Eur Respir J 2002;10:797–804.
136. Walmrath D, Gunther A, Ghofrani HA, et al. Bronchoscopic surfactant administration in patients with severe adult respiratory distress syndrome and sepsis. Am J Respir Crit Care Med 1996;154:57–62.
137. Spragg R, Gilliard N, Richman P, et al. Acute effects of a single dose of porcine surfactant on patients with the adult respiratory distress syndrome. Chest 1994; 105:195–202.
138. Wiswell TE, Smith RM, Katz LB, et al. Bronchopulmonary segmental lavage with Surfaxin (KL(4)-surfactant) for acute respiratory distress syndrome. Am J Respir Crit Care Med 1999;160:1188–95.
139. Willson DF, Jiao JH, Bauman LA, et al. Calf lung surfactant extract in acute hypoxemic respiratory failure in children. Crit Care Med 1996;24:1316–22.
140. Willson DF, Bauman LA, Zaritsky A, et al. Instillation of calf lung surfactant extract (calfactant) is beneficial in pediatric acute hypoxemic respiratory failure. Crit Care Med 1999;27:188–95.
141. Lopez-Herce J, de Lucas N, Carrillo A, et al. Surfactant treatment for acute respiratory distress syndrome. Arch Dis Child 1999;80:248–52.
142. Hermon MM, Golej J, Burda H, et al. Surfactant therapy in infants and children: three years experience in a pediatric intensive care unit. Shock 2002;17:247–51.
143. Herting E, Moller O, Schiffman JH, et al. Surfactant improves oxygenation in infants and children with pneumonia and acute respiratory distress syndrome. Acta Paediatr 2002;91:1174–8.
144. Auten RL, Notter RH, Kendig JW, et al. Surfactant treatment of full-term newborns with respiratory failure. Pediatrics 1991;87:101–7.

145. Lotze A, Knight GR, Martin GR, et al. Improved pulmonary outcome after exogenous surfactant therapy for respiratory failure in term infants requiring extracorporeal membrane oxygenation. J Pediatr 1993;122:261–8.
146. Lotze A, Mitchell BR, Bulas DI, et al. Multicenter study of surfactant (beractant) use in the treatment of term infants with severe respiratory failure. J Pediatr 1998;132:40–7.
147. Khammash H, Perlman M, Wojtulewicz J, et al. Surfactant therapy in full-term neonates with severe respiratory failure. Pediatrics 1993;92:135–9.
148. Findlay RD, Taeusch HW, Walther FJ. Surfactant replacement therapy for meconium aspiration syndrome. Pediatrics 1996;97:48–52.
149. Luchetti M, Casiraghi G, Valsecchi R, et al. Porcine-derived surfactant treatment of severe bronchiolitis. Acta Anaesthesiol Scand 1998;42:805–10.
150. Luchetti M, Ferrero F, Gallini C, et al. Multicenter, randomized, controlled study of porcine surfactant in severe respiratory syncytial virus-induced respiratory failure. Pediatr Crit Care Med 2002;3:261–8.
151. Anzueto A, Baughman RP, Guntupalli KK, et al. Aerosolized surfactant in adults with sepsis-induced acute respiratory distress syndrome. N Engl J Med 1996; 334:1417–21.
152. Gregory TJ, Steinberg KP, Spragg R, et al. Bovine surfactant therapy for patients with acute respiratory distress syndrome. Am J Respir Crit Care Med 1997;155: 109–31.
153. Seger N, Soll R. Animal derived surfactant extract for treatment of respiratory distress syndrome. Cochrane Database Syst Rev 2009;2:CD007836.
154. Soll R, Ozek E. Multiple versus single doses of exogenous surfactant for the prevention or treatment of neonatal respiratory distress syndrome. Cochrane Database Syst Rev 2009;1:CD000141.
155. Clark DA, Nieman GF, Thompson JE, et al. Surfactant displacement by meconium free fatty acids: an alternative explanation for atelectasis in meconium aspiration syndrome. J Pediatr 1987;110:765–70.
156. Tibby SM, Hatherill M, Wright SM, et al. Exogenous surfactant supplementation in infants with respiratory syncytial virus bronchiolitis. Am J Respir Crit Care Med 2000;162:1251–6.
157. Ivascu FA, Hirschl RB. New approaches to managing congenital diaphragmatic hernia. Semin Perinatol 2004;28:185–98.
158. Van Meurs K, Congenital Diaphragmatic Hernia Study Group. Is surfactant therapy beneficial in the treatment of the term newborn infants with congenital diaphragmatic hernia? J Pediatr 2004;145:312–6.
159. Moller JC, Schaible T, Roll C, et al. Treatment with bovine surfactant in severe acute respiratory distress syndrome in children: a randomized multicenter study. Intensive Care Med 2003;29:437–46.
160. Hall SB, Venkitaraman AR, Whitsett JA, et al. Importance of hydrophobic apoproteins as constituents of clinical exogenous surfactants. Am Rev Respir Dis 1992;145:24–30.
161. Hudak ML, Farrell EE, Rosenberg AA, et al. A multicenter randomized masked comparison of natural vs synthetic surfactant for the treatment of respiratory distress syndrome. J Pediatr 1996;128:396–406.
162. Bloom BT, Kattwinkel J, Hall RT, et al. Comparison of Infasurf (calf lung surfactant extract) to Survanta (beractant) in the treatment and prevention of RDS. Pediatrics 1997;100:31–8.
163. Hudak ML, Martin DJ, Egan EA, et al. A multicenter randomized masked comparison trial of synthetic surfactant versus calf lung surfactant extract in

the prevention of neonatal respiratory distress syndrome. Pediatrics 1997;100: 39–50.

164. Horbar JD, Wright LL, Soll RF, et al. A multicenter randomized trial comparing two surfactants for the treatment of neonatal respiratory distress syndrome. J Pediatr 1993;123:757–66.
165. Vermont-Oxford Neonatal Network. A multicenter randomized trial comparing synthetic surfactant with modified bovine surfactant extract in the treatment of neonatal respiratory distress syndrome. Pediatrics 1996;97:1–6.
166. Rollins M, Jenkins J, Tubman R, et al. Comparison of clinical responses to natural and synthetic surfactants. J Perinat Med 1993;21:341–7.
167. Sehgal SS, Ewing CK, Richards T, et al. Modified bovine surfactant (Survanta) vs a protein-free surfactant (Exosurf) in the treatment of respiratory distress syndrome in preterm infants: a pilot study. J Natl Med Assoc 1994;86:46–52.
168. Choukroun ML, Llanas B, Apere H, et al. Pulmonary mechanics in ventilated preterm infants with respiratory distress syndrome after exogenous surfactant administration: a comparison between two surfactant preparations. Pediatr Pulmonol 1994;18:273–98.
169. Curstedt T, Jornvall H, Robertson B, et al. Two hydrophobic low-molecular-mass protein fractions of pulmonary surfactant: characterization and biophysical activity. Eur J Biochem 1987;168:255–62.
170. Oosterlaken-Dijksterhuis MA, Haagsman HP, van Golde LM, et al. Characterization of lipid insertion into monomolecular layers mediated by lung surfactant proteins SP-B and SP-C. Biochemistry 1991;30:10965–71.
171. Oosterlaken-Dijksterhuis MA, Haagsman HP, van Golde LM, et al. Interaction of lipid vesicles with monomolecular layers containing lung surfactant proteins SP-B or SP-C. Biochemistry 1991;30:8276–81.
172. Oosterlaken-Dijksterhuis MA, van Eijk M, van Golde LMG, et al. Lipid mixing is mediated by the hydrophobic surfactant protein SP-B but not by SP-C. Biochim Biophys Acta 1992;1110:45–50.
173. Revak SD, Merritt TA, Degryse E, et al. The use of human low molecular weight (LMW) apoproteins in the reconstitution of surfactant biological activity. J Clin Invest 1988;81:826–33.
174. Seeger W, Günther A, Thede C. Differential sensitivity to fibrinogen inhibition of SP-C- vs. SP-B-based surfactants. Am J Physiol 1992;261:L286–91.
175. Wang Z, Gurel O, Baatz JE, et al. Differential activity and lack of synergy of lung surfactant proteins SP-B and SP-C in surface-active interactions with phospholipids. J Lipid Res 1996;37:1749–60.
176. Yu SH, Possmayer F. Comparative studies on the biophysical activities of the low-molecular-weight hydrophobic proteins purified from bovine pulmonary surfactant. Biochim Biophys Acta 1988;961:337–50.
177. Wang Z, Baatz JE, Holm BA, et al. Content-dependent activity of lung surfactant protein B (SP-B) in mixtures with lipids. Am J Physiol Lung Cell Mol Physiol 2002; 283:L897–906.
178. Spragg RG, Taut FJ, Lewis JF, et al. Recombinant surfactant protein C based surfactant for patients with severe direct lung injury. Am J Respir Crit Care Med 2011;183(8):1055–61.
179. Davis JM, Russ GA, Metlay L, et al. Short-term distribution kinetics in intratracheally administered exogenous lung surfactant. Pediatr Res 1992;31:445–50.
180. Espinosa FF, Shapiro AH, Fredberg JJ, et al. Spreading of exogenous surfactant in an airway. J Appl Physiol 1993;75:2028–39.

181. Grotberg JB, Halpern D, Jensen OE. Interaction of exogenous and endogenous surfactant: spreading-rate effects. J Appl Physiol 1995;78:750–6.
182. Davis JM, Richter SE, Kendig JW, et al. High frequency jet ventilation and surfactant treatment of newborns in severe respiratory failure. Pediatr Pulmonol 1992;13:108–12.
183. Davis JM, Notter RH. Lung surfactant replacement for neonatal pathology other than primary respiratory distress syndrome. In: Boynton B, Carlo W, Jobe A, editors. New therapies for neonatal respiratory failure: a physiologic approach. Cambridge: Cambridge University Press; 1994. p. 81–92.
184. Leach CL, Greenspan JS, Rubenstein SD, et al. Partial liquid ventilation with perflubron in premature infants with severe respiratory distress syndrome. N Engl J Med 1996;335:761–7.
185. Leach CL, Holm BA, Morin FC, et al. Partial liquid ventilation in premature lambs with respiratory distress syndrome: efficacy and compatibility with exogenous surfactant. J Pediatr 1995;126:412–20.
186. Chappell SE, Wolfson MR, Shaffer TH. A comparison of surfactant delivery with conventional mechanical ventilation and partial liquid ventilation in meconium aspiration injury. Respir Med 2001;95:612–7.
187. King DM, Wang Z, Kendig JW, et al. Concentration-dependent, temperature-dependent non-newtonian viscosity of lung surfactant dispersions. Chem Phys Lipids 2001;112:11–9.
188. King DM, Wang Z, Palmer HJ, et al. Bulk shear viscosities of endogenous and exogenous lung surfactants. Am J Physiol Lung Cell Mol Physiol 2002;282: L277–84.
189. Marks LB, Oberdoerster G, Notter RH. Generation and characterization of aerosols of dispersed surface active phospholipids by ultrasonic and jet nebulization. J Aerosol Sci 1983;14:683–94.
190. Marks LB, Notter RH, Oberdoerster G, et al. Ultrasonic and jet aerosolization of phospholipids and the effects on surface activity. Pediatr Res 1984;17:742–7.
191. Wojciak JF, Notter RH, Oberdoerster G. Size stability of phosphatidylcholine-phosphatidylglycerol aerosols and a dynamic film compression state from their interfacial impaction. J Colloid Interface Sci 1985;106:547–57.
192. Dijk PH, Heikamp A, Bambang-Oetomo S. Surfactant nebulization versus instillation during high frequency ventilation in surfactant-deficient rabbits. Pediatr Res 1998;44:699–704.
193. Ellyett KM, Broadbent RS, Fawcett ER, et al. Surfactant aerosol treatment of respiratory distress syndrome in the spontaneously breathing rabbit. Pediatr Res 1996;39:953–7.
194. Zelter M, Escudier BJ, Hoeffel JM, et al. Effects of aerosolized artificial surfactant on repeated oleic acid injury in sheep. Am Rev Respir Dis 1990;141:1014–9.
195. Ruppert C, Kuchenbuch T, Boensch M, et al. Dry powder aerosolization of a recombinant surfactant protein-C-based surfactant for inhalative treatment of the acutely inflamed lung. Crit Care Med 2010;38(7):1584–91.
196. Walmrath D, Grimminger F, Pappert D, et al. Bronchoscopic administration of bovine natural surfactant in ARDS and septic shock: impact on gas exchange and haemodynamics. Eur Respir J 2002;19:805–10.
197. Balaraman V, Meister J, Ku TL, et al. Lavage administration of dilute surfactants after acute lung injury in neonatal piglets. Am J Respir Crit Care Med 1998;158:12–7.
198. Balaraman V, Sood SL, Finn KC, et al. Physiologic response and lung distribution of lavage vs bolus Exosurf in piglets with acute lung injury. Am J Respir Crit Care Med 1996;153:1838–43.

199. Gommers D, Eijking EP, van't Veen A, et al. Bronchoalveolar lavage with a diluted surfactant suspension prior to surfactant instillation improves the effectiveness of surfactant therapy in experimental acute respiratory distress syndrome (ARDS). Intensive Care Med 1998;24:494–500.
200. van Der Beek J, Plotz F, van Overbeek F, et al. Distribution of exogenous surfactant in rabbits with severe respiratory failure: the effect of volume. Pediatr Res 1993;34:154–8.
201. Raghavendran K, Pryhuber GS, Chess PR, et al. Pharmacotherapy of acute lung injury and acute respiratory distress syndrome. Curr Med Chem 2008;15:1911–24.
202. Rossaint R, Falke KJ, Lopez F, et al. Inhaled nitric oxide for the acute respiratory distress syndrome. N Engl J Med 1993;328:399–405.
203. Gerlach H, Rossaint R, Pappert D, et al. Time-course and dose-response of nitric oxide inhalation for systemic oxygenation and pulmonary hypertension in patients with adult respiratory distress syndrome. Eur J Clin Invest 1993;23:499–502.
204. Young JD, Brampton WJ, Knighton JD, et al. Inhaled nitric oxide in acute respiratory failure in adults. Br J Anaesth 1994;73:499–502.
205. Rossaint R, Gerlach H, Schmidt-Ruhnke H, et al. Efficacy of inhaled nitric oxide in ARDS. Chest 1995;107:1107–15.
206. Fierobe L, Brunet F, Dhainaut J-F, et al. Effect of inhaled nitric oxide on right ventricular function in adult respiratory distress syndrome. Am J Respir Crit Care Med 1995;151:1414–9.
207. Dellinger RP, Zimmerman JL, Taylor RW, et al. Effects of inhaled nitric oxide in patients with acute respiratory distress syndrome: results of a randomized phase II trial. Crit Care Med 1998;26:15–23.
208. Troncy E, Collet JP, Shapiro S, et al. Inhaled nitric oxide in acute respiratory distress syndrome. A pilot randomized controlled study. Am J Respir Crit Care Med 1998;157:1483–8.
209. Michael JR, Barton RG, Saffle JR, et al. Inhaled nitric oxide versus conventional therapy: effect on oxygenation in ARDS. Am J Respir Crit Care Med 1998;157:1372–80.
210. Papazian L, Bregeon F, Gaillat F, et al. Respective and combined effect of prone position and inhaled nitric oxide in patients with acute respiratory distress syndrome. Am J Respir Crit Care Med 1998;157:580–5.
211. Jolliet P, Bulpa P, Ritz M, et al. Additive beneficial effects of the prone position, nitric oxide, and almitrine bismesylate on gas exchange and oxygen transport in acute respiratory distress syndrome. Crit Care Med 1997;25:786–94.
212. Gillart T, Bazin JE, Cosserant B, et al. Combined nitric oxide, prone positioning and almitrine infusion improve oxygenation in severe ARDS. Can J Anaesth 1998;45:402–9.
213. Payen D, Muret J, Beloucif S, et al. Inhaled nitric oxide, almitrine infusion, or their coadministration as a treatment of severe hypoxemic focal lung lesions. Anesthesiology 1998;89:1158–65.
214. Wysocki M, Roupie E, Langeron O, et al. Additive effect on gas exchange of inhaled nitric oxide and intravenous almitrine bismesylate in the adult respiratory distress syndrome. Intensive Care Med 1994;20:254–9.
215. Lu Q, Mourgeon E, Law-Koune J, et al. Dose-response curves of inhaled nitric oxide with and without intravenous almitrine in nitric oxide-responding patients with acute respiratory distress syndrome. Anesthesiology 1995;83:929–43.
216. Zwissler B, Gregor K, Habler O, et al. Inhaled prostacyclin (PGI_2) versus inhaled nitric oxide in adult respiratory distress syndrome. Am J Respir Crit Care Med 1996;154:1671–7.

217. Walmrath D, Schneider T, Schermuly R, et al. Direct comparison of inhaled nitric oxide and aerosolized prostacyclin in acute respiratory distress syndrome. Am J Respir Crit Care Med 1996;153:991–6.
218. Pappert D, Busch T, Gerlach H, et al. Aerosolized prostacyclin versus inhaled nitric oxide in children with severe acute respiratory distress syndrome. Anesthesiology 1995;82:1507–11.
219. Matthay MA, Calfee CS. Aerosolized β-adrenergic agonist therapy reduces pulmonary edema following lung surgery. Chest 2008;133:833–5.
220. Perkins GD, McAuley DF, Thickett DR, et al. The beta-agonist lung injury trial (BALTI): a randomized placebo-controlled clinical trial. Am J Respir Crit Care Med 2006;173:281–7.
221. Matthay MA, Abraham E. Beta-adrenergic agonist therapy as a potential treatment for acute lung injury. Am J Respir Crit Care Med 2006;173:254–5.
222. Bernard GR, Vincent JL, Laterre PF, et al. Efficacy and safety of recombinant human activated protein C for severe sepsis. N Engl J Med 2001;344:699–709.
223. Idell S. Anticoagulants for acute respiratory distress syndrome: can they work? Am J Respir Crit Care Med 2001;164:517–20.
224. Laterre PF, Wittebole X, Dhainaut JF. Anticoagulant therapy in acute lung injury. Crit Care Med 2003;31(Suppl):S329–36.
225. Abraham E, Wunderink R, Silverman H, et al. Efficacy and safety of monoclonal antibody to human tissue necrosis factor alpha in patients with sepsis syndrome: a randomized, controlled, double-blind, multicenter clinical trial. JAMA 1995;273:934–41.
226. Abraham E, Anzueto A, Gutierrez G, et al. Double-blind randomized controlled trial of monoclonal antibody to human tumour necrosis factor in treatment of septic shock. Lancet 1998;351:929–33.
227. Cohen J, Carlet J. INTERSEPT: an international, multicenter, placebo controlled trial of monoclonal antibody to human tumor necrosis factor-alpha in patients with sepsis. Crit Care Med 1996;24:1431–40.
228. Tracey K, Lowry S, Cerami A. Cachectin/TNF-alpha in septic shock and septic adult respiratory distress syndrome. Am Rev Respir Dis 1988;138:1377–9.
229. Fisher CJ, Slotman GJ, Opal SM, et al. Initial evaluation of human recombinant interleukin-1 receptor antagonist in the treatment of sepsis syndrome: a randomized open-label, placebo-controlled multicenter study. Crit Care Med 1994;22: 12–21.
230. Fisher CJ, Dhainaut JFA, Opal SM, et al. Recombinant human IL-1 receptor antagonist in the treatment of patients with sepsis syndrome. Results from a randomized, double blind, placebo-controlled trial. Phase III rhIL-1ra sepsis syndrome study group. JAMA 1994;271:1836–43.
231. Bernard GR, Luce JM, Sprung CL, et al. High dose corticosteroids in patients with the adult respiratory distress syndrome. N Engl J Med 1987;317:1565–70.
232. Luce JM, Montgomery AB, Marks JD, et al. Ineffectiveness of high-dose methylprednisolone in preventing parenchymal lung injury and improving mortality in patients with septic shock. Am Rev Respir Dis 1988;138:62–8.
233. Keel JB, Hauser M, Stocker R, et al. Established acute respiratory distress syndrome: benefit of corticosteroid rescue therapy. Respiration 1998;65: 258–64.
234. Hooper RG, Kearl RA. Established adult respiratory distress syndrome successfully treated with corticosteroids. South Med J 1996;89:359–64.
235. Biffl WL, Moore FA, Moore EE, et al. Are corticosteroids salvage therapy for refractory acute respiratory distress syndrome? Am J Surg 1995;170:591–5.

236. Meduri GU, Headley AS, Golden E, et al. Effect of prolonged methylprednisolone therapy in unresolving acute respiratory distress syndrome: a randomized controlled trial. JAMA 1998;280:159–65.
237. Staudinger T, Presterl E, Graninger W, et al. Influence of pentoxifylline on cytokine levels and inflammatory parameters in septic shock. Intensive Care Med 1996;22:888–93.
238. Bacher A, Mayer N, Klimscha W, et al. Effects of pentoxifylline on hemodynamics and oxygenation in septic and nonseptic patients. Crit Care Med 1997;25:795–800.
239. Staubach K-H, Schroder J, Stuber F, et al. Effect of pentoxifylline in severe sepsis. Arch Surg 1998;133:94–100.
240. Zeni F, Pain P, Vindimian M, et al. Effects of pentoxifylline on circulating cytokine concentrations and hemodynamics in patients with septic shock: results from a double-blind, randomized, placebo-controlled study. Crit Care Med 1996;24:207–14.
241. Lauterbach R, Zembala M. Pentoxifylline reduces plasma tumour necrosis factor-alpha concentration in premature infants with sepsis. Eur J Pediatr 1996;155:404–9.
242. Suter PM, Domenighetti G, Schaller M-D, et al. *N*-Acetyl-cysteine enhances recovery from acute lung injury in man, a randomized, double-blind, placebo-controlled clinical study. Chest 1994;105:190–4.
243. Jepsen S, Herlevsen P, Knudsen P, et al. Antioxidant treatment with *N*-acetylcysteine during adult respiratory distress syndrome: a prospective, randomized, placebo-controlled study. Crit Care Med 1992;20:918–23.
244. Bernard GR, Wheeler AP, Arons MM, et al. A trial of antioxidants *N*-acetylcysteine and procysteine in ARDS. Chest 1997;112:164–72.
245. Rosenfeld WN, Davis JM, Parton L, et al. Safety and pharmacokinetics of recombinant human superoxide dismutase administered intratracheally to premature neonates with respiratory distress syndrome. Pediatrics 1996;97:811–7.
246. Davis JM, Rosenfeld WN, Sanders RJ, et al. Prophylactic effects of recombinant human superoxide dismutase in neonatal lung injury. J Appl Physiol 1993;74:2234–41.
247. Lanzenberger-Schragl E, Donner A, Kashanipour A, et al. High frequency ventilation techniques in ARDS. Acta Anaesthesiol Scand Suppl 1996;109:157–61.
248. Fort P, Farmer C, Westerman J, et al. High-frequency oscillatory ventilation for adult respiratory distress syndrome–a pilot study. Crit Care Med 1997;25:937–47.
249. Mammel MC. High-frequency oscillation and partial liquid ventilation. Crit Care Med 2001;29:1293.
250. Bigatello LM, Patroniti N, Sangalli F. Permissive hypercapnia. Curr Opin Crit Care 2001;7:34–40.
251. Brower RG, Fessler HE. Mechanical ventilation in acute lung injury and acute respiratory distress syndrome. Clin Chest Med 2000;21:491–510.
252. Medoff BD, Harris RS, Kesselman H, et al. Use of recruitment maneuvers and high-positive end-expiratory pressure in a patient with acute respiratory distress syndrome. Crit Care Med 2000;28:1210–6.
253. Papadakos PJ, Lachmann B. The open lung concept of alveolar recruitment can improve outcome in respiratory failure and ARDS. Mt Sinai J Med 2002;69:73–7.
254. The Acute Respiratory Distress Syndrome Network. Ventilation with lower tidal volumes as compared with traditional tidal volumes for acute lung injury and the acute respiratory distress syndrome. N Engl J Med 2000;342:1301–8.

255. Eisner MD, Thompson T, Hudson LD, et al. Efficacy of low tidal volume ventilation in patients with different clinical risk factors for acute lung injury and the acute respiratory distress syndrome. Am J Respir Crit Care Med 2001;164:231–6.
256. Hess DR, Bigatello LM. Lung recruitment: the role of recruitment maneuvers. Respir Care 2002;47:308–17 [discussion: 317–8].
257. Mehta S, MacDonald R, Hallett DC, et al. Acute oxygenation response to inhaled nitric oxide when combined with high-frequency oscillatory ventilation in adults with acute respiratory distress syndrome. Crit Care Med 2003;31:383–9.
258. Steinbrook R. How best to ventilate? Trial design and patient safety in studies of the acute respiratory distress syndrome. N Engl J Med 2003;348:1393–401.
259. Marraro GA. Innovative practices of ventilatory support with pediatric patients. Pediatr Crit Care Med 2003;4:8–20.
260. Ward NS. Effects of prone position ventilation in ARDS. An evidence-based review of the literature. Crit Care Clin 2002;18:35–44.
261. Day RW, Guarin M, Lynch JM, et al. Inhaled nitric oxide in children with severe lung disease: results of acute and prolonged therapy with two concentrations. Crit Care Med 1996;24:215–21.
262. Abman SH, Griebel JL, Parker DK, et al. Acute effects of inhaled nitric oxide in children with severe hypoxemic respiratory failure. J Pediatr 1994;124:881–8.
263. Demirakca S, Dotsch J, Knotche C, et al. Inhaled nitric oxide in neonatal and pediatric acute respiratory distress syndrome: dose response, prolonged inhalation, and weaning. Crit Care Med 1996;24:1913–9.
264. Okamoto K, Hamaguchi M, Kukita I, et al. Efficacy of inhaled nitric oxide in children with ARDS. Chest 1998;114:827–33.
265. Goldman AP, Tasker RC, Hosiasson S, et al. Early response to inhaled nitric oxide and its relationship to outcome in children with severe hypoxemic respiratory failure. Chest 1997;112:752–8.
266. Nakagawa TA, Morris A, Gomez RJ, et al. Dose response to inhaled nitric oxide in pediatric patients with pulmonary hypertension and acute respiratory distress syndrome. J Pediatr 1997;131:63–9.
267. Karamanoukian HL, Glick PL, Wilcox DL, et al. Pathophysiology of congenital diaphragmatic hernia VII: inhaled nitric oxide requires exogenous surfactant therapy in the lamb model of CDH. J Pediatr Surg 1995;30:1–4.
268. Rais-Bahrami K, Rivera O, Seale W, et al. Effect of nitric oxide in meconium aspiration syndrome after treatment with surfactant. Crit Care Med 1997;25:1744–7.
269. Gommers D, Hartog A, van't Veen A, et al. Improved oxygenation by nitric oxide is enhanced by prior lung reaeration with surfactant, rather than positive end-expiratory pressure, in lung-lavaged rabbits. Crit Care Med 1997;25:1868–73.
270. Zhu GF, Sun B, Niu S, et al. Combined surfactant therapy and inhaled nitric oxide in rabbits with oleic acid-induced acute respiratory distress syndrome. Am J Respir Crit Care Med 1998;158:437–43.
271. Hartog A, Gommers D, van't Veen A, et al. Exogenous surfactant and nitric oxide have a synergistic effect in improving gas exchange in experimental ARDS. Adv Exp Med Biol 1997;428:277–9.
272. Warnecke G, Struber M, Fraud S, et al. Combined exogenous surfactant and inhaled nitric oxide therapy for lung ischemia-reperfusion injury in minipigs. Transplantation 2001;71:1238–44.
273. Zheng S, Zhang WY, Zhu LW, et al. Surfactant and inhaled nitric oxide in rats alleviate acute lung injury induced by intestinal ischemia and reperfusion. J Pediatr Surg 2001;36:980–4.

274. Sokol GM, Fineberg NS, Wright LL, et al. Changes in arterial oxygen tension when weaning neonates from inhaled nitric oxide. Pediatr Pulmonol 2001;32:14–9.
275. Uy IP, Pryhuber GS, Chess PR, et al. Combined-modality therapy with inhaled nitric oxide and exogenous surfactant in term infants with acute respiratory failure. Pediatr Crit Care Med 2000;1:107–10.
276. Hintz SR, Suttner DM, Sheehan AM, et al. Decreased use of neonatal extracorporeal membrane oxygenation (ECMO): how new treatment modalities have affected ECMO utilization. Pediatrics 2000;106:1339–43.
277. Okamoto K, Kukita I, Hamaguchi M, et al. Combined effects of inhaled nitric oxide and positive end-expiratory pressure during mechanical ventilation in acute respiratory distress syndrome. Artif Organs 2000;24:390–5.
278. Borelli M, Lampati L, Vascotto E, et al. Hemodynamic and gas exchange response to inhaled nitric oxide and prone positioning in acute respiratory distress syndrome patients. Crit Care Med 2000;28:2707–12.
279. Kendig JW, Notter RH, Cox C, et al. A comparison of surfactant as immediate prophylaxis and as rescue therapy in newborns of less than 30 weeks gestation. N Engl J Med 1991;324:865–71.
280. Willson DF, Chess PR, Notter RH. Surfactant for pediatric acute lung injury. Pediatr Clin North Am 2008;55:545–75.
281. Chess P, Finkelstein JN, Holm BA, et al. Surfactant replacement therapy in lung injury. In: Notter RH, Finkelstein JN, Holm BA, editors. Lung injury: mechanisms, pathophysiology, and therapy. Boca Raton (FL): Taylor & Francis; 2005. p. 617–63.
282. Amital A, Shitrit D, Raviv Y, et al. The use of surfactant in lung transplantation. Transplantation 2008;86:1554–9.

Inhaled Nitric Oxide and Inhaled Prostacyclin in Acute Respiratory Distress Syndrome: What is the Evidence?

Nitin Puri, MD[a,*], Richard Phillip Dellinger, MD, FCCP[b]

KEYWORDS

- Acute respiratory distress syndrome • Inhaled nitric oxide
- Inhaled prostacyclin

The mortality for acute respiratory distress syndrome (ARDS) remains unacceptably high, between 40% and 50%.[1,2] The syndrome is characterized by hypoxemia secondary to increased alveolar capillary permeability and proteinaceous extravascular lung water. Increased pulmonary artery pressures are postulated as due to subclinical microthrombi and secondary inflammatory reactions.[3] Increased pulmonary vascular resistance (PVR) in patients with acute lung injury (ALI) is independently associated with increased mortality.[4] In normal adult lungs, parenchymal shunt is usually less than 5%, whereas in the most extreme ARDS patients, the shunt fraction can be greater than 50%.[5] Inhaled vasodilators can help reverse both these physiologic dysfunctions by improving ventilation-perfusion mismatch and decreasing PVR. Use of inhaled vasodilators in ARDS has been the subject of an extensive amount of research over the past two decades. Two vasodilators, inhaled prostacyclin (IP) and inhaled nitric oxide (iNO), are reviewed in this article, albeit the bulk of the literature concerns iNO.

The authors gratefully acknowledge receiving Consulting fee and research support (materials alone) from Ikaria.

[a] Division of Pulmonary and Critical Care Medicine, Department of Medicine, Cooper University Hospital, Robert Wood Johnson Medical School, Camden, NJ 08103, USA
[b] Division of Critical Care Medicine, Department of Medicine, Cooper University Hospital, 1 Cooper Plaza, Camden, NJ 08103, USA
* Corresponding author.
E-mail address: puri-nitin@cooperhealth.edu

Crit Care Clin 27 (2011) 561–587
doi:10.1016/j.ccc.2011.05.001 **criticalcare.theclinics.com**
0749-0704/11/$ – see front matter

INHALED NITRIC OXIDE

Biology of Inhaled Nitric Oxide

The role nitric oxide (NO) plays in the human body continues to be defined. Before 1987, NO was considered a mere toxic pollutant associated with cigarette smoke and the burning of fossil fuels. The importance of this gas changed dramatically when it was discovered to be an endothelial-derived relaxing factor vital in maintaining cellular homeostasis.[6] Over the past 20 years, understanding of NO and its utility in the critically ill has expanded exponentially.

NO is a colorless gas with an unpaired electron that makes it prone to forming complexes to enhance stability.[7] It is created by the enzyme, NO synthase (NOS), which comes from neuronal, inducible (macrophages) and endothelial sources. Endothelial NOS provides the primary reservoir of NO in the pulmonary vasculature. NOS facilitates a chemical reaction between the amino acid L-arginine, oxygen, and nicotinamide adenine dinucleotide phosphate hydrogen (NADPH) to create NO in the endothelium. NO activates the enzyme guanylate cyclase in the vascular smooth muscle to create cyclic guanosine monophosphate GMP (cGMP) from guanosine triphosphate. cGMP activates cGMP-dependent protein kinase, which leads to a series of reactions that cause smooth muscle relaxation and vascular dilitation (**Fig. 1**).[8] NO enters the body through inhalation and it is engages in 1 of 3 predominant reactions (**Fig. 2**).[9]

1. NO reacts with oxyhemoglobin in the pulmonary circulation to create methemoglobin. Methemoglobin is reduced to ferrous hemoglobin and nitrate by NADPH-methemoglobin reductase from erythrocytes.[8] This reaction is thought to form the basis for iNO use in ARDS.[10] iNO only flows into the well-ventilated regions of the lung, due to its rapid transformation by oxyhemeglobin. This allows iNO to cause selective smooth muscle relaxation by the cGMP mechanism (described previously). This smooth muscle relaxation leads to selective vasodilatation of the pulmonary vasculature in well-aerated regions of the lung, which theoretically improves shunt in ARDS.[11]
2. NO reacts with oxygen in the blood to form the toxic molecule, nitrogen dioxide (NO_2).
3. NO reacts with plasma proteins to form *S*-nitrosothiols. *S*-nitrosothiols are proteins with sulfur groups that store NO and have vasodilatory properties to relieve hypoxic vasoconstriction in the pulmonary circulation. A greater understanding of these proteins has led to the trials of ethyl nitrate to lower PVR in porcine models.[12]

Immunologic Effects

Whether iNO has a predominant pro-inflammatory or anti-inflammatory effect on lung tissue is debated. Neutrophils are known mediators of ALI, and NO has been shown to down-regulate neutrophil function.[13] iNO similarly diminishes the procoagulant process in lung injury. Yet NO byproducts can cause surfactant dysfunction and toxic oxidative damage that could contribute to lung injury.[9]

The Justification for Clinical Trials Using Inhaled Nitric Oxide

In 1991, researchers showed that iNO could relieve hypoxic vasoconstriction in the pulmonary vasculature of lambs with induced pulmonary hypertension (by breathing stable thromboxane endoperoxide analog or a hypoxic gas mixture) without clinically significant systemic vasodilitation.[11] This was in contrast to intravenous (IV) nitroglycerin and IV nitroprusside, which had previously been demonstrated to relieve pulmonary vasoconstriction but lowered mean arterial pressure (MAP). iNO was shown to

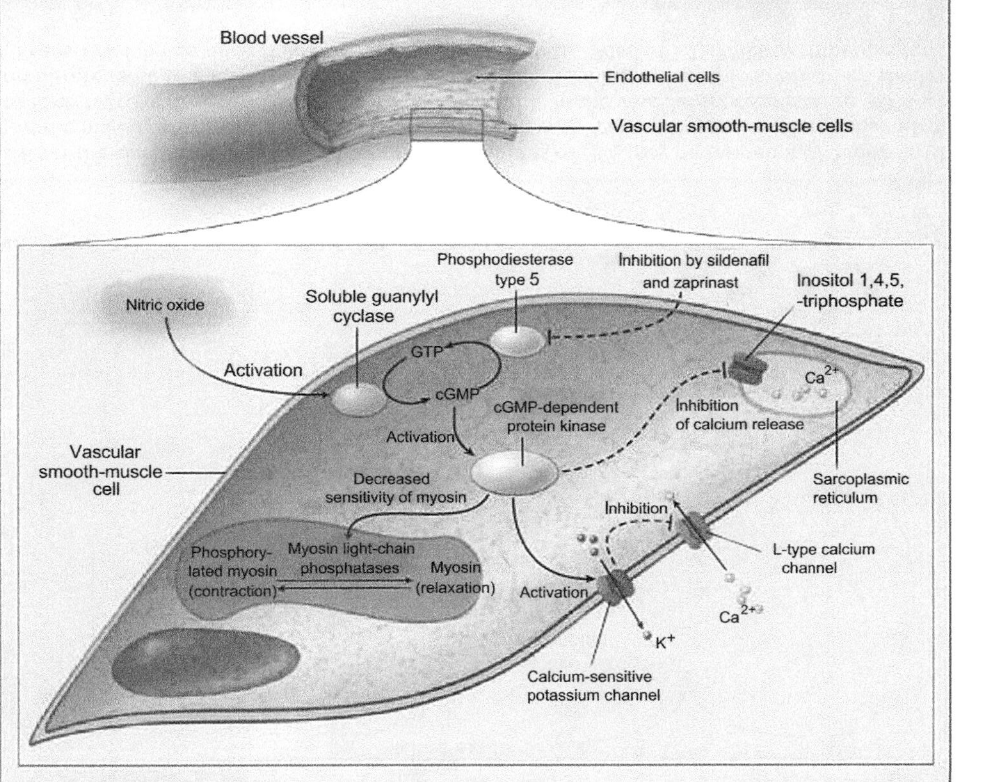

Fig. 1. Regulation of the relaxation of vascular smooth muscle by NO. NO activates soluble guanylyl cyclase, leading to the activation of cGMP-dependent protein kinase), which, in turn, decreases the sensitivity of myosin to calcium-induced contraction and lowers the intracellular calcium concentration by activating calcium-sensitive potassium channels and inhibiting the release of calcium from the sarcoplasmic reticulum. cGMP is degraded by phosphodiesterase type 5, which is inhibited by sildenafil and zaprinast. GTP denotes guanosine triphosphate. (*From* Griffiths MJ, Evans TW. Inhaled nitric oxide therapy in adults. N Engl J Med 353;25:2683; with permission.)

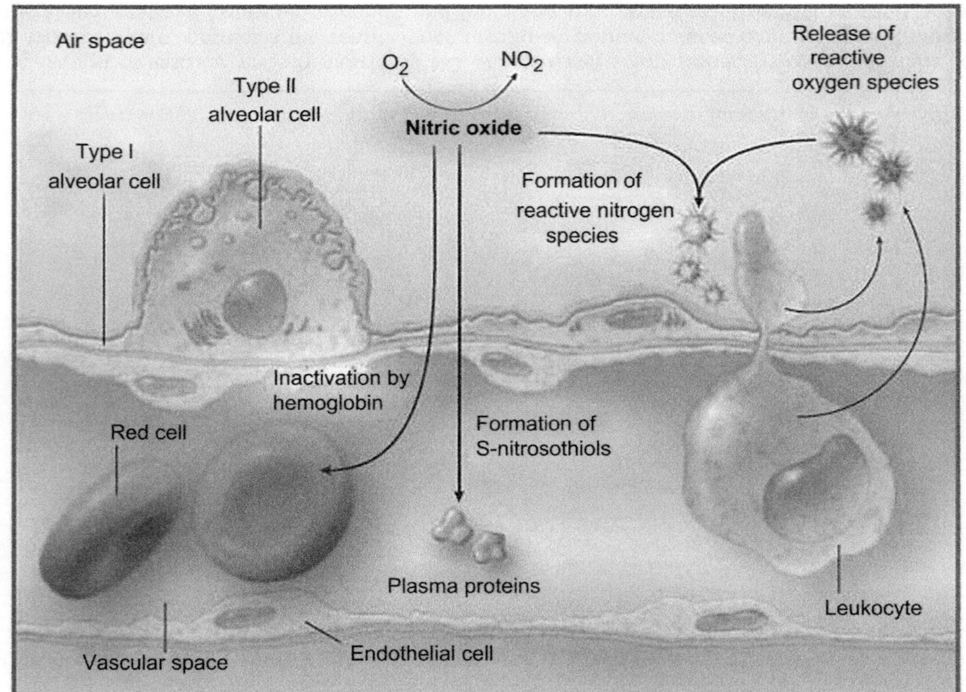

Fig. 2. Biochemical fates of iNO at the alveolar-capillary membrane. Small amounts of NO_2 may be formed if iNO mixes with high concentrations of O_2 in the air space. Depending on the milieu of the lung parenchyma, NO may react with reactive oxygen species (derived from activated leukocytes or is chemia–reperfusion injury) to form reactive nitrogen species, such as peroxynitrite. In the vascular space, dissolved NO is scavenged by oxyhemoglobin (forming methemoglobin and nitrate) and, to a lesser extent, plasma proteins (eg, forming nitrosothiols, which are stable intravascular sources of NO activity). (*From* Griffiths MJ, Evans TW. Inhaled nitric oxide therapy in adults. N Engl J Med 353;25:2683; with permission.)

decrease PVR and pulmonary arterial pressure (PAP) without causing a significant increase in NO_2.[14] In patients with primary pulmonary hypertension, iNO decreased pulmonary arterial pressures similarly to IV prostacyclin. Rossaint and colleagues[15] performed the first trial in ARDS patients on the effects of iNO and IV prostacyclin. Ten consecutive patients with ARDS received both iNO and IV prostacyclin. Both decreased the PAP, but only IV prostacyclin decreased patient's MAP. This was due to IV prostacyclin decreasing systemic vascular resistance (SVR), unlike iNO, which had no clinically significant effect on SVR. iNO and IV prostacyclin both decreased PVR, but only INO improved hypoxia as reflected by increased arterial partial pressure of oxygen to fraction of inspired oxygen ratio (Pao_2/Fio_2). It was hypothesized that iNO increased blood flow to regions of the lung with greater ventilation and distributed it away from areas of poor ventilation. IV prostacyclin worsened hypoxia reflected by decreased Pao_2/Fio_2 ratio. Roissaint tested both an 18 and 36 parts per million (ppm) doses of iNO but did not find significant differences between the 2 doses. The amount of iNO given to patients was substantially more than the amount of NO produced in humans lungs, which is only 8 parts per billion (ppb), approximately 2000 times less than the study dose.[16] Despite the significant limitations of the study, including the small number of patients, the use of extracorpeal life support, and the heterogeneous causes of ARDS, it lent credence to the vasodilatory properties of iNO and the safety of iNO in patients with ARDS. Their findings helped justify the argument for more human clinical trials using iNO to treat ARDS.

iNO in the 1990s

The hope of the beneficial effects of iNO in treating ARDS is reflected by the number of studies examining its use in the 1990s. The trials had significant limitations, including small numbers of subjects, heterogeneous patient populations, different delivery methods of iNO, lack of homogeneity in treatment of ARDS, and crossover design. These limiting factors made extrapolating any significant insight about iNO difficult. The trials did expand knowledge about iNO and more importantly helped shape the later randomized controlled trials. Four questions were addressed in a majority of these trials.

1. What dose was iNO most effective?
2. Are there clinically significant hemodynamic effects of iNO?
3. Are particular patient groups resistant to effects of iNO?
4. Is iNO safe?

The ideal dose for iNO in ARDS was the subject of 5 trials. Gerlach and colleagues[17] studied 12 patients with severe ARDS, in an attempt to determine this dose. iNO increased patient's oxygenation; a plateau was observed at 10 ppm. This was dissimilar to its linear affect on mean PAP (MPAP), which continued to decrease with progressive increases in doses of iNO. Patients had a quick physiologic response, within 3 minutes, to iNO as both oxygenation and MPAP were lowered. Gerlach and colleagues concluded that iNO worked in a dose-responsive manner and its effects on oxygenation were independent from its effects on MPAP. Puybasset and colleagues[18] studied the use of low dose iNO (doses 0.1 to 5 ppm) in 6 critically ill patients. These patients were known responders to iNO at 10 ppm. Four of the 6 patients had linear improvements in oxygenation and MPAP with increased doses of iNO. This study lent credibility to the dose-dependant theory of iNO and the effectiveness of even smaller doses of iNO. These results were in contrast to 2 other small trials, which showed that iNO had a curvilinear response in ARDS patients.[19,20] The conflicting results from these studies made it difficult to draw conclusions about the ideal dose of iNO in ARDS.

McIntyre and colleagues[21] performed iNO trials in 14 surgical patients with ARDS and MPAP greater than 30 mm Hg. They used iNO at variable doses (20 ppm and 40 ppm) and both caused significant decreases in MPAP. In contrast, a study ALI patients with MPAP less than 30 mm Hg treated with iNO showed minimal decrease in MPAP.[22] It was hypothesized that patients with greater degree of pulmonary hypertension in the presence of ARDS were more likely to respond to iNO.[23] Even among patients with severe pulmonary hypertension, however, response to iNO was not uniform.

In a prospective trial of 27 patients, researchers tried to quantify either structural (CT scan appearance), inflammatory (bronchial alveolar lavage results), oxygenation (Pao_2/Fio_2 ratio), and vasculopathy (PVR) as predisposing factors to response to iNO.[24] They were unable to identify any reliable and reproducible correlations. From previous research, septic shock patients were postulated as resistant to iNO due to pulmonary vasculature under the influence of endogenous and exogenous catecholamine vasopressors.[25] This hypothesis was explored by Kraft and colleagues,[26] who studied 25 consecutive patients with septic shock and ARDS. Responders to iNO therapy were those who had an increase in arterial oxygenation of 20% or a decrease in the MPAP by 15%. They tested 18 and 36 PPPM doses of iNO. Ten of the 25 patients were classified as responders and these patients had lower overall mortality. This study supported the hypothesis that patients with ARDS who had septic shock were less likely to respond to iNO therapy. Manktelow and colleagues[27] further explored this question when they reviewed 88 ARDS patients who received iNO. Overall there was a 58% response rate to iNO, but only 33% patients with septic shock responded to iNO. Patients with fewer than 7 days of respiratory failure had a relatively significant ($P<.06$) clinical response defined as 20% improvement in Pao_2/Fio_2 and/or 20% decrease PVR.

Randomized Controlled Trials of Inhaled Nitric Oxide in Acute Respiratory Distress Syndrome

Two single-center, randomized controlled trials were published in 1998. Michael and colleagues[28] randomized 40 patients with ARDS to either conventional therapy or 5 to 20 ppm iNO plus conventional therapy to examine the primary endpoint of an improvement in oxygenation at 72 hours. Improvement in oxygenation was defined as a decrease in the Fio_2 by 0.15 (or 15%). The iNO dose was determined by an attending physician with a suggested starting dose at 5 ppm. At 1, 12, and 24 hours, the iNO group had statistically significant improvement in their Pao_2/Fio_2 ratio, but this finding did not persist. At 72 hours, there was no significant difference in Pao_2, Fio_2, and Pao_2/Fio_2 ratio. Sepsis had no effect on the Pao_2/Fio_2ratio response to iNO in this trial. Troncy and colleagues[29] randomized 30 ARDS patients to determine the efficacy of iNO on lung function and its impact on morbidity and mortality. Their primary endpoint was extubation prior to 30 days. The dose of iNO varied between 2.5 and 40 ppm with an increase in iNO mandated by protocol if a 5% increase in Pao_2 occurred in 10 minutes with a higher iNO dose. iNO could be restarted if a patient's pulmonary status declined as defined by a Fio_2 greater than 0.4, a positive end-expiratory pressure (PEEP) greater than 10 mm Hg, or Pao_2 less than 60 mm Hg. The iNO group had a higher Acute Physiology and Chronic Health Evaluation (APACHE) II score (27.4 vs 23.2) and lower Pao_2/Fio_2 ratios (119 $\pm$ 13.6 vs 152 $\pm$ 18.5). Initially, Pao_2 increased (statistically significantly) in the iNO group, but the 30-day mortality and days of mechanical ventilation were not significantly different between groups. Twenty-five patients were septic and 5 had direct lung injury–induced ARDS. Again, iNO improved oxygenation in the short term but over an extended period of time did not affect mortality or length of mechanical ventilation. One encouraging sign was noted as survivors who were treated with iNO had a 20% reduction in length of mechanical ventilation versus the control group (10.8 ± 1.2 vs 12.8 ± 4.2). The investigators suggested the utility of iNO might be proved if future studies changed their focus. They recommended treating ARDS patients earlier in their course, limiting the patient population to direct lung injury–induced ARDS patients, and using only patients who were responsive to iNO therapy. Both of these studies had similar limitations, including the variable treatment doses of iNO, small patient populations, the lack of blinding of investigators, and the lack of a placebo gas. Both studies showed iNO increased oxygenation immediately but did not effect long-term outcome defined by mortality and Pao_2/Fio_2 ratio.[23,28,29]

The third trial, from 1998, was a phase II, randomized controlled multicenter trial, which recruited patients from 30 academic centers.[30] This phase II trial recruited 177 patients and randomized them to at varying iNO doses (1.25 ppm, 5 ppm, 20 ppm, 40 ppm, and 80 ppm) or nitrogen gas. The primary endpoints examined were the dose effects of iNO on mortality, the number of days alive and ventilator-free, and days alive after meeting oxygenation criteria for extubation. A response to iNO was defined as a greater than 20% increase in Pao_2. The placebo group had 57 patients and the pooled iNO group had 120 patients. The iNO groups had between 22 and 34 patients except for the 80 ppm group, which had 8 patients due to that dose deemed unnecessarily high by an international consensus conference after the trial was begun.[31] Patients were allowed into the trial if they met American-European Consensus Conference (AECC) definition of ARDS within the prior 72 hours, had a pulmonary source of infection causing ARDS, were not immune compromised, and had no vasopressor requirements. After the initiation of iNO, clinicians could not change ventilator settings for 4 hours. This novel element of the study allowed for evaluation of the true effect of iNO without obfuscation of results by ventilator manipulation. Sixty percent of patients responded in the pooled iNO group, but 24% also responded in the placebo group. After 24 hours, the Fio_2 used was lower in the pooled iNO group than the placebo group, but by day 2 this effect disappeared. The mortality rate for the placebo and pooled iNO group were both 30%. A post hoc analysis suggested potential benefit of the 5-ppm group showing a percentage of patients alive and free of mechanical ventilation compared with the placebo group. The phase II part of this trial was important because it was the largest performed to date and it was well designed. This multicenter study had strong design, including the standard use of ventilator practices, the standardization of iNO delivery, and strict inclusion criteria. Although the quality of the study was better, the results were not significantly different from the single center trials. This analysis was the basis for the phase III trial by the same group.

Two multicenter randomized trials from Europe were published in 1999. A multicenter randomized trial from France (only published in abstract form) demonstrated that iNO improved oxygenation but did not affect clinical outcomes.[32] Lundin and colleagues[33] performed a multicenter, randomized controlled trial in Europe. Their study tested whether 268 patients with ALI treated with titratable doses of iNO (1–40 ppm) at baseline would have an increased reversal of ALI. The secondary endpoints examined were the frequency of development of severe respiratory failure ($Fio_2 > 0.9$ and $Pao_2 < 8$ kPa in 3 blood gas analyses 4 hours apart, PEEP >10 mm Hg), mortality at 30 and 90 days, and time to reversal of ALI. The primary importance of their work was their separation of iNO responders from nonresponders. Patient response to iNO was tested at doses of 1 ppm, 20 ppm, and 40 ppm and if they did not have an acute increase in oxygenation or decrease in MPAP they entered the nonresponder group. One hundred and eighty responders were randomized to iNO plus conventional therapy versus conventional therapy alone. Outcomes in responders were compared with nonresponders. There was no significant difference in frequency of reversal of ALI, mortality at 30 or 90 days, and the time to reversal of ALI. The iNO group had less severe respiratory failure events, however, than the conventional treatment group (2 vs 9). A post hoc analysis suggested the conventional treatment group had more days alive and free of mechanical ventilation than the iNO treatment group. The investigators attributed this to a non–statistically significant increase in mortality in the intervention group. iNO patients developed renal dysfunction significantly more ($P<.025$) and had renal replacement therapy initiated more frequently even though it was by individual provider discretion. This study dispelled the theory that nonresponders caused previous trials to be negative. It also raised the question of a link between iNO and renal dysfunction. Other randomized trials of iNO in ARDS have not shown this finding.

A meta-analysis in 2003 analyzed the 5 randomized controlled trials available and determined iNO had no effect on mortality or ventilator-free days.[34] The validity of the meta-analysis was questioned for a multitude of reasons but further making results uninterpretable were the wide CIs. Metaanalysis did provide further impetus for researchers to discover why iNO was not working in ARDS patients. Gerlach and colleagues[35] attempted to answer this question by building on their previous work on dose-response curves. They randomized 40 patients with severe ARDS to a conventional therapy group or a conventional therapy plus iNO 10-ppm treatment group for 4 days. The primary endpoint for this study was the effect of iNO on Pa_{O_2}/F_{IO_2} ratio and MPAP. In actuality, their primary interest was subjects' response to iNO with repeated dose-responsive curves. The trial's secondary endpoints results were similar to previous trials with a reduction in use of extracorporeal membrane oxygenation in the iNO group and no difference in length of mechanical ventilation. Patients on initial treatment with iNO improved their oxygenation significantly. The subjects also became responsive to lower doses of iNO therapy over time (96 hours), offering an explanation to previous negative trials. Prior randomized control trials did perform daily dose-response curves and possibly used excessive doses of iNO in ARDS patients.

Unfortunately, this trial was not available to Taylor and colleagues[36] when they were recruiting for the phase III part of their study on iNO in ARDS patients. They recruited patients from 43 hospitals in the United States and randomized 385 patients to receive either conventional therapy or conventional therapy plus iNO at 5PPM. Strict eligibility criteria were used in this phase, similar to their previous phase II trial.[31] The primary endpoint assessed was days alive without the need for mechanical ventilation through day 28. Secondary endpoints were being alive and meeting extubation criteria, days alive after a successful unassisted ventilation test, and mortality. The 2 study groups were statistically equal except the iNO group had a higher MPAP. There was no difference in the primary or secondary endpoints. There was no difference in renal disease, but the iNO group had a higher incidence of nosocomial infections. The editorial accompanying the study opined that iNO be regulated to salvage therapy only for ARDS.[37] A follow-up on study patients done at hospital discharge and at 1 year showed no difference in mortality or quality of life between groups.[38] The major contribution this study provided to understanding of iNO was that a fixed dose of 5 ppm did not show clinical benefit and it crystallized the need for a randomized control trial that used dose-response curves. **Table 1** summarizes the data from randomized controlled trials in ARDS.

Inhaled Nitric Oxide Added to Adjunctive Therapies in Acute Respiratory Distress Syndrome

Positive end-expiratory pressure, recruitment, prone positioning, and high-frequency oscillatory ventilation

Researchers theorized if iNO improved perfusion and ventilation to well-aerated regions of the lung in ARDS, then using maneuvers to open atelectatic alveoli in ARDS might improve the utility of iNO. These hypotheses have been tested in multiple trials using PEEP, prone positioning, and alternative modes of ventilation. The use of PEEP plus iNO improved shunt fraction and oxygenation in canines [39] Puybasset and colleagues[40] followed this with a prospective trial of PEEP and iNO in human ALI patients. Using CT scans of the lungs they showed an association between PEEP induced recruitment and response to iNO. This theory was further tested in 9 trauma patients with ARDS whose oxygenation did not improve with iNO.[41] Researchers added PEEP, which optimized patient's compliance and improved their Pao_2/Fio_2 ratio. Adding iNO created a further improvement in Pao_2/Fio_2. Furthermore, 6 of 9 patients responded to the use of PEEP and became responsive to iNO, converting them from nonresponders to responders.

Patients refractory to conventional modes of ventilation may be subjected to prone positioning to increase oxygenation based the reversal of gravitation forces.[42] Several studies looking at the additive effects of prone positioning and iNO were done between 1998 and 2001. Papazian and colleagues[43] showed that both iNO and prone positioning increased the Pao_2/Fio_2 ratio in ARDS but did not have a synergistic effect. A retrospective review of the short-term oxygenation effects of iNO versus prone positioning concluded both prone positioning and iNO increased Pao_2/Fio_2 ratio, but prone positioning improved hypoxemia more substantially.[44] The study was fraught with design flaws, including its retrospective nature and selection bias. It was impossible to draw definitive conclusions about the superiority of either therapy. Johannigman and colleagues[45] prospectively studied 16 ARDS trauma patients recruited over 2 years and treated with prone positioning and iNO at 1 ppm. Oxygenation increased with both prone positioning and iNO. The effects of combining the two methods were additive on Pao_2/Fio_2 ratio and increased the number of responders to iNO therapy. Patients who responded to iNO had decreases in their PVR. The study was limited by its small sample size but offered the hypothesis that prone positioning and iNO could be synergistic if used together. No randomized controlled trial exists to test this theory and is unlikely to be done due to difficulty in trial design.[46,47] Another postulated mechanism to open atelectatic alveoli to improve oxygenation in ARDS is the recruitment maneuver (RM). The RM has a multitude of variations, but Park and colleagues[48] used 30 mm Hg for 30 to 35 seconds in ARDS patients combined with iNO to see if the combination of therapies would improve oxygenation. In their prospective trial, they enrolled 23 patients with ARDS and divided them into 3 groups: RM group, iNO group plus RM group, and iNO alone group. The RM converted 3 nonresponding iNO patients into responders, but the Pao_2/Fio_2 in the combined therapy group was not statistically different. Again, it is difficult to draw conclusions from this trial due to its small size and design flaws, including not increasing PEEP after the RM maneuver. RM changed 3 patients not responsive to iNO to responders.

A similar physiologic principle has been demonstrated by those who have used high-frequency oscillatory ventilation (HFOV) in ARDS to recruit atelectatic alveoli. Using iNO plus HFOV in animals significantly improved oxygenation in an ARDS

Table 1
Randomized controlled trials of iNO use in adults in acute respiratory distress syndrome

Study	Year	Number of Patients/ Center	Patient Details	Control	Dose of Inhaled Nitric Oxide	Primary Outcome Measured	Results	Comments
Michael et al[28]	1998	40/1	ARDS with PFR <150 and chest radiograph with infiltrates	Usual care	5, 10, 15, and 20 ppm every 6 h for 24 h, then clinically adjusted	Oxygenation improvement to allow decrease in F_{IO_2}	No improvement in oxygenation at 72 h	Improvement oxygenation 1, 12, and 24 h, but not at 72 h; significant study design limitations
Troncy et al[29]	1998	30/1	Lung injury score >2.5	Usual care	Initial titration (2.5, 5, 10, 20, 30, and 40 ppm every 10 minutes) daily retitration	Extubation before 30 days	No difference in length of MV	Improved oxygenation in the short term; significant study design limitations
Dellinger et al[30]	1998	177/30	AECC ARDS within 72 h, excluded severe sepsis or nonpulmonary organ failure	Nitrogen	1.25–80 ppm	Dose effect on mortality, days alive and ventilator-free, days alive after meeting oxygen criteria for extubation	No significant differences between control and intervention groups	Strong study design, standard ventilator practices, standard iNO delivery and strict inclusion criteria
Payen et al[32]	1999	203/23	AECC ARDS	Nitrogen	10 ppm	Weaning from MV	No improvement	Published only in abstract form

Lundin et al[33]	1999	268/43	Chest radiograph infiltrates and ARDS with PFR <165 mm Hg with MV for 18 to 96 h	Usual care	2,10, or 40 ppm (lowest effective dose)	Reversal of ALI	No significant difference in reversal of ALI	Study dispelled theory of nonresponders causing iNO trials to be negative. An association between iNO treatment and renal dysfunction in post hoc subset analysis
Gerlach et al[35]	2003	40/1	AECC ARDS, F_{IO_2} $\geq$0.6, PFR $\leq$150, PEEP $\geq$10 cm H_2O, PAOP $\leq$18 mm Hg, duration of MV <48 h	Usual care	10 ppm (with daily dose-response analysis)	iNO effect on Pa_{O_2}/F_{IO_2} ratio and MPAP	No significant effect on oxygenation or MPAP	Patients became responsive to lower doses of iNO over time; showed importance of daily dose response curves
Park et al[48]	2003	23/1	AECC and duration of ARDS $\leq$2 days	Usual care	5 ppm $\pm$ recruitment maneuvers	Oxygenation	No improvement	RM may improve response to iNO; study with significant design limitations
Taylor et al[36]	2004	385/46	ARDS with PFR <250, excluded sepsis cause ALI and any nonpulmonary organ failure	Nitrogen	5 ppm in the intervention group (192 patients)	Survival without needs for MV during the first 28 days	No difference between groups	Well-designed study, showed need for dose response curve trial in ARDS

Abbreviations: MV, mechanical ventilation; PAOP, pulmonary arterial occlusion pressure; PFR, Pa_{O_2}/F_{IO_2} ratio.

Data from Creagh-Brown BC, Griffiths MJ, Evans TW. Bench-to-bedside review: inhaled nitric oxide therapy in adults. Crit Care 2009;212:1–8.

model.[49] In another trial, neonates seemed to have responded to this combination therapy, too.[50] Mehta and colleagues[51] performed an observational, unblinded trial on 23 ARDS patients who had failed conventional and HFOV ventilation. They added iNO to HFOV as a rescue therapy and 83% patients responded with an increase in Pao_2/Fio_2 (≥20%). These trials using PEEP, RM, prone positioning, and HFOV are hypothesis generating, but prospective trials are needed to truly evaluate if combination therapy with iNO is indicated.

Delivery of Inhaled Nitric Oxide

Ambient iNO has been reported as a contaminant in compressed hospital air and its effect on critically ill patients has never been determined.[52] This fact added to the scientist's inability to determine the exact dose of iNO given in research studies has always troubled iNO trials.[53] Delivery methods have changed dramatically and eventually the INOvent trademark (INO Therapeutics LLC) was proved a reliable method of delivery.[54] It delivers a constant preset amount of iNO with different modes of ventilation. It also produces low concentrations of NO_2.[51] In 1999, the Food and Drug Administration approved iNO to treat persistent pulmonary hypertension and hypoxia in term or near-term infants (>34 weeks), which led to the standardization of delivery of iNO to all patients.[55] This standardization included the off-label use of the gas to treat ARDS with the INOMAX system (Ikaria), formerly INOvent). GeNO LLC is developing alternative methods of iNO delivery, which could broaden the use of iNO in the critically ill.[56]

Cost

The price of iNO has been anything but consistent. Before being Food and Drug Administration approved, iNO was a relatively cheap option for hypoxemia in ARDS. This patent was sold to the industry and the price went up from approximately $2 per hour to $125 per hour in the United Kingdom.[57] The expense of iNO ($3000 daily with a 96-hour price limit of $12,000 in the United States) allowed the proliferation of aerosolized prostacylins ($275 daily) in treatment of ARDS and other causes of pulmonary hypertension.[58] In the United States, iNO is now sold in bulk to hospitals through a multitier pricing system, which has reduced the cost. Unless allotted usage of iNO is exceeded, then iNO is billed hourly (Kathy Lofland, RRT, personal communication, 2011).

Safety and Rebound Phenomenon

The safety of using iNO in ARDS patients has been monitored since the beginning of its use. The standardization of delivery has made concerns about accidental overdoses negligible. A few definitive conclusions can be drawn from the 20 years of research. It should not be used in patients with methemoglobin reductase deficiency because patients may develop unsafe levels of methemoglobinemia.[8] Patients without this deficiency have a low risk of developing methemoglobinemia at recommended doses.[59] Twelve trials were part of a meta-analysis of the use of iNO in ARDS patients and no increased risk of methemoglobinemia (>5%) was found.[60]

Taylor and colleagues[36] had 3 patients with increased NO_2 levels only in the group that received 80 ppm iNO, but otherwise no significant risk of NO_2 toxicity has been demonstrated. The concern about iNO inducing renal dysfunction was only shown in one study.[33] A Cochrane meta-analysis combined analysis of this study and 3 others with low risk of bias and showed the risk of renal dysfunction is not significantly increased ($P = .23$).[61] This same meta-analysis found no increased risk of bleeding in the 5 trials reviewed. The risks of using iNO in ARDS seems minimal, but due to lack of understanding of the pathogenesis of ARDS, unforeseen risks may exist.

Inhaled Nitric Oxide Rebound Phenomenon

One documented risk has been rebound pulmonary hypertension in patients weaned too quickly from iNO.[62] This phenomenon was described in infants after corrective heart surgery who were treated with iNO for pulmonary hypertension and subsequently took 28 hours to be weaned from the gas.[63] The rebound phenomenon generally occurs when patients have been on the gas for greater than 6 hours. Down-regulation of endothelial NOS was previously thought to be the cause of this phenomenon, but now it is understood that endothelial NOS is reversibly inhibited by iNO.[64]

Why Inhaled Nitric Oxide Does Not Decrease Mortality in Acute Respiratory Distress Syndrome

There are many reasons that iNO has not has not decreased mortality in ARDS. The primary reason is likely that mortality from ARDS secondary to hypoxemia is rare.[59] Multiorgan dysfunction is a more common cause of death in ARDS patients. The temporary increase in oxygenation caused by iNO is likely less important than its effects on PVR.[4] Extensive research has been done on iNO in ARDS, but perhaps scientists have not been asking the right questions. The large randomized controlled trials have not used dose-response curves to define treatment doses creating a possible bias in studies and similarly exposing patients to the ill effects of too much iNO.[35] More trials on iNO in ARDS need to be done to understand its effect on mortality.

Summary of Inhaled Nitric Oxide Use in Acute Respiratory Distress Syndrome

Over the past 20 years, iNO has gone from being a toxic pollutant to one of the most studied gases in critical care medicine. Initial studies showed tremendous promise in helping ARDS patients, but randomized controlled trials have not borne significant improvements in outcome. The results are summarized in a recent review by the Cochrane collaborators (**Figs. 3** and **4**).[61] Researchers know more about iNO and its dosing mechanisms, which perhaps will allow them to ask the appropriate questions to find its utility in ARDS. It remains a safe option for salvage therapy in ARDS patients with refractory hypoxemia, until those questions can be answered.

INHALED PROSTACYCLIN

Biology of Inhaled Prostacyclin

Part of the normal physiology of the lung is the constant process of formation and release of prostaglandins. Any significant disturbance in normal pulmonary physiology can easily upset this balance. A significant development in understanding Prostaglandins was made in 1976 when prostaglandin I_2 (PGI_2) was discovered.[64] PGI_2 is a naturally occurring prostanoid (complex group of fatty acids) derived from arachadonic acid in the vascular endothelium. It stimulates the enzyme, adenylate cyclase, in smooth muscle to allow the creation of cyclic adenosine monophosphate (cAMP) from ATP. This leads to a cAMP-mediated decrease in intracellular calcium by protein kinases and subsequent smooth muscle relaxation (**Fig. 5**).[65,66] PGI_2 has a short half-life (3–6 minutes) at physiologic pH, making it an ideal pulmonary vasodilator in ARDS because it does not have time to spill over into poorly ventilated regions of the lung. It spontaneously degrades into 6-ketoprostaglandin F1α, a stable metabolite that is cleared by the kidneys. Besides its vasodilator effect, PGI_2 has potent antiplatelet effects, including dissolving existing thrombi and inhibiting platelet aggregation. As discussed previously, this is important in ARDS due to the subclinical microthrombi that form in the pulmonary vasculature and increase MPAP.[3] IV PGI_2 was tried before inhaled PGI_2 in ARDS patients, but its use was limited due to unwanted physiologic

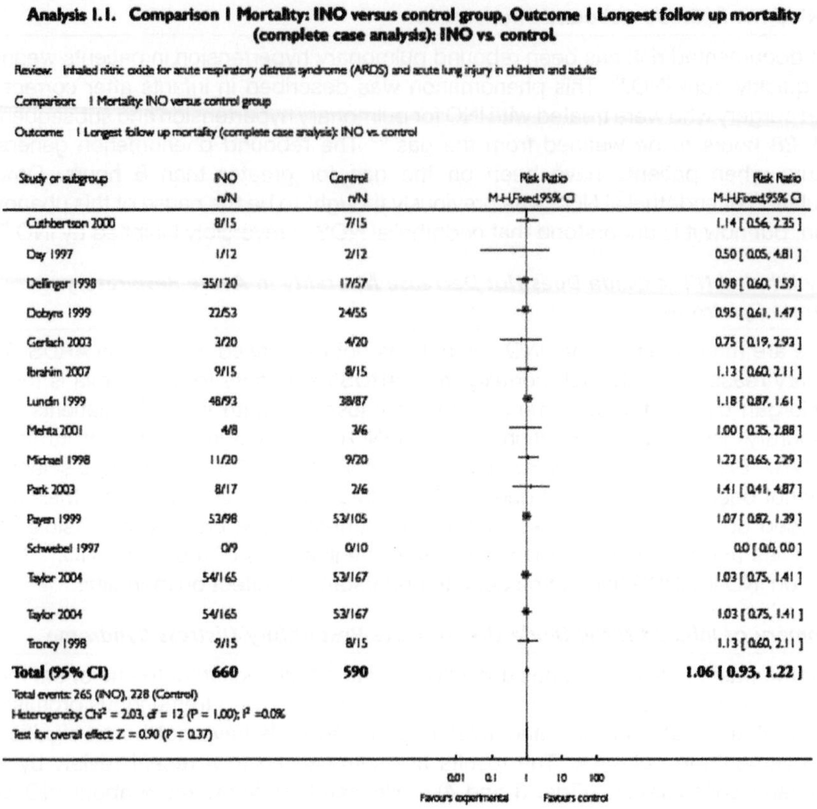

Analysis 1.1. Comparison 1 Mortality: INO versus control group, Outcome 1 Longest follow up mortality (complete case analysis): INO vs. control.

Review: Inhaled nitric oxide for acute respiratory distress syndrome (ARDS) and acute lung injury in children and adults

Comparison: 1 Mortality: INO versus control group

Outcome: 1 Longest follow up mortality (complete case analysis): INO vs. control

Study or subgroup	INO n/N	Control n/N	Risk Ratio M-H,Fixed,95% CI
Cuthbertson 2000	8/15	7/15	1.14 [0.56, 2.35]
Day 1997	1/12	2/12	0.50 [0.05, 4.81]
Dellinger 1998	35/120	17/57	0.98 [0.60, 1.59]
Dobyns 1999	22/53	24/55	0.95 [0.61, 1.47]
Gerlach 2003	3/20	4/20	0.75 [0.19, 2.93]
Ibrahim 2007	9/15	8/15	1.13 [0.60, 2.11]
Lundin 1999	48/93	38/87	1.18 [0.87, 1.61]
Mehta 2001	4/8	3/6	1.00 [0.35, 2.88]
Michael 1998	11/20	9/20	1.22 [0.65, 2.29]
Park 2003	8/17	2/6	1.41 [0.41, 4.87]
Payen 1999	53/98	53/105	1.07 [0.82, 1.39]
Schwebel 1997	0/9	0/10	0.0 [0.0, 0.0]
Taylor 2004	54/165	53/167	1.03 [0.75, 1.41]
Taylor 2004	54/165	53/167	1.03 [0.75, 1.41]
Troncy 1998	9/15	8/15	1.13 [0.60, 2.11]
Total (95% CI)	**660**	**590**	**1.06 [0.93, 1.22]**

Total events: 265 (INO), 228 (Control)

Heterogeneity: Chi^2 = 2.03, df = 12 (P = 1.00); I^2 =0.0%

Test for overall effect: Z = 0.90 (P = 0.37)

0.01 0.1 1 10 100

Favours experimental Favours control

Fig. 3. This forest plot graph compares mortality between the control groups and intervention groups of iNO therapy in adults and children in ARDS. No statistical difference in mortality was noted with iNO therapy versus controls in this compilation of trials. (*From* Ashfari A, Brok J, Moller AM, et al. Inhaled nitric oxide for acute respiratory distress syndrome [ARDS] and acute lung injury in children and adults. Cochrane Database Syst Rev 2010;7:CD002787. doi:10.1002/14651858; with permission.)

effects.[67] IV PGI_2 decreases MAP and increases lung parenchymal shunting, which can worsen hypoxia in ARDS. Inhaled PGI_2 has pulmonary vasoselectivity and, therefore, lacks these unintended consequences; aerosolized prostaglandins have become the focus of research in ARDS. Four inhaled prostaglandin derivatives exist:

1. Prostaglandin E_1 (alprostadil)
2. PGI_2 (Flolan, prostacyclin, and epoprostenol)
3. Iloprost (a longer-acting synthetic derivative of PGI_2)
4. Treprostinil (a long-acting, stable PGI_2, Tyvaso).

IP has been the most widely used and studied aerosolized prostaglandin derivative in ARDS patients and therefore is the focus of this review.

Justification for Use of Inhaled Prostacyclin

The first trial of IP in a human was in 1978.[68] A plethora of case series and small clinical trials with significant limitations have been published.[69] Before trying IP in ARDS

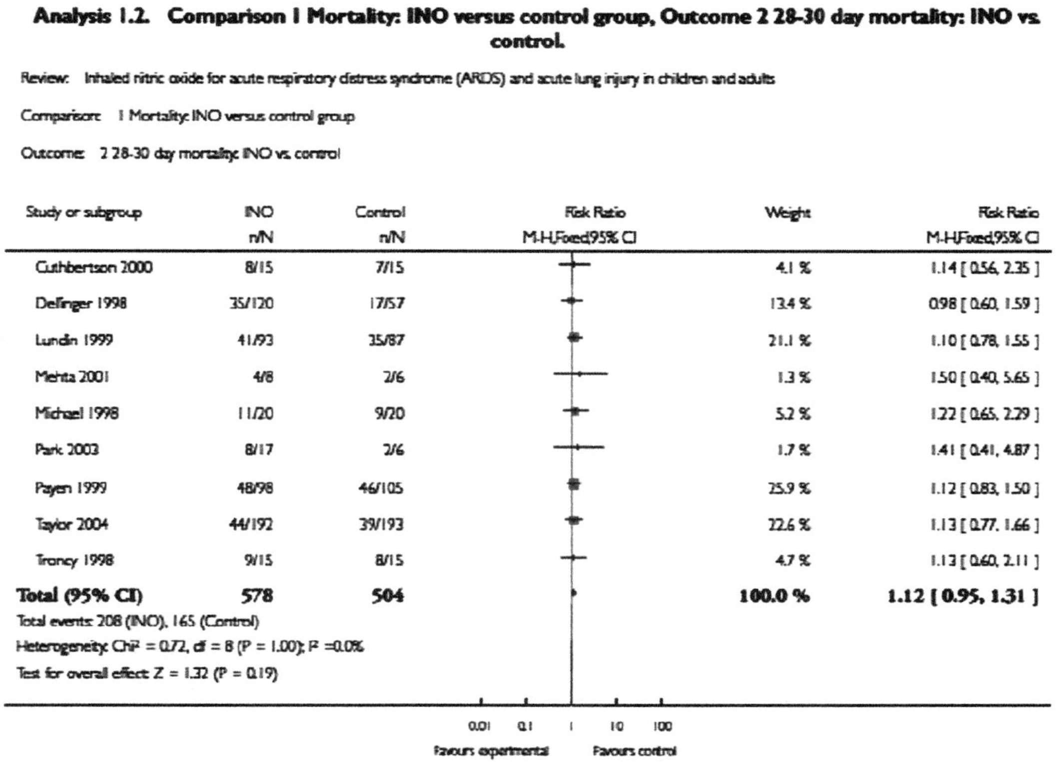

Analysis 1.2. Comparison 1 Mortality: INO versus control group, Outcome 2 28-30 day mortality: INO vs. control.

Review: Inhaled nitric oxide for acute respiratory distress syndrome (ARDS) and acute lung injury in children and adults

Comparison: 1 Mortality: INO versus control group

Outcome: 2 28-30 day mortality: INO vs. control

Study or subgroup	INO n/N	Control n/N	Risk Ratio M-H,Fixed,95% CI	Weight	Risk Ratio M-H,Fixed,95% CI
Cuthbertson 2000	8/15	7/15		4.1 %	1.14 [0.56, 2.35]
Dellinger 1998	35/120	17/57		13.4 %	0.98 [0.60, 1.59]
Lundin 1999	41/93	35/87		21.1 %	1.10 [0.78, 1.55]
Mehta 2001	4/8	2/6		1.3 %	1.50 [0.40, 5.65]
Michael 1998	11/20	9/20		5.2 %	1.22 [0.65, 2.29]
Park 2003	8/17	2/6		1.7 %	1.41 [0.41, 4.87]
Payen 1999	48/98	46/105		25.9 %	1.12 [0.83, 1.50]
Taylor 2004	44/192	39/193		22.6 %	1.13 [0.77, 1.66]
Troncy 1998	9/15	8/15		4.7 %	1.13 [0.60, 2.11]
Total (95% CI)	**578**	**504**		**100.0 %**	**1.12 [0.95, 1.31]**

Total events: 208 (INO), 165 (Control)

Heterogeneity: $Chi^2 = 0.72$, $df = 8$ ($P = 1.00$); $I^2 = 0.0\%$

Test for overall effect: $Z = 1.32$ ($P = 0.19$)

0.01 0.1 1 10 100

Favours experimental Favours control

Fig. 4. This forest plot graph compares 28-day to 30-day mortality between the control groups and intervention groups of iNO therapy in adults and children in ARDS. No statistical difference in 28-day to 30-day mortality was noted with iNO therapy versus controls in this compilation of trials. (*From* Ashfari A, Brok J, Moller AM, et al. Inhaled nitric oxide for acute respiratory distress syndrome [ARDS] and acute lung injury in children and adults. Cochrane Database Syst Rev 2010;7:CD002787. doi:10.1002/14651858; with permission.)

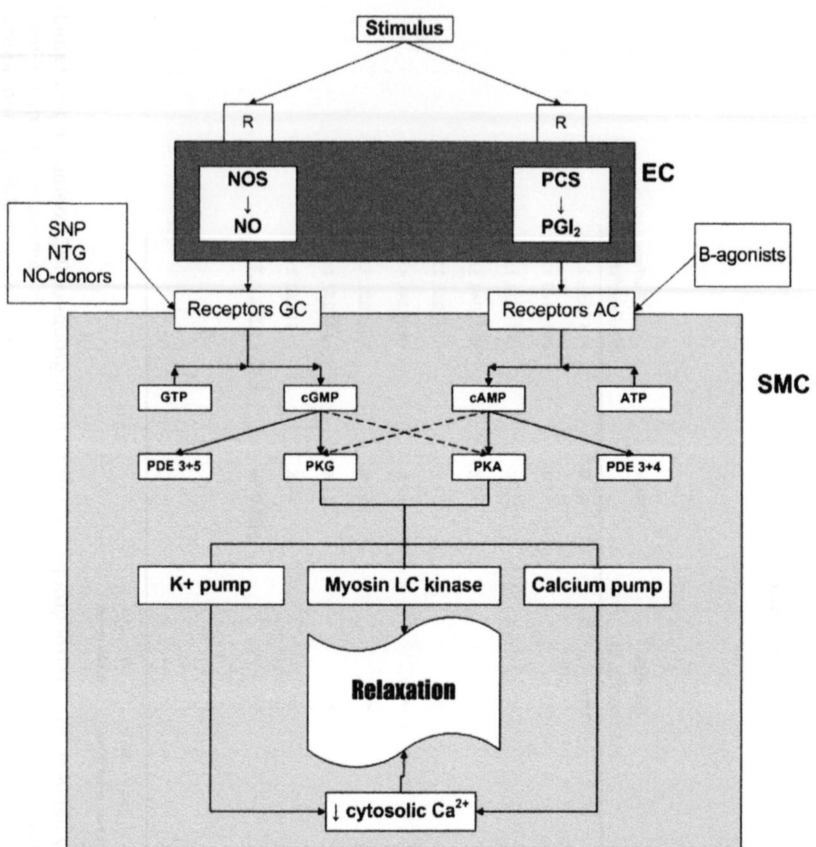

Fig. 5. Physiologic effect of nitric oxide (NO) and prostacyclin (PGI2) production by the endothelial cell (EC) on the vascular smooth muscle cell (SMC). Cyclic guanosine monophosphate (cGMP) activates protein kinase G (PKG) and, to a lesser extent, protein kinase A (PKA) and is metabolized predominantly by phosphodiesterase (PDE) type-5. Cyclic adenosine monophosphate (cAMP) activates PKA and, to a lesser extent, PKG and is metabolized predominantly by PDE type-3. Both protein kinase A and G act via the sarcolemmal potassium (K) and calcium (Ca2) pumps to decrease cytosolic calcium and thereby induce smooth muscle relaxation. R, receptor; NOS, nitric oxide synthase; PCS, prostacyclin synthase; SNP, sodium nitroprusside; NTG, nitroglycerin; GC, guanylate cyclase; AC, adenylate cyclase; GTP, guanosine triphosphate; ATP, adenosine triphosphate. (*From* Lowson SM. Inhaled alternatives to nitric oxide. Crit Care Med 2005;33(Suppl 3):S190; with permission.)

patients, IP was shown to have significant effects on platelet aggregation in healthy human volunteers and alleviate induced hypoxic pulmonary vasoconstriction in dogs.[70,71] The first case series in ARDS patients was from 1993, in which IP decreased PVR by 30%, increased the Pao_2/Fio_2 ratio from 120 to 173, and decreased shunt fraction. The investigators first tried IV prostacyclin in all 3 patients and PVR decreased, but shunt fraction increased.[72] The unsuccessful use of IV vasodilators in ARDS and the successful trial with iNO in 1993 encouraged researchers to do more research on alternatives to iNO due to concerns about its toxicity.[15,73]

Trials of Inhaled Prostacyclin

Animals

Most of the animal trials tested the effect of IP in models of hypoxic pulmonary vasoconstriction and evaluated parameters that are relevant to ARDS, such as pulmonary hypertension and right ventricular ejection fraction. Zwissler and colleagues[74] induced pulmonary hypertension in 6 canines by making them hypoxic (same subjects they tested iNO and IP effect on MPAP), then tested fixed doses of iNO and IP to evaluate their effect on right ventricular function. Both iNO and IP decreased hypoxic vasoconstriction decreasing the stress on the right ventricle, but only iNO increased right ventricular ejection fraction. This study had significant limitations, including its small size and the use of fixed doses of IP and iNO without knowledge of their clinical equivalence. Zobel and colleagues[75] were the only researchers in the 1990s to test iNO and IP in an ALI and a pulmonary hypertension model. iNO was more effective in decreasing pulmonary shunt, but both IP and INO were equivalent in decreasing MPAP. The rest of the trials in animals had similar findings showing iNO was more effective than IP at fixed dosing, but due to trial flaws, insight from these studies were limited.[69] It was concluded, however, that IP was safe to use due to limited side effects seen in these trials and its pulmonary vasoselectivity similar to iNO.

Human trials

Van Heerden and colleagues[76] in a crossover trial design exposed 5 ARDS patients to both iNO (10 ppm) and IP (50 ng/kg/min) and allowed 30 minutes between exposures as a washout period for each gas. IP caused a decreased shunt fraction and MPAP in all patients as opposed to iNO, which only caused a decrease in shunt fraction and MPAP in 3 patients. It was difficult to interpret these findings due to the small trial size and crossover design. Van Heerden and colleagues felt confident their results meant iNO and IP had similar effects in ARDS. This theory was further explored by researchers who showed that IP improved oxygenation in mechanically ventilated patients with severe pneumonia.[77] Their group used a crossover trial design and exposed 16 ARDS patients to both iNO and IP with a 60-minute washout period.[78] As opposed to previous studies, the inhalation gases were titrated to maximal effect. Patients increased their Pao_2/Fio_2 ratios with both iNO (29 mm Hg) and IP (21 mm Hg) exposure. After termination of iNO, patients returned to their baseline Pao_2/Fio_2 ratio in 5 minutes and IP in 25 minutes. Shunt fraction reduction was identical (7%) with each gas, but MPAP decreased more significantly in the IP group (IP 35.0 to 31.9 vs iNO 34.8 to 33.0) These results implied IP worked as well, if not better than, iNO in reducing MPAP in ARDS and equally as well as in improving Pao_2/Fio_2 ratio. Another study was published in the same year using crossover trial design and the AECC criteria for ARDS in 8 patients.[79] The difference in this study was comparison of the 3 fixed doses of iNO (1, 4, and 8 ppm) and IP (1, 10, and 25 ng/kg/min). IP was administered first due to concerns about lingering cardiopulmonary effects of iNO. The Pao_2/Fio_2 ratio improved with IP at the 2 higher doses (10 and 25 ng/kg/min) and iNO at all 3 doses. MPAP decreased by a minimum of 10% in all patients treated with 25 ng/kg/min of IP, but only a few patients responded to iNO (5/8) at all doses. Patients in this study had significant variability in their responses to both gases and researchers postulated that the primary mechanism of developing ARDS may influence IP therapeutic effect. This was addressed in another study where investigators compared IP's effect in ARDS due to primary lung injury versus secondary lung injury.[80] Fifteen consecutive patients were randomized due to their mechanism of ARDS and exposed to a mean dose of 34 ng/kg/min of IP. The 6 patients with primary lung injury had a statistically significant decrease in their Pao_2/Fio_2 ratio ($P<.05$). Of the 9 patients who had secondary causes for ARDS, 8 had a statistically significant increase in their Pao_2/Fio_2 ratio ($P<.05$) and all 9 had statistically significant decrease in their MPAP ($P<.02$). The investigators performed CT scans on all the patients and hypothesized the homogenous consolidations in primary lung ARDS caused IP not to be effective because it likely vasodilated vasculature to consolidated lung. This was opposed to patients with secondary lung injury where the majority of consolidated lung was in gravity dependent regions, allowing IP to vasodilate the vasculature in regions with well-aerated alveoli. **Table 2** summarizes the clinical studies with IP in ARDS.

Efficacy of Inhaled Prostacyclin in Acute Respiratory Distress Syndrome

Despite the conflicting data about the utility of IP in ARDS, its use in critically ill patients has increased. A retrospective review of its use at a tertiary teaching hospital over 1 year showed that 27 patients received either IP or PGE_1 for ARDS.[81] Neither therapy significantly improved Pao_2/Fio_2 ratio at the 3 endpoints (2 hours, 4 hours, and end of therapy) selected by the investigators.

A Cochrane Database review in 2010 of IP in ARDS determined that none of the trials of IP in adults was appropriate for consideration for meta-analysis due to methodologic limitations.[82] A randomized, double-blind placebo controlled safety and efficacy study started in 2006 that tested IP in ARDS and pulmonary hypertension is finished and has been submitted for publication (Shala Siddiqui, personal communication, 2010) This trial would be the first randomized controlled trial of IP in ARDS and hopefully provide insight into its utility. Currently, IP and other inhaled prostaglandins are used in ARDS without any randomized controlled trials to guide the medical community. They seem to have limited efficacy if used in the correct patient population.

Delivery of Inhaled Prostacyclin

The science of delivery of IP to mechanically ventilated patients is imprecise. Unlike iNO, IP lacks a single delivery device. The devices that are used to deliver IP in the United States vary between hospitals.[83] This lack of standardization is a limitation to IP trials in ARDS. Aersolized delivery of medications is notoriously ineffective with as little as 3% delivered to the lungs.[84] Effective alveolar deposition can only occur when particles are 1 to 2 μm in diameter.[85] Due to advancements in ultrasonic nebulization, it is more effective at concentrating IP than jet nebulization.[86] For example, jet nebulizers operate at different flow rates leading to wide ranges of particle size and large variability of dose delivery. Van Heerdan and colleagues[87] studied 9 patients, trying to determine the appropriate dose of IP ARDS patients should receive using a jet nebulizer. Their study determined that up to 50 ng/kg/min was safe to use in humans, but they admit the actual mass of IP actually deposited in the respiratory tract was not known. This variability in dose delivery can be avoided by electronic nebulizers. Electronic nebulizers do not use heat, allowing them to produce a reliable volume of small aerosol particles and they do not use an external flow source, which can alter the amount of aerosol particles delivered.[88] Currently, they remain unapproved for continuous nebulization.

Safety of Inhaled Prostacyclin

Inhaled prostacylin is made from a freeze-dried sodium salt, which is dissolved in a glycine solvent. The created solution needs to be maintained at a narrow pH range (10–11). Concern exists about it being a tracheal irritant due to its alkaline pH. In a porcine model, evidence of sterile tracheitis existed at doses that are 9 times greater (normal human dose 5 to 50 ng/kg/min) than those used in human trials.[89] There is scant literature on worsening bronchospasm in patients exposed to high doses of IP (up to 500 μg), but caution is advised by experts when using IP in patients with reactive airway disease.[85,90,91] The primary safety concerns with IP are its effects on SVR and platelets. A well-designed study on the effects of exposure to IP (28 ng/kg/min) for 8 hours in 14 lambs evenly divided between control and treatment groups found no significant effects of pulmonary toxicity, platelet dysfunction, or decreased MAP.[92] The findings are important because IP is not metabolized in the pulmonary system and theoretically could cause hypotension with systemic absorption. The lack of platelet dysfunction as measured by platelet aggregation and bleeding time was in direct contrast to prior studies where subjects were exposed to much higher doses of IP (200–450 μg).[68,70] Experts hesitate to use IP in patients at risk for bleeding, but significant problems have not been described in trials involving ARDS patients.[83,87]

Other Inhaled Prostaglandins

A majority of PGE_1 is metabolized in the lung, which reduces the possibility of clinically significant side effects including decreased MAP. Putensen and colleagues[93] compared the selective vasodilatory effects of iNO, aerosolized PGE_1 and IV PGE_1 in 10 ARDS patients who met the AECC on ARDS criteria. The trial was a crossover design with patients receiving both gases (30-minute washout period) and only patients who were responders to both gases were included in the trial. The lowest concentration, which increased Pao_2 by both gases, was used. The Pao_2, PVR, and right ventricular ejection fraction improved significantly ($P<.05$) compared with baseline with all 3 interventions. IV prostacyclin infusion was the only intervention that significantly decreased SVR ($P<.05$) and significantly ($P<.05$) increased cardiac index compared with baseline. Another study in 15 ARDS patients showed that PGE_1 increased Pao_2, Pao_2/Fio_2 ratio and decreased venous admixture at 4-hour, 1-hour to 2-hour and 24-hour intervals.[94] Both of these trials were too small to draw any conclusions about PGE_1, but they seem to imply that PGE_1 is as effective as IP. Randomized controlled trials are needed to test PGE_1 efficacy, but currently it is used regularly in some tertiary care centers in the United States.[81] Other inhaled prostaglandins exist and are used in patients for pulmonary hypertension, but the literature is scant about their effectiveness in ARDS.

Combination Therapy of Inhaled Nitric Oxide and Inhaled Prostacyclin

There is not significant literature describing combination therapy with IP in ARDS. The use of any inhaled prostaglandin with iNO would make sense because both cause vasodilatation through different pathways. The combination therapy has proved effective in improving oxygenation after lung transplantation but has yet to be described in ARDS patients.[95] A case report about a patient with refractory hypoxemia started on IP while ventilated with high-frequency percussive ventilation describes a significant improvement in Pao_2/Fio_2 ratio.[96] The case report uses the same principle that more recruited lung leads to more area for IP to vasodilate. Phosphodiesterase inhibitors and endothelin receptor antagonists have been combined with IP in other patient populations, but no such trial exists for ARDS patients.

Cost of Inhaled Prostacyclin

The cost of IP is $275 daily.[83] The delivery systems are nonstandardized and the cost of each system is different. IP benefited from the high cost of iNO, but like iNO its use in ARDS is not Food and Drug Administration approved (**Table 3**).

Table 2
Adult trials of inhaled prostacyclin and aloprostadil in acute respiratory distress syndrome

Study	Year	Number Patients/ Centers	Patient Details	Trial Design	Primary Outcome	Results	Comment
Walmrath et al[72]	1993	3/1	ARDS with P/F <150 mm Hg	Case series	Improved P/F ratio	Improved P/F ratio and decreased MPAP	First human evidence that IP may improve oxygenation and MPAP in ARDS
Van Heerden et al[76]	1996	5/1	AECC ARDS with lung injury score >2.0	Crossover trial design not RCT	IP was as effective as iNO in improving hypoxemia and reducing MPAP	IP worked in all patients and iNO worked in 3 patients	Difficult to interpret results due to small trial and crossover design; seems IP is effective
Walmrath et al[78]	1996	16/1	Lung injury score 2.75 ± 0.05	Crossover trial design not RCT	IP was as effective as iNO in selective pulmonary vasodilatation and improving oxygenation	IP improved MPAP more than iNO. Shunt fraction improvement was equal and iNO improved P/F ratio more than IP	Difficult to interpret results due to small trial and crossover design; seems IP is effective
Zwissler et al[79]	1996	8/1	B/l infiltrates on chest radiograph, PAOP <18 mm Hg, P/F ratio <155 mm Hg, MPAP >30 mm Hg	Crossover trial design not RCT	Characterize IP effectiveness in improving P/F ratio and MPAP at fixed doses in comparison with fixed doses iNO	IP improved P/F ratio at 2 higher doses and iNO improved it at all doses; IP at highest dose improved MPAP in all patients; iNO at all doses only improved MPAP in 5/8	Difficult to interpret results due to small trial and crossover design; seems IP is effective and may have more effect on MPAP

Meyer et al[94]	1998	15/1	P/F ratio <160 mm Hg	Case series	Aloprostadil improves oxygenation in ALI	Aloprostadil improved oxygenation	Difficult to interpret due to trial design
Putensen et al[93]	1998	10/1	AECC ARDS	Prospective nonrandomized observational trial	iNO and aloprostadil are equivalent in improving gas exchange	iNO and aloprostadil both improved gas exchange as opposed to IV aloprostadil, which worsened it	Difficult to interpret results due to small trial; aloprostadil can improve gas exchange in ARDS
Van Heerden et al[87]	2000	9/1	Lung injury score >2.5	Unblinded, prospective interventional trial	Efficacy and dose-responsive relationship of IP in ARDS	IP is efficacious in improving oxygenation in ARDS	Difficult to interpret due to small trial, IP seems safe and optimal starting dose 10 ng/kg/min
Domenighetti et al[80]	2001	15/1	AECC ARDS and P/F <150 mm Hg	Prospective nonrandomized observational trial	Mechanism of ARDS influences usefulness of IP	IP is effective in increasing P/F ratio and decreasing MPAP in ARDS from nonpulmonary causes	Difficult to interpret results due to small trial; however, IP seems ineffective in lung injury induced ARDS

Abbreviations: B/l, bilateral; P/F, oxygen content/fractional oxygen concentration; RCT, randomized controlled trial.

Table 3
Comparison of inhaled nitric oxide and inhaled nitric oxide and inhaled prostacyclin in ARDS

	Inhaled Nitric Oxide	Inhaled Prostacyclin
Randomized Controlled Trials[61,82]	5	0
Cost[83]	$1880/day	$275/day
Delivery[83]	Standardized single mode	Multiple modes
Possible Clinical Benefit	No effect on mortality, temporary increase in oxygenation, decrease MPAP	No effect on mortality, temporary increase in oxygenation, decrease MPAP
Side Effects	Insignificant	Insignificant

Summary of Inhaled Prostacyclin

Knowledge of IP has grown substantially in the past 30 years.[83] It seems a safe alternative to iNO in ARDS patients, but less research exists about its utility. IP and other prostaglandin derivatives are used in ARDS with increasing frequency. Randomized controlled trials with consistent dosing methods need to be developed to define its role in ARDS, to help guide clinicians.

ACKNOWLEDGMENTS

We would like to thank Harold Pavlesky, MD for his help in preparing this article. We are also grateful to Karen Mitchell and Marita Malone at Cooper University Hospital, New Jersey.

REFERENCES

1. Esteban A, Anzueto A, Frutos F, et al. Characteristics and outcomes in adult patients receiving mechanical ventilation. JAMA 2002;287:345–55.
2. Zambano M, Vincent JL. Mortality rates for patients with acute lung injury/ARDS have decreased over time. Chest 2008;133:1120–7.
3. Zapol WM, Kobayashi K, Snider MT, et al. Vascular obstruction causes pulmonary hypertension in severe acute respiratory failure. Chest 1977;71:306–7.
4. Bull TM, Clark B, McFann K, et al. Pulmonary vascular dysfunction is associated with poor outcomes in patients with acute lung injury. Am J Respir Crit Care Med 2010;182:1123–8.
5. Bigatello LM, Zapol WM. New approaches to acute lung injury. Br J Anaesth 1996;77:99–109.
6. Moncada S, Palmer RM, Higgs EA. Nitric oxide: physiology, pathophysiology, and pharmacology. Pharmacol Rev 1991;43:109–42.
7. Coggins MP, Block KD. Nitric oxide in the pulmonary vasculature. Arterioscler Thromb Vasc Biol 2007;27:1877–85.
8. Griffiths MJ, Evans TW. Inhaled nitric oxide therapy in adults. N Engl J Med 2005; 353(25):2683–95.
9. Creagh-Brown BC, Griffiths MJ, Evans TW. Bench-to-bedside review: inhaled nitric oxide therapy in adults. Crit Care 2009;212:1–8.
10. Rimar S, Gillis C. Selective pulmonary vasodilitation by inhaled nitric oxide is due to hemoglobin inactivation. Circulation 1993;88:2884–7.
11. Frostell C, Fratacci MD, Wain JC, et al. Inhaled nitric oxide. A selective pulmonary vasodilator reversing hypoxic pulmonary vasoconstriction. Circulation 1991;83:2038–47.

12. Brandler MD, Powell SC, Craig DM, et al. A novel inhaled organic nitrate that affects pulmonary vascular tone in a piglet model of hypoxia-induced pulmonary hypertension. Pediatr Res 2005;58:531–6.
13. Koh Y, Hurford WE. Inhaled nitric oxide in acute respiratory distress syndrome: from bench to bedside. Int Anesthesiol Clin 2003;41(1):91–102.
14. Pepke-Zeba J, Higenbottam TW, Dinh-Xuan AT, et al. Inhaled nitric oxide as a cause of selective pulmonary vasodilitation in pulmonary hypertension. Lancet 1991;338:1173–4.
15. Rossaint R, Falke KF, Lopez F, et al. Inhaled nitric oxide for the adult respiratory distress syndrome. N Engl J Med 1993;328:399–405.
16. Gustafsson LE, Leone AM, Persson MG. Endogenous nitric oxide is present in the exhaled air of rabbits, guinea pigs and humans. Biochem Biophys Res Commun 1991;181:852–7.
17. Gerlach H, Rossaint R, Pappert D, et al. Time-course and dose-response of nitric oxide inhalation for systemic oxygenation and pulmonary hypertension in patients with adult respiratory distress syndrome. Eur J Clin Invest 1993;80:761–70.
18. Puybasset L, Rouby JJ, Mourgeon E, et al. Inhaled nitric oxide in acute respiratory failure: dose-response curves. Intensive Care Med 1994;20:319–27.
19. Bigatello LM, Hurford WE, Kacmarek RM, et al. Prolonged inhalation of low concentration of nitric oxide in patients with severe adult respiratory syndrome. Anesthesiology 1994;80:761–70.
20. Lu Q, Mourgeon E, Law-Kourne JD, et al. Dose-response curves of inhaled nitric oxide with and without intravenous almitrine in nitric oxide-responding patients with acute respiratory distress syndrome. Anesthesiology 1995;83:929–43.
21. McIntyre R, Moore F, Piedalue F, et al. Inhaled nitric oxide variably improves oxygenation and pulmonary hypertension in patients with acute respiratory distress syndrome. J Trauma 1995;39(3):418–25.
22. Lundin S, Wesfelt UN, Stenqvist O, et al. Response to nitric oxide inhalation in early acute lung injury. Intensive Care Med 1996;22:728–34.
23. Klinger JR. Inhaled nitric oxide in ARDS. Crit Care Clin 2002;18:45–68.
24. Brett SJ, Hansell DM, Evans TW. Clinical correlates in acute lung injury response to inhaled nitric oxide. Chest 1998;114:1397–404.
25. Puybasset L, Rouby JJ, Mourgeon E, et al. Inhaled nitric oxide in reverses the increase in pulmonary vascular resistance induced by permissive hypercapnia in patients with acute respiratory distress syndrome. Anesthesiology 1994;80: 1254–67.
26. Kraft P, Fridrich P, Fitzgerald RD, et al. Effectiveness of nitric oxide inhalation in septic ARDS. Chest 1996;109:486–93.
27. Manktelow C, Bigatellow LM, Hess D, et al. Physiologic determinants of the response to inhaled nitric oxide in patients with acute respiratory distress syndrome. Anesthesiology 1997;87:297–307.
28. Micheal JR, Barton RG, Saffle JR, et al. Inhaled nitric oxide versus conventional therapy. Am J Respir Crit Care Med 1998;157:1372–80.
29. Troncy E, Collet JP, Shapiro S, et al. Inhaled nitric oxide in acute respiratory distress syndrome. Am J Respir Crit Care Med 1998;157:1483–8.
30. Dellinger RP, Zimmerman JL, Taylor RW, et al. Effects of inhaled nitric oxide in patients with acute respiratory distress syndrome: results of a randomized phase II trial. Crit Care Med 1998;26:15–23.
31. Bernard GR, Artigas K, Brigham J, et al. Report of the American-European Consensus Conference on ARDS: definitions, mechanisms, relevant outcomes, and clinical trial coordination. Am J Respir Crit Care Med 1994;149:818–24.

32. Payen D, Vallet B. Groupe d'Etude sur le NO inhale au cours de l'ARDS (GENOA). Results of the French prospective multicentric randomized double-blind placebo-controlled trial on inhaled nitric oxide (NO) in ARDS. Intensive Care Med 1999; 25(suppl 1):S166 [abstract 645].
33. Lundin S, Mang H, Smithies M, et al. Inhalation of nitric oxide in acute lung injury: results of a European multicentre study. The European Study Group of Inhaled Nitric Oxide. Intensive Care Med 1999;25(9):911–9.
34. Sokol J, Jacobs SE, Bohn D. Inhaled nitric oxide for acute hypoxic respiratory failure in children and adults: a meta-analysis. Anesth Analg 2003;97:989–98.
35. Gerlach H, Keh D, Semmerow A, et al. Dose-response characteristics during long-term inhalation of nitric oxide in patients with severe acute respiratory distress syndrome. Am J Respir Crit Care Med 2003;167:1008–15.
36. Taylor RW, Zimmerman JL, Dellinger RP, et al. Low-dose inhaled nitric oxide in patients with acute lung injury: a randomized controlled trial. JAMA 2004;291:1603–9.
37. Adhikari N, Granton JT. Inhaled nitric oxide for acute lung injury: no place for NO? JAMA 2004;291:1629–31.
38. Angus DC, Clermont GC, Linde-Zwirble WT, et al. Healthcare costs and long-term outcomes after acute respiratory distress syndrome: a phase III trial of inhaled nitric oxide. Crit Care Med 2006;34:2883–90.
39. Putensen C, Ransanen J, Lopez FA, et al. Continuous positive airway pressure modulates effect of inhaled nitric oxide on the ventilation-perfusion distributions in canine lung injury. Chest 1994;106:1563–7.
40. Puybasset L, Rouby J, Mourgeon E, et al. Factors influencing cardiopulmonary effects of inhaled nitric oxide. Am J Respir Crit Care Med 1995;152:318–28.
41. Johannigman JA, Davis K, Campbell RS, et al. Positive end-expiratory pressure and response to inhaled nitric oxide: changing nonresponders to responders. Surgery 2000;127:390–4.
42. Gattinoni I, Pelosi P, Vitale G, et al. Body position changes redistribute lung computed tomographic density in patients with acute respiratory failure. Anesthesiology 1991;74:15–23.
43. Papazian L, Bregeon F, Gaillat F, et al. Respective and combined effects of prone position and inhaled nitric oxide in patients with acute respiratory distress syndrome. Am J Respir Crit Care Med 1998;167:580–5.
44. Dupont H, Mentec H, Cheval C, et al. Short-term effect of inhaled nitric oxide and prone positioning on gas exchange in patients with severe acute respiratory distress syndrome. Crit Care Med 2000;28:304–8.
45. Johannigman JA, Davis K, Miller SL, et al. Prone positioning and inhaled nitric oxide:synergistic therapies for acute respiratory distress syndrome. J Trauma 2001; 50:589–96.
46. Borelli M, Lampati L, Vascotto E, et al. Hemodynamic and gas exchange response to inhaled nitric oxide and prone positioning in acute respiratory distress syndrome patients. Crit Care Med 2000;28:2707–12.
47. Martinez M, Diaz E, Joseph D, et al. Improvement in oxygenation by prone position and nitric oxide in patients with acute respiratory distress syndrome. Intensive Care Med 1999;25:29–36.
48. Park KJ, Lee YJ, Oh YJ, et al. Combined effects of inhaled nitric oxide and a recruitment maneuver in patients with acute respiratory distress syndrome. Yonsei Med J 2003;44:219–26.
49. Kinsella JP, Truog WE, Walsh WF, et al. Randomized, multicenter trial of inhaled nitric oxide and high frequency oscillatory ventilation in severe, persistant pulmonary hypertension of the newborn. J Pediatr 1997;131:55–62.

50. Kinsella JP, Parker TA, Galan H, et al. Independent and combined effects of inhaled nitric oxide, liquid perfluorchemical, and high-frequency oscillatory ventilation in premature lambs with respiratory distress syndrome. Am J Respir Crit Care Med 1999;159:1220–7.
51. Mehta S, MacDonald R, Hallet DC, et al. Acute oxygenation response to inhaled nitric oxide when combined with high-frequency oscillatory ventilation in adults with acute respiratory distress syndrome. Crit Care Med 2003;31:383–9.
52. Pinsky MR, Fidan G, Lee KH, et al. Contamination of hospital compressed air with nitric oxide. Chest 1997;111:1759–63.
53. Imanaka H, Hess D, Kirmse M, et al. Inaccuracies of nitric oxide delivery systems during adult mechanical ventilation. Anesthesiology 1997;87:1591–3.
54. Kirmse M, Hess D, Fujino Y, et al. Delivery of inhaled nitric oxide using the Ohmeda INOvent Delivery System. Chest 1998;113:1650–7.
55. The Neonatal Inhaled Nitric Oxide Study Group. Inhaled nitric oxide and persistent pulmonary hypertension in the newborn. N Engl J Med 1997;336:605–10.
56. Available at: http://www.genollc.com. Accessed April 3, 2011.
57. Pierce CM, Peters MJ, Cohen G, et al. Cost of nitric oxide is exorbitant. BMJ 2002; 325:336.
58. Lowson SM. Inhaled alternatives to nitric oxide. Crit Care Med 2005;33:S188–95.
59. Adhikari NK, Burns KE, Friedrich JO, et al. Effect of nitric oxide on oxygenation and mortality in acute lung injury: systemic review and meta-analysis. BMJ 2007;334:779.
60. Greenbaum R, Bay J, Hargreaves ND, et al. Effects of higher oxides of nitrogen on the anaesthetized dog. Br J Anaesth 1967;39:393–404.
61. Ashfari A, Brok J, Moller AM, et al. Inhaled nitric oxide for acute respiratory distress syndrome (ARDS) and acute lung injury in children and adults. Cochrane Database Syst Rev 2010;7:CD002787.
62. Miller O, Tang S, Keech A, et al. Rebound pulmonary hypertension on withdrawal from inhaled nitric oxide. Lancet 1995;346:51–2.
63. Aranda M, Pearl RG. Inhaled nitric oxide and pulmonary vasoreactivity. J Clin Monit 2000;16:393–401.
64. Moncada S, Gryglewski R, Bunting S, et al. An enzyme isolated from arteries transforms prostaglandins endoperoxides to an unstable substance that inhibits platelet aggregation. Nature 1976;263:663–5.
65. Kerins DM, Murray R, Fitzgerald GA. Prostacyclin and prostaglandin E1: molecular mechanisms and therapeutic utility. Prog Hemost Thromb 1991;10:307–37.
66. Siobal MS. Pulmonary vasodilators. Respir Care 2007;52:885–99.
67. Schreen T, Radermacher P. Prostacyclin (PGI_2): new aspects of an old substance in treatment of critically ill patients. Intensive Care Med 1997;23:146–58.
68. Szczekilk A, Gryglewski R, Nizankowska E, et al. Pulmonary and anti-platelet effects of intravenous and inhaled prostacyclin in man. Prostaglandins 1978;16: 651–60.
69. Lowson SM. Inhaled alternatives to nitric oxide. Anesthesiology 2002;96:1504–13.
70. Burghuber OC, Silberbauer K, Haber P, et al. Pulmonary and antiaggregatory effects of prostacyclin after inhalation and intravenous infusion. Respiration 1984;45:450–5.
71. Welte M, Zwissler B, Habazettl H, et al. PGI_2 Aerosol versus nitric oxide for selective pulmonary vasodilation in hypoxic pulmonary vasoconstriction. Eur Surg Res 1993;25:329–40.
72. Walmrath D, Schneider T, Pilch J, et al. Aerosolised prostacyclin in adult respiratory distress syndrome. Lancet 1993;342:961–2.

73. Radermacher P, Santak B, Wust HJ, et al. Prostacyclin for the treatment of pulmonary hypertension in the adult respiratory distress syndrome: effects on pulmonary capillary pressure and ventilation-perfusion distributions. Anesthesiology 1990;72:238–44.
74. Zwissler B, Welte M, Messmer K. Effects of inhaled prostacyclin as compared to inhaled nitric oxide on right ventricular performance in hypoxic pulmonary vasoconstriction. J Cardiothorac Vasc Anesth 1995;9:283–9.
75. Zobel G, Dacar D, Rodl S, et al. Inhaled nitric oxide versus inhaled prostacyclin in acute respiratory failure with pulmonary hypertension in piglets. Pediatr Res 1995;38:198–204.
76. Van Heerden PV, Blythe D, Webb SA. Inhaled aerosolized prostacyclin and nitric oxide as selective pulmonary vasodilators in ARDS—a pilot study. Anaesth Intensive Care 1996;24(5):564–8.
77. Walmrath D, Schneider T, Pilch J, et al. Effects of aerosolized prostacyclin in severe pneumonia impact of fibrosis. Am J Respir Crit Care Med 1995;151:724–30.
78. Walmrath D, Schneider T, Schermuly R, et al. Direct comparison of inhaled nitric oxide and aerosilized prostacyclin in acute respiratory distress syndrome. Am J Respir Crit Care Med 1996;153(3):991–6.
79. Zwissler B, Kemming G, Habler O, et al. Inhaled prostacyclin versus inhaled nitric oxide in adult respiratory distress syndrome. Am J Respir Crit Care Med 1996;154:1671–7.
80. Domenighetti G, Stricker H, Waldispuehl B, et al. Nebulized prostacyclin in acute respiratory distress syndrome: Impact of primary (pulmonary injury) and secondary (extrapulmonary) disease on gas exchange response. Crit Care Med 2001;26:15–23.
81. Camamo JM, McCoy RH, Erstad BL. Retrospective evaluation of inhaled prostaglandins in patients with acute respiratory distress syndrome. Pharmacotherapy 2005;25:184–90.
82. Afshari A, Brok J, Moller AM, et al. Aerosolized prostacyclin for acute lung injury (ALI) and acute respiratory distress syndrome (ARDS). Cochrane Database Syst Rev 2010;8:CD007733.
83. Siobal MS, Hess DR. Are inhaled vasodilators useful in acute lung injury and acute respiratory distress syndrome. Respir Care 2010;55:144–57.
84. MacIntyre NR, Silver RM, Miller CW, et al. Aerosol deliver in intubated, mechanically ventilated patients. Crit Care Med 1985;13:81–4.
85. Siobal M. Aerosolized prostacyclins. Respir Care 2004;49:640–52.
86. Katial RK, Reisner C, Buchmeier A, et al. Comparison of three commercial ultrasonic nebulizers. Ann Allergy Asthma Immunol 2000;84:225–61.
87. Van Heerden P, Barden A, Michalopoulos N, et al. Dose-response to inhaled aerosilized prostacyclin for ARDS. Chest 2000;117:819–27.
88. Dhand R. Nebulizers that use a vibrating mesh or plate with multiple apertures to generate aerosol. Respir Care 2002;47:1406–16.
89. Van Heerdan PV, Caterina P, Filion P, et al. Pulmonary toxicity of inhaled aersolized prostacyclin therapy: an observational study. Anaesth Intensive Care 2000;28:161–6.
90. Parsargiklian M, Bianco S. Ventilatory and cardiovascular effects of prostacyclin and 6-oxo-PGF1 alpha by inhalation. Adv Prostaglandin Thromboxane Res 1980;7:943–51.
91. Hardy CC, Bradding P, Robinson C, et al. Bronchoconstrictor and Antibronchoconstrictor Properties of Inhaled Prostacyclin in Asthma. J Appl Physiol 1988;64:1567–74.

92. Habler O, Kleen M, Zissler, et al. Inhalation of Prostacyclin for 8 hours does not produce sign of acute pulmonary toxicity in healthy lambs. Intensive Care Med 1996;22:426–33.
93. Putensen C, Hormann C, Kleinsasser A, et al. Cardiopulmonary effects of aerosolized prostaglandin E_1 and nitric oxide inhalation in patients with acute respiratory distress syndrome. Am J Respir Crit Care Med 1998;157:1743–7.
94. Meyer J, Theilmeier G, Van Aken H, et al. Inahled prostaglandin E_1 for treatment of acute lung injury in severe multiple organ failure. Anesth Analg 1998;86:753–8.
95. Della Rocca G, Coccia C, Pompei L, et al. Hemodynamic and oxygenation changes of combined therapy with inhaled nitric oxide and inhaled aerosolized prostacyclin. J Cardiothorac Vasc Anesth 2001;15:224–7.
96. Allan PF, Codispoti CA, Womble SG, et al. Inhaled prostacyclin in combination with high frequency percussive ventilation. J Burn Care Res 2010;31:347–52.

Glucocorticoid Treatment in Acute Lung Injury and Acute Respiratory Distress Syndrome

Paul E. Marik, MD[a,*], G. Umberto Meduri, MD[b], Patricia R.M. Rocco, MD, PhD[c], Djillali Annane, MD, PhD[d]

KEYWORDS

- Acute respiratory distress syndrome • Glucocorticoid
- Intensive care unit • Mechanical ventilation
- Secondary prevention • Systemic inflammation

The acute respiratory distress syndrome (ARDS) is a common and vexing problem faced by critical care providers worldwide. Despite extensive investigation over the past 3 decades, the impact of ARDS in terms of morbidity, mortality, and health care costs remains very high.[1,2] Except for glucocorticoids, no pharmacologic therapy has yet been shown to decrease the mortality of ARDS independent of treating the underlying cause. This article outlines the scientific rationale for glucocorticoid treatment in ARDS, discusses the factors affecting response to treatment, reviews the results of recent experimental and controlled clinical trials, debunks some of the myths concerning glucocorticoid-related side effects in critically ill patients, and outlines a protocol for glucocorticoid treatment based on the best available data.

Conflicts of Interest: None of the authors have a conflict of interest to declare.
[a] Division of Pulmonary and Critical Care Medicine, Department of Medicine, Eastern Virginia Medical School, Norfolk, VA, USA
[b] Division of Pulmonary, Critical Care, and Sleep Medicine, Departments of Medicine, University of Tennessee Health Science Center and Memphis Veterans Affairs Medical Center, Memphis, TN, USA
[c] Laboratory of Pulmonary Investigation, Carlos Chagas Filho Biophysics Institute, Federal University of Rio de Janeiro, Rio de Janeiro, Brazil
[d] General Intensive Care Unit, Université de Versailles SQY (UniverSud Paris), Garches, France
* Corresponding author.
E-mail address: MarikPE@EVMS.EDU

Crit Care Clin 27 (2011) 589–607
doi:10.1016/j.ccc.2011.05.007 **criticalcare.theclinics.com**
0749-0704/11/$ – see front matter

PROGRESSIVE ARDS, PERSISTENT INFLAMMATION, AND INADEQUATE GLUCOCORTICOID ACTIVITY

Experimental and clinical evidence have shown a strong cause-and-effect relationship between persistence of systemic inflammation and the progression (unresolving) of ARDS. At the cellular level, patients with unresolving ARDS have inadequate glucocorticoid-glucocorticoid receptor (GC-GR)–mediated down-regulation of inflammatory transcription factor nuclear factor-κB (NF-κB) despite elevated levels of circulating cortisol, a condition recently defined as *critical illness–related corticosteroid insufficiency* (CIRCI).[3,4] Patients with unresolving ARDS have persistent elevation of both systemic and bronchoalveolar lavage (BAL) levels of inflammatory mediators, markers of fibrogenesis, and alveolar-capillary membrane (ACM) permeability (BAL albumin, total protein, and percentage neutrophils). At the tissue level, uninhibited increased NF-κB activation leads to ongoing tissue injury, intra- and extravascular coagulation, and proliferation of mesenchymal cells, resulting in maladaptive lung repair and ultimately end-organ dysfunction and failure.[3] The ability of activated GC-GR to downregulate systemic inflammation and restore tissue homeostasis can be significantly enhanced with exogenous glucocorticoid treatment.[5]

In a randomized trial,[6] longitudinal measurements of biomarkers provided compelling evidence that prolonged methylprednisolone treatment modifies CIRCI and positively affects all aspects of ARDS.[7] Treatment with prolonged methylprednisolone was associated with increased GC-GRα activity and reduced NF-κB DNA binding and transcription of inflammatory mediators.[5] In ARDS, methylprednisolone treatment led to rapid and sustained reduction in plasma and BAL levels of proinflammatory mediators,[5,8] chemokines and adhesion molecules, and markers of fibrogenesis[9] and ACM permeability,[8] while increasing the antiinflammatory cytokine interleukin (IL)-10 and ratios of antiinflammatory to proinflammatory cytokines.

FACTORS AFFECTING RESPONSE TO PROLONGED GLUCOCORTICOID TREATMENT

Duration of treatment is an important determinant of efficacy and toxicity. Optimization of glucocorticoid treatment is affected by three factors: (1) actual biologic duration of the disease process (systemic inflammation and CIRCI), (2) recovery time of the hypothalamic-pituitary-adrenal (HPA) axis, and (3) cumulative risk associated with prolonged treatment (risk) and the essential role of secondary prevention (risk reduction).

Longitudinal measurements of plasma and BAL inflammatory cytokine levels in ARDS showed that inflammation extends well beyond resolution of respiratory failure.[3,10,11] One uncontrolled study found that, despite prolonged methylprednisolone administration, local and systemic inflammation persisted for at least 14 days (limit of study).[8] Similar findings were reported in a randomized controlled trial on day 10 of methylprednisolone treatment.[5] Recently, two longitudinal studies in patients with severe community-acquired pneumonia (CAP) found high levels of circulating inflammatory cytokines 3 weeks after clinical resolution of sepsis.[12,13] These data suggest that patients with ARDS or pulmonary sepsis may have prolonged immune dysregulation (even after clinical recovery), and that a longer course of corticosteroids may be required.

Prolonged glucocorticoid treatment is associated with downregulation of glucocorticoid receptor levels and suppression of the HPA axis, affecting systemic inflammation after discontinuing treatment. Experimental and clinical literature[14] underscores the importance of continuing glucocorticoid treatment beyond clinical resolution of acute respiratory failure (extubation). In the recent ARDS network trial, methylprednisolone was discontinued within 12 to 36 hours of extubation and, as acknowledged by the authors, likely contributed to the deterioration in the PaO_2:FiO_2 ratio, higher rate of reintubation, and loss of the significant initial survival benefit found during treatment.[14,15] In two other ARDS trials,[6,16] glucocorticoid treatment was continued for up to 18 days after extubation to maintain reduction in inflammation.[6,16] This prolonged glucocorticoid treatment was not associated with relapse of ARDS. The extent of improvement in systemic and pulmonary inflammation during prolonged methylprednisolone administration is superior to any other investigated intervention in ARDS.[7]

A short course of steroid treatment is associated with suppression of adrenal response to adrenocorticotropic hormone in 45% of patients, which may persist of 10 to 14 days.[17] In the recent HYPOLYTE study, a corticotropin stimulation test was performed before treatment with hydrocortisone and after a 7-day course.[18] On repeat testing, the patients with CIRCI treated with hydrocortisone had a blunted response compared with those who received placebo. These studies provide compelling supportive data that short-term glucocorticoids suppress the HPA axis and that the sudden and premature withdrawal of corticosteroids may result in inadequate glucocorticoid activity and a rebound effect. For this reason, the recommendation to discontinue methylprednisolone treatment in those for whom no response occurs after 3 days[19] goes against published literature[20] and is potentially harmful, as described later.

Table 1 shows potential complications masked by or associated with prolonged glucocorticoid treatment and secondary prevention measures.[6,16] Although the risk for infection and neuromuscular weakness is not increased during low-to-moderate–dose prolonged glucocorticoid treatment (reviewed later), implementation of secondary prevention measures is still crucial for several reasons.

Infection Surveillance

Failed or delayed recognition of nosocomial infections in the presence of a blunted febrile response represents a serious threat to the recovery of patients undergoing prolonged glucocorticoid treatment. In two randomized trials[6,16] that incorporated infection surveillance, nosocomial infections were frequently identified in the absence of fever. The infection surveillance protocol incorporated bronchoscopy with bilateral BAL at 5- to 7-day intervals in intubated patients (without contraindication), and a systematic diagnostic protocol when patients developed clinical and laboratory signs suggestive of infection in the absence of fever.[21] It is important to emphasize (as discussed later) that contrary to popular opinion "stress-dose" corticosteroids actually reduce the acquisition of secondary (nosocomial) infections.[18]

Increased Risk for Neuromuscular Weakness With Neuromuscular Blocking Agents

The combination of glucocorticoids and neuromuscular blocking agents versus glucocorticoids alone significantly increases the risk for prolonged neuromuscular weakness.[22,23] Therefore, using neuromuscular blocking agents is strongly discouraged in patients undergoing concomitant glucocorticoid treatment, particularly when other risk factors are present (eg, sepsis, aminoglycosides).

Glucocorticoid Treatment Can Impair Glycemic Control

The use of a continuous infusion of a glucocorticoid has been reported to result in better glycemic control with less variability of blood glucose concentration.[24,25] This finding may be clinically relevant because studies have shown that an oscillating blood glucose level is associated with greater oxidative injury than sustained

Table 1
Potential complications associated with prolonged glucocorticoid treatment and secondary prevention measures

Potential Complications	Secondary Preventative Measures
Glucocorticoids blunt the febrile response, leading to failed or delayed recognition of nosocomial infections	Surveillance BAL sampling at 5- to 7-day intervals in intubated patients Systematic diagnostic protocol if patient develops signs of infection
Glucocorticoids given in combination with neuromuscular blocking agents increase the risk of prolonged neuromuscular weakness	Avoid concomitant use of neuromuscular blocking agents
Glucocorticoids given as an intermittent bolus produce glycemic variability	After an initial bolus, administer glucocorticoids as a constant infusion
Rapid glucocorticoid tapering is associated with rebound inflammation and clinical deterioration	Slow taper over 9–12 days During and after taper, monitor C-reactive protein and clinical variables; if patient deteriorates escalate to prior dosage or restart treatment
Suppression of endogenous cortisol synthesis	Avoid concomitant use of etomidate, which causes further suppression of cortisol synthesis

Abbreviation: BAL, bronchoalveolar lavage.

hyperglycemia.[26] Several reports indicate that glucose variability may be an independent predictor of outcome in critically ill patients.[27] A continuous infusion of glucocorticoid may, however, result in greater suppression of the HPA axis, necessitating a slower taper.

Avoidance of Rebound Inflammation

Ample evidence[9,28–34] shows that early removal of glucocorticoid treatment may lead to rebound inflammation and an exaggerated cytokine response to endotoxin.[35] Experimental work has shown that short-term exposure of alveolar macrophages[36] or animals to dexamethasone is followed by enhanced inflammatory cytokine response to endotoxin.[37] Similarly, normal human subjects pretreated with hydrocortisone had significantly higher tumor necrosis factor α (TNF-α) and IL-6 response after endotoxin challenge compared with controls.[38] Two potential mechanisms may explain rebound inflammation: homologous downregulation and glucocorticoid-induced adrenal insufficiency. Glucocorticoid treatment downregulates the glucocorticoid receptor levels in most cell types, thereby decreasing efficacy of the treatment.[39] Downregulation occurs at both the transcriptional and translational level, and hormone treatment decreases receptor half-life by approximately 50%.[39] In experimental animals, overexpression of glucocorticoid receptors improves resistance to endotoxin-mediated septic shock, whereas blockade increases mortality.[40] No study to date has investigated recovery of glucocorticoid receptor levels and function after prolonged glucocorticoid treatment in patients with sepsis or ARDS.

REVIEW OF EXPERIMENTAL STUDIES

Several studies using animal models of lung injury have shown that glucocorticoids, if given simultaneously with or before the experimental insult, decrease morbidity and mortality.[41] Although systemic methylprednisolone or dexamethasone improved pulmonary inflammation,[42] prophylactic treatment (30 min before injury) did not attenuate acute lung injury (ALI).[43] Methylprednisolone at a dose of 10 mg/kg, starting on day 5 after infection with reovirus, and given daily until the end of the time course of the disease, also did not attenuate the infiltration of inflammatory leukocytes, cytokine/chemokine expression, or the development of fibrotic changes in the lungs.[44] Conversely, Rocco and colleagues[45] observed that an early single dose of corticosteroid was able to adequately regulate the remodeling process in paraquat-induced ALI resulting in improved lung mechanics.

Additionally, in experimental ALI, prolonged glucocorticoid administration decreases edema and lung collagen formation, whereas early withdrawal rapidly negates the positive effects of therapy in experimental ALI.[28–30] Limiting steroid treatment to the first 6 days after ALI enhances accumulation of collagen after discontinuing therapy, whereas continuing treatment through day 12 has an alleviating effect.[29] In contrast, Silva and colleagues[46] reported that early short-term, low-dose methylprednisolone is as effective as prolonged therapy in inducing lung parenchyma repair in ALI. These conflicting results may be attributed to the experimental ALI model, the intensity of lung injury, and the type or modes of steroid delivery.

Many factors trigger ALI/ARDS, and differences in the initial insult combined with underlying conditions may result in the activation of different inflammatory mechanisms.[47] For example, Leite-Junior and colleagues[48] hypothesized that steroid treatment might act differently in models of pulmonary or extrapulmonary ALI, with similar mechanical compromise. They observed that methylprednisolone is effective at inhibiting fibrogenesis independent of the cause of ALI, but its ability to attenuate inflammatory responses and lung mechanical changes varies according to the cause of ALI. Overall, these experimental studies suggest that glucocorticoids may be used in specific conditions, such as in a small dose early in the course of ALI/ARDS and (in pulmonary ALI/ARDS. Additionally, these studies show that premature discontinuation of treatment leads to rebound inflammation and fibroproliferation.

PROLONGED GLUCOCORTICOID TREATMENT IN ALI/ARDS

Controlled trials have prospectively evaluated whether early initiation of glucocorticoid treatment prevents progression of the temporal continuum of systemic inflammation in patients with or at risk for ARDS.[49,50] A prospective controlled study (N = 72) found that the intraoperative intravenous administration of 250 mg of methylprednisolone just before pulmonary artery ligation during pneumonectomy reduced the incidence of postsurgical ARDS (0% vs 13.5%; $P<.05$) and duration of hospital stay (6.1 vs 11.9 days; $P = .02$).[49] Early treatment with hydrocortisone in patients with severe CAP prevented progression to septic shock (0% vs 43%; $P = .001$) and ARDS (0% vs 17%; $P = .11$),[51] and in patients with early ARDS, prolonged methylprednisolone treatment prevented progression to respiratory failure requiring mechanical ventilation (42% vs 100%; $P = .02$)[50] or to unresolving ARDS (8% vs 36%; $P = .002$).[16] These results contrast with the negative findings of older trials investigating a time-limited (24–48 h) massive daily dose of glucocorticoids.[52]

REVIEW OF CONTROLLED CLINICAL STUDIES

Eight controlled studies (five randomized controlled trials and three cohorts) have evaluated the effectiveness of prolonged glucocorticoid treatment initiated before day 14 of early ALI/ARDS (N = 334)[16,50,51,53] and late ARDS (N = 235),[6,15,54–56] and were the subject of two recent meta-analyses (limited to studies that have investigated prolonged treatment).[14,57] The methodologic quality of these studies was fair.[14,57] **Table 2** shows the effect on inflammation and important patient-centered outcome variables. These trials consistently reported that treatment-induced reduction in systemic inflammation[6,15,16,51,53,54,56] was associated with significant improvement in P_{AO_2}:F_{IO_2},[6,15,16,51,53,54,56] and significant reductions in multiple organ dysfunction score,[6,15,16,51,54,56] duration of mechanical ventilation,[6,15,16,50,51,53] and intensive care unit (ICU) length of stay (all with *P* values <.05).[6,15,16,50,51] The aggregate of these consistently reproducible findings shows that desirable effects (see **Table 2**) clearly outweigh undesirable effects and provide a strong (grade 1B) level of evidence that the sustained antiinflammatory effect achieved during prolonged glucocorticoid treatment accelerates resolution of ARDS, leading to earlier removal of mechanical ventilation. The low cost of off-patent methylprednisolone (approximately $240 for 28 days of intravenous therapy in the United States[16]) makes this treatment globally and equitably available.

Four of the five randomized trials provided Kaplan-Meier curves for continuation of mechanical ventilation, and each showed a twofold or greater rate of extubation in the first 5 to 7 days of treatment.[6,15,16,51] In the ARDS Network trial, the treated group had a 9.5-day reduction in duration of mechanical ventilation before treatment discontinuation (14.1 ± 1.7 vs 23.6 ± 2.9; $P = .006$) and more patients discharged home after initial weaning (62% vs 49%; $P = .006$).[15] Meta-analysis of randomized trials[58] showed a sizable increase in mechanical ventilation–free days (weighted mean difference, 6.58 days; 95% CI, 2.93–10.23; $P<.001$) and ICU-free days (weighted mean difference, 7.02 days; 95% CI, 3.20–10.85; $P<.001$) that was threefold greater than the one reported with low tidal volume ventilation[59] or conservative fluid management.[60] Little or no evidence of heterogeneity was seen across the studies. Reduction in duration of mechanical ventilation and ICU stay translates into tangible cost savings.

As shown in **Fig. 1**, glucocorticoid treatment initiated before day 14 of ARDS was associated with a marked reduction in the risk of death (RR, 0.68; 95% CI: 0.56–0.81; $P<.001$; degree of heterogeneity [I^2], 56%). Although the pooled studies had significant heterogeneity, subgroup and meta-regression analyses showed that heterogeneity had minimal effect on treatment efficacy.[14] Nevertheless, as a result of the marked differences in study design and patient characteristics and the limited size of the studies (<200 patients), the cumulative mortality summary of these studies should be interpreted with some caution. Therefore, a recent consensus statement recommended early initiation of prolonged glucocorticoid treatment for patients with severe ARDS (P_{AO_2}:F_{IO_2}<200 on positive end-expiratory pressure 10 cm H_2O) and before day 14 for patients with unresolving ARDS, grading the evidence for a survival benefit as weak (grade 2B).[4] The ARDS Network trial reported that treated patients had increased mortality when randomized after day 14 of ARDS (8% vs 35%; $P = .01$).[15] This subgroup (n = 48), however, had large differences in baseline characteristics, and the mortality difference lost significance ($P = .57$) when the analysis was adjusted for these imbalances.[61] Therefore, evidence is lacking that treatment initiated after 14 days is associated with worse outcome, and therefore this treatment should not be negated in the subgroup of patients with physiologic evidence of unresolving ARDS.

MYTHS ABOUT COMPLICATIONS OF PROLONGED GLUCOCORTICOID TREATMENT

The most commonly cited and propagated myths that might temper enthusiasm for glucocorticoid treatment include increased risks of infection and neuromuscular weakness.[62,63] Substantial evidence has accumulated showing that systemic

Table 2
Prolonged glucocorticoid treatment initiated before day 14 of acute lung injury/acute respiratory distress syndrome

Study	Hospital Mortality[a]	Reduction in Inflammation	Improvement in PaO_2:FiO_2	Reduction in Duration of MV	Reduction in ICU stay	Rate of Infection
Early ALI/ARDS (≤3 d)	38% vs 62%	3 of 3	4 of 4	4 of 4	3 of 3	.30 vs .39
Confalonieri et al,[51] 2005 (n = 46)	0.0% vs 30%[b]	Yes	Yes	Yes	Yes	0 vs .17
Lee et al,[50] 2005 (n = 20)	8% vs 88%[b]	NR	Yes	Yes	Yes	.33 vs 0
Annane et al,[53] 2006[c] (n = 177)	64% vs 73%[c]	Yes	Yes	Yes	NR	14 vs .13
Meduri et al,[16] 2007 (n = 91)	24% vs 43%[b]	Yes	Yes	Yes	Yes	.63 vs 1.43
Unresolving ARDS (≥5 d)	26% vs 45%	5 of 5	5 of 5	2 of 3	2 of 3	.48 vs .51
Meduri et al,[6] 1998 (n = 22)	13% vs 57%[b]	Yes	Yes	Yes	Yes	0 vs NR
Varpula et al,[56] 2000 (n = 31)	19% vs 20% (30 days)	Yes	Yes	No	No	.56 vs .33
Huh et al,[54] 2002 (n = 48)	43% vs 74%[b]	Yes	Yes	NR	NR	NR
Steinberg et al,[15] 2006 (n = 132)	27% vs 36% (60 days)	Yes	Yes	Yes	Yes	.31 vs .47
Early and Unresolving ARDS	34% vs 55%	8 of 8	9 of 9	6 of 7	5 of 6	.38 vs .44

Abbreviations: ALI, acute lung injury; ARDS, acute respiratory distress syndrome; ICU, intensive care unit; MV, mechanical ventilation; NR, not reported.
Comparisons are reported as glucocorticoid-treated versus control.
[a] Mortality is reported as hospital mortality unless specified otherwise in parenthesis.
[b] Statistically significant reduction in mortality.
[c] Significant reduction in hospital mortality (P = .02) only for the subgroup of patients (n = 129) with relative adrenal insufficiency.

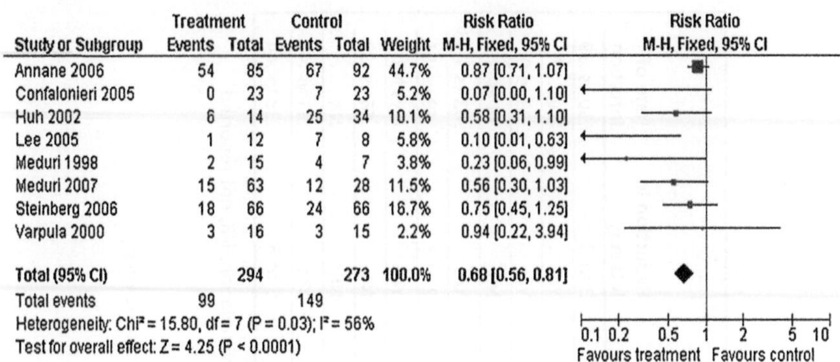

Study or Subgroup	Treatment Events	Treatment Total	Control Events	Control Total	Weight	Risk Ratio M-H, Fixed, 95% CI
Annane 2006	54	85	67	92	44.7%	0.87 [0.71, 1.07]
Confalonieri 2005	0	23	7	23	5.2%	0.07 [0.00, 1.10]
Huh 2002	6	14	25	34	10.1%	0.58 [0.31, 1.10]
Lee 2005	1	12	7	8	5.8%	0.10 [0.01, 0.63]
Meduri 1998	2	15	4	7	3.8%	0.23 [0.06, 0.99]
Meduri 2007	15	63	12	28	11.5%	0.56 [0.30, 1.03]
Steinberg 2006	18	66	24	66	16.7%	0.75 [0.45, 1.25]
Varpula 2000	3	16	3	15	2.2%	0.94 [0.22, 3.94]
Total (95% CI)		**294**		**273**	**100.0%**	**0.68 [0.56, 0.81]**
Total events	99		149			

Heterogeneity: Chi² = 15.80, df = 7 (P = 0.03); I² = 56%
Test for overall effect: Z = 4.25 (P < 0.0001)

Fig. 1. Effects of prolonged glucocorticoid treatment on ARDS survival. Df, degree of freedom; I^2, degree of heterogeneity; M-H, Mantel-Haenszel test.

inflammation is also implicated in the pathogenesis of these complications,[64–66] suggesting that treatment-induced downregulation of systemic inflammation could theoretically prevent, or partly offset, their development or progression.

Glucocorticoid Treatment Does Not Increase Infection Risk

Contrary to older studies investigating a time-limited (24–48 h) massive daily dose of glucocorticoids (methylprednisolone, up to 120 mg/kg/d),[67,68] recent trials investigating "stress-dose" glucocorticoids have not reported an increased rate of nosocomial infections.[69–71] The effect of glucocorticoids on immune suppression is critically dose-dependent. Experience with organ transplants has proven that high-dose corticosteroids effectively abolish T-cell–mediated immune responsiveness and are very effective in preventing/treating graft rejection. However, although stress-doses of corticosteroids downregulate (but do not suppress) systemic inflammation with decreased transcription of proinflammatory mediators, they maintain innate and Th1 immune responsiveness and prevent an overwhelming compensatory antiinflammatory response.[34,72]

In fact, new cumulative evidence indicates that downregulation of life-threatening systemic inflammation with prolonged low-to-moderate dose glucocorticoid treatment improves innate immunity[34,72] and provides an environment less favorable to the intracellular and extracellular growth of bacteria.[73] At stress doses, corticosteroids have been shown to increase neutrophil activity,[72] increase the homing of dendritic cells with preservation of monocyte function,[74] preserve IL-12 function, and attenuate the overwhelming inflammatory response. In the ARDS Network study, corticosteroid treatment was associated with a reduction in nosocomial pneumonia.[15] These data are supported by the HYPOLYTE study,[18] which randomized patients with multiple trauma to hydrocortisone or placebo. The major end point of this study, hospital-acquired pneumonia, was significantly reduced in the patients randomized to hydrocortisone (35.6% vs 51.3%; *P* = .007).

Glucocorticoid Treatment Does Not Increase the Risk of Neuromuscular Weakness

The incidence of neuromuscular weakness is similar in patients treated with or without prolonged glucocorticoids (17% vs 18%).[57] Two recent studies found no association between prolonged glucocorticoid treatment and electrophysiologically or clinically proven neuromuscular dysfunction.[75,76] Given that neuromuscular dysfunction is an independent predictor of prolonged weaning,[77] and ARDS randomized trials have consistently reported a significant reduction in duration of mechanical ventilation,[6,15,16,51,53] clinically relevant neuromuscular dysfunction caused by glucocorticoid or glucocorticoid-induced hyperglycemia seems highly unlikely. The combination of glucocorticoids and neuromuscular blocking agents significantly increases the risk for prolonged neuromuscular weakness compared with steroids alone.[22]

GLUCOCORTICOIDS IN CAP

Similar to ALI/ARDS, current pathophysiologic understanding places dysregulated systemic inflammation, characterized by persistent elevation in circulating inflammatory cytokine levels over time, as the key pathogenetic process contributing to morbidity and mortality in CAP. Two research findings are relevant to the rationale for prolonged glucocorticoid treatment in CAP. First, higher levels of inflammatory cytokines at hospital admission (acute phase of hospitalized pneumonia) correlate with worse short-term (hospital) and long-term[13,78] morbidity and mortality. Second, even when patients survive hospital admission, inflammatory cytokines remain elevated for weeks after clinical resolution of pneumonia, and IL-6 levels at hospital discharge correlate with subsequent 1-year mortality.[78]

A limited number of trials have investigated glucocorticoid treatment in patients with pneumonia (not severe)[79–82] and severe pneumonia (**Fig. 2**). Preliminary small trials[16,51,83,84] have shown evidence of efficacy in patients with severe pneumonia admitted to the ICU (CAP subgroup with high mortality), and a large Cooperative Study Program Study (CSP #574 ESCAPe) is currently studying the effect of prolonged (20 days) methylprednisolone in patients with severe pneumonia admitted to the ICU. The literature for patients without severe pneumonia, however, is limited to small inconclusive trials (n = 469) conducted over a span of 54 years.[79–82] Because these small studies included patients with low acute mortality risk (6%), evidence of a short-term mortality benefit is lacking.[79–82] Two older trials (involving treatment for 5–7 days)[79,81] and a more recent one (3-day treatment)[82] reported faster clinical

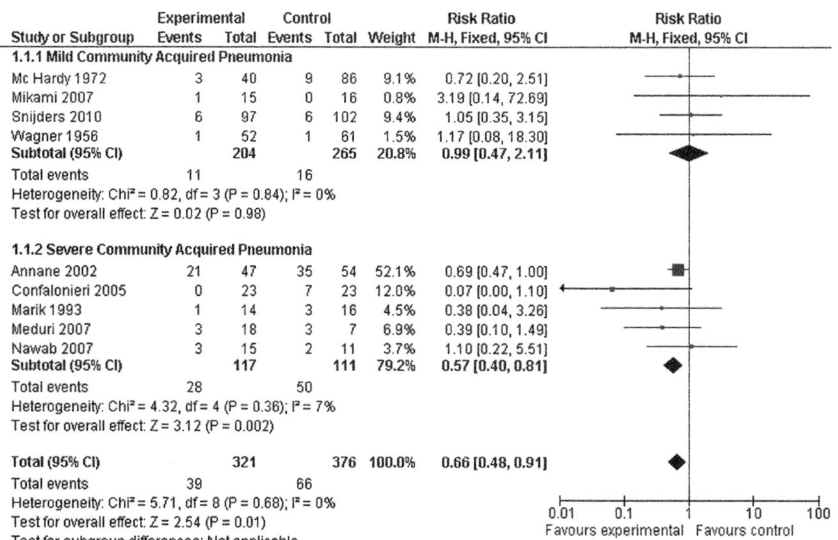

Study or Subgroup	Experimental Events	Experimental Total	Control Events	Control Total	Weight	Risk Ratio M-H, Fixed, 95% CI
1.1.1 Mild Community Acquired Pneumonia						
Mc Hardy 1972	3	40	9	86	9.1%	0.72 [0.20, 2.51]
Mikami 2007	1	15	0	16	0.8%	3.19 [0.14, 72.69]
Snijders 2010	6	97	6	102	9.4%	1.05 [0.35, 3.15]
Wagner 1956	1	52	1	61	1.5%	1.17 [0.08, 18.30]
Subtotal (95% CI)		**204**		**265**	**20.8%**	**0.99 [0.47, 2.11]**
Total events	11		16			
Heterogeneity: Chi² = 0.82, df = 3 (P = 0.84); I² = 0%						
Test for overall effect: Z = 0.02 (P = 0.98)						
1.1.2 Severe Community Acquired Pneumonia						
Annane 2002	21	47	35	54	52.1%	0.69 [0.47, 1.00]
Confalonieri 2005	0	23	7	23	12.0%	0.07 [0.00, 1.10]
Marik 1993	1	14	3	16	4.5%	0.38 [0.04, 3.26]
Meduri 2007	3	18	3	7	6.9%	0.39 [0.10, 1.49]
Nawab 2007	3	15	2	11	3.7%	1.10 [0.22, 5.51]
Subtotal (95% CI)		**117**		**111**	**79.2%**	**0.57 [0.40, 0.81]**
Total events	28		50			
Heterogeneity: Chi² = 4.32, df = 4 (P = 0.36); I² = 7%						
Test for overall effect: Z = 3.12 (P = 0.002)						
Total (95% CI)		**321**		**376**	**100.0%**	**0.66 [0.48, 0.91]**
Total events	39		66			
Heterogeneity: Chi² = 5.71, df = 8 (P = 0.68); I² = 0%						
Test for overall effect: Z = 2.54 (P = 0.01)						
Test for subgroup differences: Not applicable						

Fig. 2. Forrest plot of survival in patients with mild versus severe CAP.

resolution[79,81] and less antibiotic use[82] but no impact on mortality. The most recent trial[80] included 213 patients but had serious limitations, including: (1) an uncommon and vague primary end point, (2) antibiotic coverage not in agreement with recent guidelines,[85] and (3) unusual daily glucocorticoid dosage.

Six studies have compared long-term outcomes in hospitalized patients with CAP versus a control population.[78,86–90] These studies consistently reported a decreased long-term survival among the patients with CAP compared with the control group, and mortality estimates were unchanged after adjusting for age and comorbidities.[78,87–89] Using a large dataset (Genetic and Inflammatory Markers of Sepsis Study) that included 1886 patients, Kellum and colleagues[12] and Yende and colleagues[78] reported that high levels of the circulating inflammatory cytokines TNF-α and IL-6 persisted 3 weeks after clinical resolution of CAP, and that degree of IL-6 elevation at hospital discharge predicted subsequent 90-day and 1-year mortality (one-third caused by cardiovascular disease).[78] Although glucocorticoids may have a limited role in decreasing acute mortality in patients without severe sepsis who are at a low risk of dying, reduction of systemic inflammation at hospital admission and discharge may positively affect long-term outcome and requires urgent research.

GLUCOCORTICOIDS AND *PNEUMOCYSTIS JIROVECI* PNEUMONIA

Pneumocystis jiroveci pneumonia (PCP) is the most common opportunistic pneumonia in patients with AIDS. Similar to CAP and ALI/ARDS, lung injury and respiratory impairment during pneumocystis pneumonia are mediated by marked host inflammatory responses to the organism.[91] Severe PCP is characterized by neutrophilic lung inflammation, and respiratory impairment and death are more closely correlated with the degree of lung inflammation than with the organism burden in pneumonia.[92] A meta-analysis of six randomized controlled trials (n = 489) investigating prolonged glucocorticosteroid treatment in patients with AIDS with PCP and hypoxemia provided evidence of safety and a mortality benefit. Mortality at 1 month (treated vs control) was 13% versus 21% (RR, 0.56, 95% CI, 0.32–0.98; *P* = .04; I^2, 43%); mortality at 3 months was 18% versus 27% (RR, 0.68, 95% CI, 0.50–0.94; *P* = .02; I^2, 0%).[93] Consensus guidelines, based on the findings of these trials, recommended a 21-day oral regimen of prednisone in patients with PCP and hypoxemia ($Po_2 \leq 70$ mm Hg).[94] After the introduction of prolonged glucocorticoid treatment in PCP, the long-term prognosis for patients with AIDS substantially improved, leading to reinstatement of life support in medical ICUs.[93]

GLUCOCORTICOIDS AND SEVERE H1N1 PNEUMONIA

The use of corticosteroids in patients with severe H1N1 pneumonia is controversial. The rationale for using glucocorticoids is that H1N1 pneumonia is associated with a cytokine storm with severe pulmonary inflammation.[95,96] The main cause of death in patients with H1N1 is severe respiratory failure with extensive diffuse alveolar damage (DAD), necrotizing bronchiolitis, and DAD with intense alveolar hemorrhage.[97] Furthermore, corticosteroids do not seem to increase the viral load when patients are concomitantly treated with antiviral agents (oseltamivir).[98] Despite the World Health Organization (WHO) statement that for severely ill patients with H1N1, "high dose systemic corticosteroids…are not recommended for use outside of the context of clinical trials,"[99] recent data suggest that approximately 30% of patients admitted to an ICU with ARDS from H1N1 are treated with corticosteroids.[100] An initial report of 13 patients with suspected H1N1 pneumonia and ARDS reported a significant improvement in lung injury and multiple organ dysfunction scores after initiation of prospectively designed protocol-driven glucocorticoid treatment.[101] However, three large cohort retrospective studies from Europe and Asia suggest that in patients with severe H1N1 infection, nonprotocolized treatment with corticosteroids may increase mortality.[102–104] The only proper method for assessing the efficacy and safety of any drug for any disease is a randomized, double-blind trial. Registries and retrospective cohorts usually have the goal of describing the natural history of a disease rather than investigating interventions that may otherwise vary widely. They cannot allow an adequate minimization of selection and confusion biases in the evaluation of drug efficacy or safety, even when based on propensity score analysis.[105] After more than half a century of using corticosteroids for severe infections or ARDS, no single randomized trial has shown increased mortality or increased superinfection. Therefore, in the absence of a randomized controlled trial, an evidence-based recommendation cannot to made.

GLUCOCORTICOIDS AND ACID-ASPIRATION PNEUMONITIS

Aspiration pneumonitis is best defined as acute lung injury following the aspiration of regurgitated gastric contents.[106] This syndrome occurs in patients with a marked disturbance of consciousness such as drug overdose, seizures, massive cerebrovascular accident, following head trauma and anesthesia. Corticosteroids have been used in the management of aspiration pneumonitis since 1955.[107] However, limited data exists on which to evaluate the role of these agents, with only a single prospective, placebo-controlled study having been performed. In this study, Sukumaran and colleagues[108] randomized 60 patients with "aspiration pneumonitis" to methylprednisolone (15 mg/kg/d for 3 days) or placebo. Patients were subdivided into two groups; a younger group with drug overdose as the predominant diagnosis and an older group with neurologic disorders. Radiographic changes improved quicker in the steroid group, as did oxygenation. The number of ventilator and ICU days was significantly shorter in the overdose patients who received corticosteroids, however, these variables were longer in the neurologic group. There was no significant difference in the incidence of complications or outcome. The results of this study are somewhat difficult to interpret as it is likely that the patients in the overdose group had true "acid aspiration pneumonitis" while many patients in the neurologic group probably developed "aspiration pneumonia."[106] Wolfe and colleagues[109] performed a case controlled study of 43 patients with aspiration pneumonitis of whom 25 received high dose corticosteroids (approximately 600 mg prednisolone/day) for 4 days. While there was no difference in mortality, secondary gram-negative pneumonia was reported to be more frequent in the steroid group (7/20 vs 0/13); however, ventilator days tended to be less in this group (4.3 vs 9.8 days). Based on this limited data it is not possible to make evidence based recommendations on the use of corticosteroids in patients with acid aspiration pneumonia.

RECOMMENDATIONS FOR GLUCOCORTICOID TREATMENT OF ARDS

The authors have reviewed data showing that the drug dosage, timing and duration of administration, weaning protocol, and implementation of secondary preventive measures largely determine the risk/benefit profile of glucocorticoid treatment in ARDS. **Table 3** shows treatment regimens for early and unresolving ARDS. In agreement with a recent consensus statement from the American College of Critical Care Medicine,[4] the results of one randomized trial in patients with early severe ARDS[16] indicate that 1 mg/kg/d of methylprednisolone given as an infusion and tapered over 4 weeks is associated with a favorable risk/benefit profile when secondary

Table 3
Methylprednisolone treatment of early ARDS and unresolving ARDS

Time	Administration form	Dosage
Early severe ARDS (PaO_2:FiO_2 <200 on positive end-expiratory pressure 10 cm H_2O)		
Loading	Bolus over 30 min	1 mg/kg
Days 1–14[abc]	Infusion at 10 mL/h	1 mg/kg/d
Days 15–21[ac]	Infusion at 10 mL/h	0.5 mg/kg/d
Days 22–25[ac]	Infusion at 10 mL/h	0.25 mg/kg/d
Days 26–28[ac]	Infusion at 10 mL/h	0.125 mg/kg/d
Unresolving ARDS (less than one-point reduction in lung injury score by day 7 of ARDS)		
Loading	Bolus over 30 min	2 mg/kg
Days 1–14[abc]	Infusion at 10 mL/h	2 mg/kg/d
Days 15–21[ac]	Infusion at 10 mL/h	1 mg/kg/d
Days 22–25[ac]	Infusion at 10 mL/h	0.5 mg/kg/d
Days 26–28[ac]	Infusion at 10 mL/h	0.25 mg/kg/d
Days 29–30[ac]	Bolus over 30 min	0.125 mg/kg/d

The dosage is adjusted to ideal body weight and rounded up to the nearest 10 mg (ie, 77 mg rounded up to 80 mg). The infusion is obtained by adding the daily dosage to 240 mL of normal saline.

[a] Five days after the patient is able to ingest medications, methylprednisolone is administered by mouth in one single daily equivalent dose. Enteral absorption of methylprednisolone is compromised for days after extubation. Prednisone (available in 1-mg, 5-, 10-, and 20-mg strengths) can be used in place of methylprednisolone.

[b] If between days 1 and 14 the patient is extubated, the patient is advanced to day 15 of drug therapy and tapered according to schedule.

[c] When the patient leaves the ICU, if still not tolerating enteral intake for at least 5 days, the dosage specified should be given but divided into two doses and given every 12 hours via intravenous push until tolerating ingestion of medications by mouth.

preventive measures are implemented. For patients with unresolving ARDS, beneficial effects were shown for treatment (methylprednisolone, 2 mg/kg/d) initiated before day 14 of ARDS and continued for at least 2 weeks after extubation.[6,15] If treatment is initiated after day 14, no evidence has shown either benefit or harm.[14,61] Treatment response should be monitored with daily measurement of lung injury and multiple-organ dysfunction syndrome scores and C-reactive protein level.

Secondary prevention is important to minimize complications. Glucocorticoid treatment should be administered as a continuous infusion (while the patient is in the ICU) to minimize glycemic variations.[25,110] When given concurrently with glucocorticoids, two medications are strongly discouraged and, when possible, should be avoided: neuromuscular blocking agents for minimizing the risk of neuromuscular weakness[22] and etomidate to suppress cortisol synthesis.[111] Glucocorticoid treatment blunts the febrile response; therefore, infection surveillance is essential to promptly identify and treat nosocomial infections. Finally, in agreement with a recent consensus statement from the American College of Critical Care Medicine,[4] a slow glucocorticoid dosage reduction (9–12 days) after a complete course allows recovery of the number of glucocorticoid receptors and the HPA axis, thereby reducing the risk of rebound inflammation. Laboratory evidence of physiologic deterioration (ie, worsening PaO_2:FiO_2) associated with rebound inflammation (increased serum C-reactive protein) after the completion of glucocorticoid treatment may require its reinstitution.

SUMMARY

This article presented a rationale for the use of glucocorticoid treatment in ARDS. Based on molecular mechanisms and physiologic data, a strong association between dysregulated inflammation and progression of ARDS has been established. Furthermore, these data support a strong association between prolonged treatment with exogenous glucocorticoids leading to downregulation of the inflammatory response, improvement in organ physiology (lung injury and multiple-organ dysfunction syndrome scores), and resolution of ARDS. The available clinical trials of prolonged glucocorticoid treatment show favorable effects on clinical outcomes, including ventilator-free days, ICU-free days, and mortality. Currently, glucocorticoids are not recommended in patients with CAP who are at a low risk of dying and those with severe H1N1 infection. Research investment is needed to identify subgroup of patients with ALI/ARDS who are more likely to respond to treatment and to improve on active monitoring of the inflammatory response.

REFERENCES

1. Rubenfeld GD, Caldwell E, Peabody E, et al. Incidence and outcomes of acute lung injury. N Engl J Med 2005;353:1685–93.
2. Angus DC, Clermont G, Linde-Zwirble WT, et al. Healthcare costs and long-term outcomes after acute respiratory distress syndrome: a phase III trial of inhaled nitric oxide. Crit Care Med 2006;34:2883–90.
3. Meduri GU, Muthiah MP, Carratu P, et al. Nuclear factor-kappaB- and glucocorticoid receptor alpha- mediated mechanisms in the regulation of systemic and pulmonary inflammation during sepsis and acute respiratory distress syndrome. Evidence for inflammation-induced target tissue resistance to glucocorticoids. Neuroimmunomodulation 2005;12:321–38.
4. Marik PE, Pastores SM, Annane D, et al. Recommendations for the diagnosis and management of corticosteroid insufficiency in critically ill adult patients: consensus statements from an international task force by the American College of Critical Care Medicine. Crit Care Med 2008;36:1937–49.
5. Meduri GU, Tolley EA, Chrousos GP, et al. Prolonged methylprednisolone treatment suppresses systemic inflammation in patients with unresolving acute respiratory distress syndrome: evidence for inadequate endogenous glucocorticoid secretion and inflammation-induced immune cell resistance to glucocorticoids. Am J Respir Crit Care Med 2002;165:983–91.
6. Meduri GU, Headley S, Golden E, et al. Effect of prolonged methylprednisolone therapy in unresolving acute respiratory distress syndrome. A randomized controlled trial. JAMA 1998;280:159–65.
7. Meduri GU, Yates CR. Systemic inflammation-associated glucocorticoid resistance and outcome of ARDS. Ann N Y Acad Sci 2004;1024:24–53.
8. Meduri GU, Headley S, Tolley E, et al. Plasma and BAL cytokine response to corticosteroid rescue treatment in late ARDS. Chest 1995;108:1315–25.
9. Meduri GU, Tolley EA, Chinn A, et al. Procollagen types I and III aminoterminal propeptide levels during acute respiratory distress syndrome and in response to methylprednisolone treatment. Am J Respir Crit Care Med 1998;158:1432–41.
10. Meduri GU, Headley S, Kohler G, et al. Persistent elevation of inflammatory cytokines predicts a poor outcome in ARDS. Plasma IL-1 beta and IL-6 levels are consistent and efficient predictors of outcome over time. Chest 1995;107:1062–73.

11. Meduri GU, Kohler G, Headley S, et al. Inflammatory cytokines in the BAL of patients with ARDS. Persistent elevation over time predicts poor outcome. Chest 1995;108:1303–14.
12. Kellum JA, Kong L, Fink MP, et al. Understanding the inflammatory cytokine response in pneumonia and sepsis: results of the Genetic and Inflammatory Markers of Sepsis (GenIMS) Study. Arch Intern Med 2007;167:1655–63.
13. Lekkou A, Karakantza M, Mouzaki A, et al. Cytokine production and monocyte HLA-DR expression as predictors of outcome for patients with community-acquired severe infections. Clin Diagn Lab Immunol 2004;11:161–7.
14. Meduri GU, Marik PE, Chrousos GP, et al. Steroid treatment in ARDS: a critical appraisal of the ARDS network trial and the recent literature. Intensive Care Med 2008;34:61–9.
15. Steinberg KP, Hudson LD, Goodman RB, et al; The Acute Respiratory Distress Syndrome Network. Efficacy and safety of corticosteroids for persistent acute respiratory distress syndrome. N Engl J Med 2006;354:1671–84.
16. Meduri GU, Golden E, Freire AX, et al. Methylprednisolone infusion in patients with early severe ARDS: results of a randomized trial. Chest 2007;131:954–63.
17. Henzen C, Suter A, Lerch E, et al. Suppression and recovery of adrenal response after short-term high-dose glucocorticoid treatment. Lancet 2000; 355:542–5.
18. Roquilly A, Mahe PJ, Seguin P, et al. Hydrocortisone therapy for corticosteroid insufficiency related to trauma. The HYPOLYT study. JAMA 2011;305:1201–9.
19. Diaz JV, Brower R, Calfee CS, et al. Therapeutic strategies for severe acute lung injury. Crit Care Med 2010;38:1644–50.
20. Meduri GU, Chinn AJ, Leeper KV, et al. Corticosteroid rescue treatment of progressive fibroproliferation in late ARDS. Patterns of response and predictors of outcome. Chest 1994;105:1516–27.
21. Meduri GU, Mauldin GL, Wunderink RG, et al. Causes of fever and pulmonary densities in patients with clinical manifestations of ventilator-associated pneumonia. Chest 1994;106:221–35.
22. Leatherman JW, Fluegle WL, David WS, et al. Muscle weakness in mechanically ventilated patients with severe asthma. Am J Respir Crit Care Med 1996;153: 1686–90.
23. Behbehani NA, al Mane F, D'yachkova Y, et al. Myopathy following mechanical ventilation for acute severe asthma: the role of muscle relaxants and corticosteroids. Chest 1999;115:1627–31.
24. Weber-Carstens S, Deja M, Bercker S, et al. Impact of bolus application of low-dose hydrocortisone on glycemic control in septic shock patients. Intensive Care Med 2007;33:730–3.
25. Loisa P, Parviainen I, Tenhunen J, et al. Effect of mode of hydrocortisone administration on glycemic control in patients with septic shock: a prospective randomized trial. Crit Care 2007;11:R21.
26. Ceriello A, Esposito K, Piconi L, et al. Oscillating glucose is more deleterious to endothelial function and oxidative stress than mean glucose in normal and type 2 diabetic patients. Diabetes 2008;57:1349–54.
27. Egi M, Bellomo R, Stachowski E, et al. Variability of blood glucose concentration and short-term mortality in critically ill patients. Anesthesiology 2006;105: 244–52.
28. Hesterberg TW, Last JA. Ozone-induced acute pulmonary fibrosis in rats. Prevention of increased rates of collagen synthesis by methylprednisolone. Am Rev Respir Dis 1981;123:47–52.

29. Hakkinen PJ, Schmoyer RL, Witschi HP. Potentiation of butylated-hydroxytoluene-induced acute lung damage by oxygen. Effects of prednisolone and indomethacin. Am Rev Respir Dis 1983;128:648–51.
30. Kehrer JP, Klein-Szanto AJ, Sorensen EM, et al. Enhanced acute lung damage following corticosteroid treatment. Am Rev Respir Dis 1984;130:256–61.
31. Ashbaugh DG, Maier RV. Idiopathic pulmonary fibrosis in adult respiratory distress syndrome. Diagnosis and treatment. Arch Surg 1985;120:530–5.
32. Hooper RG, Kearl RA. Established ARDS treated with a sustained course of adrenocortical steroids. Chest 1990;97:138–43.
33. Briegel J, Jochum M, Gippner-Steppert C, et al. Immunomodulation in septic shock: hydrocortisone differentially regulates cytokine responses. J Am Soc Nephrol 2001;12(Suppl 17):S70–4.
34. Keh D, Boehnke T, Weber-Cartens S, et al. Immunologic and hemodynamic effects of "low-dose" hydrocortisone in septic shock: a double-blind, randomized, placebo-controlled, crossover study. Am J Respir Crit Care Med 2003; 167:512–20.
35. Barber AE, Coyle SM, Fischer E, et al. Influence of hypercortisolemia on soluble tumor necrosis factor receptor II and interleukin-1 receptor antagonist responses to endotoxin in human beings. Surgery 1995;118:406–10.
36. Broug-Holub E, Kraal G. Dose- and time-dependent activation of rat alveolar macrophages by glucocorticoids. Clin Exp Immunol 1996;104:332–6.
37. Fantuzzi G, Demitri MT, Ghezzi P. Differential effect of glucocorticoids on tumour necrosis factor production in mice: up-regulation by early pretreatment with dexamethasone. Clin Exp Immunol 1994;96:166–9.
38. Barber AE, Coyle SM, Marano MA, et al. Glucocorticoid therapy alters hormonal and cytokine responses to endotoxin in man. J Immunol 1993;150:1999–2006.
39. Schaaf MJ, Cidlowski JA. Molecular mechanisms of glucocorticoid action and resistance. J Steroid Biochem Mol Biol 2002;83:37–48.
40. Cooper MS, Stewart PM. Adrenal insufficiency in critical illness. J Intensive Care Med 2007;22:348–62.
41. Fernandes AB, Zin WA, Rocco PR. Corticosteroids in acute respiratory distress syndrome. Braz J Med Biol Res 2005;38:147–59.
42. Cheney FW Jr, Huang TH, Gronka R. Effects of methylprednisolone on experimental pulmonary injury. Ann Surg 1979;190:236–42.
43. Kuwabara K, Furue S, Tomita Y, et al. Effect of methylprednisolone on phospholipase A(2) activity and lung surfactant degradation in acute lung injury in rabbits. Eur J Pharmacol 2001;433:209–16.
44. London L, Majeski EI, Altman-Hamamdzic S, et al. Respiratory reovirus 1/L induction of diffuse alveolar damage: pulmonary fibrosis is not modulated by corticosteroids in acute respiratory distress syndrome in mice. Clin Immunol 2002;103:284–95.
45. Rocco PR, Souza AB, Faffe DS, et al. Effect of corticosteroid on lung parenchyma remodeling at an early phase of acute lung injury. Am J Respir Crit Care Med 2003;168:677–84.
46. Silva PL, Garcia CS, Maronas PA, et al. Early short-term versus prolonged low-dose methylprednisolone therapy in acute lung injury. Eur Respir J 2009;33: 634–45.
47. Rocco PR, Pelosi P. Pulmonary and extrapulmonary acute respiratory distress syndrome: myth or reality? Curr Opin Crit Care 2008;14:50–5.
48. Leite-Junior JH, Garcia CS, Souza-Fernandes AB, et al. Methylprednisolone improves lung mechanics and reduces the inflammatory response in pulmonary

but not in extrapulmonary mild acute lung injury in mice. Crit Care Med 2008;36: 2621–8.

49. Cerfolio RJ, Bryant AS, Thurber JS, et al. Intraoperative solumedrol helps prevent postpneumonectomy pulmonary edema. Ann Thorac Surg 2003;76: 1029–33.
50. Lee HS, Lee JM, Kim MS, et al. Low-dose steroid therapy at an early phase of postoperative acute respiratory distress syndrome. Ann Thorac Surg 2005;79: 405–10.
51. Confalonieri M, Urbino R, Potena A, et al. Hydrocortisone infusion for severe community-acquired pneumonia: a preliminary randomized study. Am J Respir Crit Care Med 2005;171:242–8.
52. Peter JV, John P, Graham PL, et al. Corticosteroids in the prevention and treatment of acute respiratory distress syndrome (ARDS) in adults: meta-analysis. BMJ 2008;336:1006–9.
53. Annane D, Sebille V, Bellissant E. Effect of low doses of corticosteroids in septic shock patients with or without early acute respiratory distress syndrome. Crit Care Med 2006;34:22–30.
54. Huh J, Lim C, Jegal Y. The effect of steroid therapy in patients with late ARDS. Tuberculosis Respir Dis 2002;52:376–84.
55. Keel JB, Hauser M, Stocker R, et al. Established acute respiratory distress syndrome: benefit of corticosteroid rescue therapy. Respiration 1998;65: 258–64.
56. Varpula T, Pettila V, Rintala E, et al. Late steroid therapy in primary acute lung injury. Intensive Care Med 2000;26:526–31.
57. Tang BM, Craig JC, Eslick GD, et al. Use of corticosteroids in acute lung injury and acute respiratory distress syndrome: a systematic review and meta-analysis. Crit Care Med 2009;37:1595–603.
58. Meduri GU, Annane D, Chrousos G, et al. Activation and regulation of systemic inflammation in ARDS. Rationale for prolonged glucocorticoid therapy. Chest 2009;136:1631–44.
59. Ventilation with lower tidal volumes as compared with traditional tidal volumes for acute lung injury and the acute respiratory distress syndrome. The Acute Respiratory Distress Syndrome Network. N Engl J Med 2000;342:1301–8.
60. Wiedemann HP, Wheeler AP, Bernard GR, et al; National Heart, Lung, and Blood Institute Acute Respiratory Distress Syndrome (ARDS) Clinical Trials Network. Comparison of two fluid-management strategies in acute lung injury. N Engl J Med 2006;354:2564–75.
61. Thompson BT, Ancukiewics M, Hudson LD, et al. Steroid treatment for persistent ARDS: a word of caution [letter]. Crit Care 2007;11:425.
62. Sprung CL, Brezis M, Goodman S, et al. Corticosteroid therapy for patients in septic shock: some progress in a difficult decision. Crit Care Med 2011;39: 571–4.
63. Sprung CL, Goodman S, Weiss YG. Steroid therapy of septic shock. Crit Care Clin 2010;25:825–34.
64. Pustavoitau A, Stevens RD. Mechanisms of neurologic failure in critical illness. Crit Care Clin 2008;24:1–24.
65. Headley AS, Tolley E, Meduri GU. Infections and the inflammatory response in acute respiratory distress syndrome. Chest 1997;111:1306–21.
66. Meduri GU. Clinical review: a paradigm shift: the bidirectional effect of inflammation on bacterial growth. Clinical implications for patients with acute respiratory distress syndrome. Crit Care 2002;6:24–9.

67. Weigelt JA, Norcross JF, Borman KR, et al. Early steroid therapy for respiratory failure. Arch Surg 1985;120:536–40.
68. Bernard GR, Luce JM, Rinaldo JE, et al. High-dose corticosteroids in patients with the adult respiratory distress syndrome. N Engl J Med 1987;317:1565–70.
69. Sligl WI, Milner DA, Sundarr S, et al. Safety and efficacy of corticosteroids for the treatment of septic shock: a systematic review and meta-analysis. Clin Infect Dis 2009;49:93–101.
70. Annane D, Bellissant E, Bollaert P, et al. Corticosteroids in the treatment of severe sepsis and septic shock in adults: a systematic review. JAMA 2009; 301:2349–61.
71. Moran JL, Graham PL, Rockliff S, et al. Updating the evidence for the role of corticosteroids in severe sepsis and shock: a Bayesian meta-analytic perspective. Crit Care 2010;14:R134.
72. Kaufmann I, Briegel J, Schliephake F, et al. Stress doses of hydrocortisone in septic shock: beneficial effects on opsonization-dependent neutrophil functions. Intensive Care Med 2008;34:344–9.
73. Meduri GU, Kanangat S, Bronze M, et al. Effects of methylprednisolone on intracellular bacterial growth. Clin Diagn Lab Immunol 2001;8:1156–63.
74. Webster JI, Tonelli L, Sternberg EM. Neuroendocrine regulation of immunity. Annu Rev Immunol 2002;20:125–63.
75. Stevens RD, Dowdy DW, Michaels RK, et al. Neuromuscular dysfunction acquired in critical illness: a systematic review. Intensive Care Med 2007;33:1876–91.
76. Hough CL, Steinberg KP, Taylor Thompson B, et al. Intensive care unit-acquired neuromyopathy and corticosteroids in survivors of persistent ARDS. Intensive Care Med 2009;35:63–8.
77. De Jonghe B, Bastuji-Garin S, Sharshar T, et al. Does ICU-acquired paresis lengthen weaning from mechanical ventilation? Intensive Care Med 2004;30: 1117–21.
78. Yende S, DAngelo G, Kellum JA, et al. Inflammatory markers at hospital discharge predict subsequent mortality after pneumonia and sepsis. Am J Respir Crit Care Med 2008;177:1242–7.
79. Wagner HN, Bennett IL, Lasagna L, et al. The effect of hydrocortisone upon the course of pneumococcal pneumonia treated with penicillin. Bull Johns Hopkins Hosp 1956;98:197–215.
80. Snijders D, Daniels JM, de Graaff CS, et al. Efficacy of corticosteroids in community-acquired pneumonia: a randomized double-blinded clinical trial. Am J Respir Crit Care Med 2010;181:975–82.
81. McHardy VU, Schonell ME. Ampicillin dosage and use of prednisolone in treatment of pneumonia: co-operative controlled trial. Br Med J 1972;4:569–73.
82. Mikami K, Suzuki M, Kitagawa H, et al. Efficacy of corticosteroids in the treatment of community-acquired pneumonia requiring hospitalization. Lung 2007; 185:249–55.
83. Nawab Q, Golden E, Confalonieri M, et al. Glucocorticoid treatment in severe community-acquired pneumonia. Am J Respir Crit Care Med 2007;175:A594.
84. Annane D, Sebille V, Charpentier C, et al. Effect of treatment with low doses of hydrocortisone and fludrocortisone on mortality in patients with septic shock. JAMA 2002;288:862–71.
85. Niederman MS, Mandell LA, Anzueto A, et al. Guidelines for the management of adults with community-acquired pneumonia. Diagnosis, assessment of severity, antimicrobial therapy, and prevention. Am J Respir Crit Care Med 2001;163: 1730–54.

86. Koivula I, Sten M, Makela PH. Prognosis after community-acquired pneumonia in the elderly: a population-based 12-year follow-up study. Arch Intern Med 1999;159:1550–5.
87. Bordon J, Wiemken T, Peyrani P, et al. Decrease in long-term survival for hospitalized patients with community-acquired pneumonia. Chest 2010;138:279–83.
88. Yende S, Angus DC, Ali IS, et al. Influence of comorbid conditions on long-term mortality after pneumonia in older people. J Am Geriatr Soc 2007;55:518–25.
89. Kaplan V, Clermont G, Griffin MF, et al. Pneumonia: still the old man's friend? Arch Intern Med 2003;163:317–23.
90. Mortensen EM, Kapoor WN, Chang CC, et al. Assessment of mortality after long-term follow-up of patients with community-acquired pneumonia. Clin Infect Dis 2003;37:1617–24.
91. Thomas CF Jr, Limper AH. Pneumocystis pneumonia. N Engl J Med 2004;350: 2487–98.
92. Limper AH, Offord KP, Smith TF, et al. Pneumocystis carinii pneumonia. Differences in lung parasite number and inflammation in patients with and without AIDS. Am Rev Respir Dis 1989;140:1204–9.
93. Briel M, Bucher HC, Boscacci R, et al. Adjunctive corticosteroids for Pneumocystis jiroveci pneumonia in patients with HIV-infection. Cochrane Database Syst Rev 2006;3:CD006150.
94. Consensus statement on the use of corticosteroids as adjunctive therapy for pneumocystis pneumonia in the acquired immunodeficiency syndrome. The National Institutes of Health-University of California Expert Panel for Corticosteroids as Adjunctive Therapy for Pneumocystis Pneumonia. N Engl J Med 1990; 323:1500–4.
95. Bermejo-Martin JF, de Lejarazu RO, Pumarola T, et al. Th1 and Th17 hypercytokinemia as early host response signature in severe pandemic influenza. Crit Care 2009;13:R201.
96. de Jong MD, Simmons CP, Thanh TT, et al. Fatal outcome of human influenza A (H5N1) is associated with high viral load and hypercytokinemia. Nat Med 2006; 12:1203–7.
97. Mauad T, Hajjar LA, Callegari GD, et al. Lung pathology in fatal novel human influenza A (H1N1) infection. Am J Respir Crit Care Med 2010;181:72–9.
98. Confalonieri M, D'Agaro P, Campello C. Corticosteroids do not cause harmful increase of viral load in severe H1N1 virus infection. Intensive Care Med 2010;36(10):1780–1.
99. World Health Organization. Clinical management of human infection with pandemic (H1N1) 2009: revised guidance. Available at: http://www.who.int/csr/resources/publications/swineflu/clinical_management_h1n1.pdf. Accessed April 13, 2011.
100. Delaney JW, Fowler RA. 2009 Influenza A (H1N1): a clinical review. Hosp Pract 2010;38:74–81.
101. Quisepe-Laime AM, Bracco JD, Barberio PA, et al. H1N1 influenza A virus-associated acute lung injury: response to combination oseltamivir and prolonged corticosteroid treatment. Intensive Care Med 2010;36:33–41.
102. Brun-Buisson C, Richard JC, Mercat A, et al. Early corticosteroids in severe influenzae A/H1N1 pneumonia and acute respiratory distress syndrome. Am J Respir Crit Care Med 2011;183(9):1200–6.
103. Martin-Loeches I, Lisboa T, Rhodes A, et al. Use of corticosteroid therapy in patients affected by severe pandemic H1N1v Influenzae A infection. Intensive Care Med 2011;37(2):272–83.

104. Kim SH, Hong SB, Yun SC, et al. Corticosteroid treatment in critically ill patients with pandemic influenza A/H1N1 infection: analytic strategy using propensity scores. Am J Respir Crit Care Med 2011;183(9):1207–14.
105. Annane D. Pro: the illegitimate crusade against corticosteroids for severe H1N1 pneumonia. Am J Respir Crit Care Med 2011;183(9):1125–6.
106. Marik PE. Aspiration Pneumonitis and Pneumonia: a clinical review. N Engl J Med 2001;344:665–72.
107. Haussmann W, Lunt RL. Problem of treatment of peptic aspiration pneumonia following obstetric anesthesia (Mendelson's syndrome). J Obstet Gynaecol Br Commonw 1955;62:509–12.
108. Sukumaran M, Granada MJ, Berger HW, et al. Evaluation of corticosteroid treatment in aspiration of gastric contents: a controlled clinical trial. Mt Sinai J Med 1980;47:335–40.
109. Wolfe JE, Bone RC, Ruth WE. Effects of corticosteroids in the treatment of patients with gastric aspiration. Am J Med 1977;63:719–22.
110. Weber-Carstens S, Keh D. Bolus or continuous hydrocortisone—that is the question. Crit Care 2007;11:113.
111. Cuthbertson BH, Sprung CL, Annane D, et al. The effects of etomidate on adrenal responsiveness and mortality in patients with septic shock. Intensive Care Med 2009;35:1868–76.

Extracorporeal CO_2 Removal in ARDS

James E. Lynch, MD[a], Don Hayes Jr, MD, MS[b], Joseph B. Zwischenberger, MD[c,*]

KEYWORDS

• Acute respiratory distress syndrome • Carbon dioxide removal
• Mechanical ventilation • Gas exchange

Currently, the only therapeutic maneuver shown to decrease mortality in acute respiratory distress syndrome (ARDS) is low tidal volume ventilation.[1,2] Conversely, high tidal volume ventilation is associated with increased mortality. The primary goal of respiratory support should be therapies that can minimize the requirement for high tidal volumes and airway pressures and provide lung rest. Extracorporeal membrane oxygenation (ECMO) provides near-total gas exchange (oxygen [O_2] and carbon dioxide [CO_2]) in both infants and adults[3–5]; however, application of this technology involves significant blood-surface interactions that may exacerbate lung injury.[5,6] In addition, ECMO is labor intensive, time limited, costly, and requires expensive equipment and a highly sophisticated team.

This article discusses the functional properties and management techniques of CO_2 removal and intracorporeal membrane oxygenation and provides a glimpse into the future of long-term gas-exchange devices. Recent trends in ventilator management dictated limited inflation pressure and tidal volume often at the cost of increasing systemic arterial CO_2 levels. This technique, often synonymous with permissive hypercapnia, has been shown to reduce the incidence of baro/volutrauma and high airway pressures and improve survival in ARDS.[7–12] Unfortunately, permissive hypercapnia is limited by respiratory acidosis causing substantial changes in hemodynamics and organ blood flow unless arterial pH is controlled.[8–13]

Financial disclosure: Drs Lynch and Hayes have nothing to disclose. Dr Zwischenberger currently receives grant monies from Ikaria, MC3, and the National Institutes of Health; receives royalties from Avalon for his patent for a double-lumen cannula; and is a consultant to Novalung.
Funding statement: No funding was required to complete this work.

[a] Division of General Surgery, Department of Surgery, University of Kentucky College of Medicine, University of Kentucky Medical Center, 800 Rose Street, C-226, Lexington, KY 40517, USA
[b] Department of Pediatrics, University of Kentucky College of Medicine, University of Kentucky Medical Center, 800 Rose Street, C-424, Lexington, KY 40536, USA
[c] Department of Surgery, University of Kentucky College of Medicine, University of Kentucky Medical Center, 800 Rose Street, MN-264, Lexington, KY 40536-0298, USA
* Corresponding author.
E-mail address: jzwis2@email.uky.edu

Crit Care Clin 27 (2011) 609–625
doi:10.1016/j.ccc.2011.05.002 **criticalcare.theclinics.com**

HISTORY OF EXTRACORPOREAL CO_2 REMOVAL FOR ARDS

Investigations into extracorporeal CO_2 removal ($ECCO_2R$) began in the late 1970s. Kolobow and Gattinoni introduced $ECCO_2R$ using a modified form of ECMO with venovenous (VV) perfusion.[14–16] Their focus was CO_2 removal allowing for a reduction in ventilatory support. Oxygenation was maintained by simple diffusion across the patient's alveoli, called *apneic oxygenation*, using low-frequency positive pressure ventilation. Unfortunately, the $ECCO_2R$ system required all of the components of a standard ECMO circuit. Studies in animals[14,15] and in humans[17–19] demonstrated $ECCO_2R$'s effectiveness in reducing ventilatory requirements. Despite the early success shown by $ECCO_2R$, a small randomized study conducted at a single center comparing $ECCO_2R$ with mechanical ventilation showed no difference in mortality.[20] Although the results of this study were disappointing for some investigators, others began to look for simpler CO_2 removal devices that would offer the benefits of gentle ventilation without all of the risks of ECMO or $ECCO_2R$.

The use of a simple arteriovenous (AV) shunt for extracorporeal gas exchange significantly reduces the complexity of conventional ECMO yet allows sufficient gas exchange to achieve near-total removal of CO_2 produced. By reducing and eliminating circuit length and complexity, several complications associated with conventional ECMO are eliminated.[21] The use of an AV shunt with fewer circuit components allows for less-intensive monitoring and avoidance of an extracorporeal pump, substantially lowers cost, and improves safety compared with conventional ECMO.[22–24]

Our lab developed a technique of simplified extracorporeal $AVCO_2$ removal ($AVCO_2R$) with a new-generation, low-resistance, commercially available, hollow fiber gas exchanger to provide lung rest in the setting of severe respiratory failure.[25] The extremely low resistance of the $AVCO_2R$ gas exchange device (<10 mm Hg pressure difference) allows blood flows of as much as 25% of an animal's cardiac output (>1300 mL/min). The cannulae used became the determinants of flow and are small in comparison to those required for typical adult ECMO patients (12F arterial and 16F venous). Groin access to the common femoral artery and femoral vein is the preferred route of vascular access. Commercially available kits allow for percutaneous insertion of these small cannulae. The prime volume of the circuit is only 200 mL and allows for crystalloid priming, avoiding the need for blood priming a circuit that is typically necessary in ECMO. Based on large animal short-term studies, $AVCO_2R$ seemed be a simple and effective treatment to achieve lung rest while minimizing ventilatory support.[26,27] Likewise, despite a 20% to 26% cardiac shunt through the $AVCO_2R$ circuit for 7 days, there was no instability in the hemodynamic profile, specifically in heart rate, cardiac output, mean arterial pressure, pulmonary arterial pressure, or Qb.[28,29]

$AVCO_2R$, however, does not provide substantial oxygen transfer when the Pao_2 level is adequate because inflow to the device is already saturated (>90%) with an O_2 carrying capacity close to maximum. There is a small direct transfer (<10%) and some benefit related to the increased $AVCO_2R$ content of the mixed venous blood reaching the pulmonary precapillary bed, which may result in a slight alteration in the normal vasoconstrictive response to local hypoxia with a resultant reduction in the pulmonary shunt.[30]

ANIMAL MODEL OF EXTRACORPOREAL CO_2 REMOVAL FOR ARDS

To establish a clinically relevant model of severe respiratory failure in adult sheep with a 40% total body surface area, full-thickness cutaneous flame burn, and smoke inhalation injury, we developed a smoke dose-dependent model of ARDS of predictable severity.[31] Using the combined smoke inhalation injury and cutaneous burn model of severe respiratory failure, we evaluated percutaneous $AVCO_2R$ and its effect on ventilator dependent days and survival. When animals met entry criteria for ARDS (Pao_2/fraction of inspired oxygen [Fio_2] <200 within 40–48 hours of injury), they were randomized to either $AVCO_2R$ or sham. With percutaneous $AVCO_2R$ removing 90% of the CO_2 produced, significant reductions were allowed in minute ventilation (13 to 1.6 L/min), tidal volume (450 to 270 mL), peak inspiratory pressure (25 to 14 cm H_2O), respiratory rate (25 to 16 breaths/min), and FiO_2 (0.86 to 0.34) whereas normocapnia was maintained.

Along with the decreased ventilatory requirements associated with $AVCO_2R$, there was a concomitant improvement in arterial oxygenation (**Fig. 1**). The Pao_2/FiO_2 ratio improved to greater than 300 by 72 hours. $AVCO_2R$ also allowed animals to be weaned from mechanical ventilation almost 3 times earlier than SHAM survivors (2.4 days of mechanical ventilation vs 6.2 days, respectively). All animals receiving $AVCO_2R$ and only 3 in the SHAM group survived the 7-day study.

Clinical Trials—$AVCO_2R$

In our initial clinical experience with $AVCO_2R$,[32] 5 patients were treated for ARDS and CO_2 retention at the University of Texas Medical Branch and the Louisiana State University Medical Center. Feasibility and safety of $AVCO_2R$ by percutaneous femoral cannulation (10–12 Fr arterial and 12–15 Fr venous) was evaluated in a 72-hour trial. Mean $AVCO_2R$ flow at 24, 48, and 72 hours was 837.4 ± 73.9 mL/min, 873 ± 83.6 mL/min, and 750 ± 104.5 mL/min, respectively, without vascular complications and no significant change in heart rate or mean arterial pressure. $AVCO_2R$ proved capable of removing a maximum of 208 mL/min of CO_2, at a Qb of 1086 mL/min. This allowed a decrease in minute ventilation from 7.2 ± 2.3 L/min, at baseline, to 3.4 ± 0.8 L/min at 24 hours. $PaCO_2$ at baseline was 93.6 ± 9.0 mm Hg and on initiation of $AVCO_2R$ decreased to 69.0 ± 10.0 mm Hg. $AVCO_2R$ removed approximately 70% of total

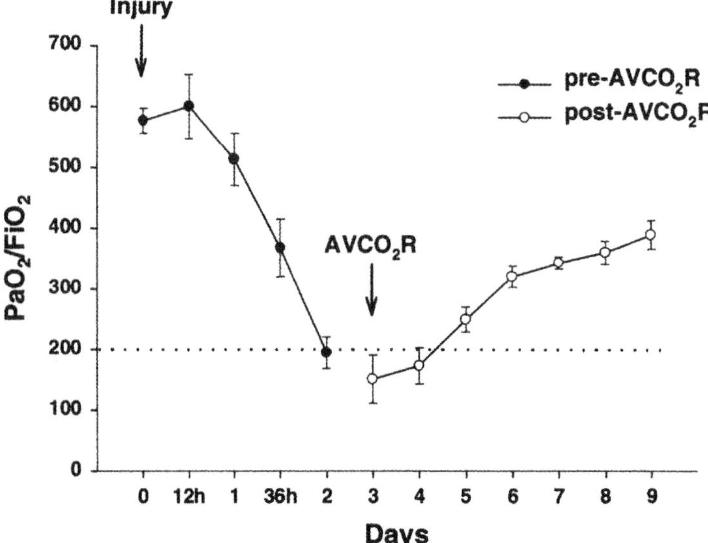

Fig. 1. Pao_2/FiO_2 ratio after smoke inhalation and cutaneous flame burn injury and after placement of $AVCO_2R$. Entry criteria (P/F <200) were met at 48 hours (194.8 ± 25.9). At the time, $AVCO_2R$ was initiated P/F was 151.5 ± 40.0. After 36 hours, P/F had improved to >200 and after 72 hours P/F was >300 (320.0 ± 17.8).

CO_2 production throughout the 72 hours of the study (**Fig. 2**). Oxygenation was successfully managed with gentle ventilation and near-apneic oxygenation. All patients survived the procedure without adverse sequelae and only minor complications. This initial study demonstrated that percutaneous $AVCO_2R$ can achieve approximately 70% CO_2 removal in adults with ARDS and CO_2 retention without hemodynamic compromise or instability.

Pumpless Extracorporeal Lung Assist and Novalung

The success of these early $AVCO_2R$ studies led to a steady increase in the interest and use of $AVCO_2R$ devices in Europe: the pumpless extracorporeal lung assist (PECLA), Novalung, and interventional lung assist (ILA).

To test the ability of the Novalung to be used in a situation where near-complete lung rest is needed, in vivo experiments using the Novalung with a bronchoalveolar lavage lung injury pig model and apneic oxygenation were performed. ILA showed a marked decrease in $PaCO_2$ and increase in Pao_2 without a significant difference in systolic and mean blood pressure from the control group (ILA clamped).[33–35]

Clinical Trials—PECLA and Novalung

The PECLA device was applied in 1800 patients for artificial lung assistance with relative ease of use and low cost.[36] It was proved clinically effective at oxygenation and CO_2 removal in a study of 70 patients with severe respiratory failure of various etiologies.[37] One institution completed a 10-year review study of patients who had been treated with PECLA for severe respiratory insufficiency. The study resulted in 159 total patients, between 7 and 78 years of age, and a cumulative experience of over 1300 days on the ILA device. During therapy, the overall mortality was 48.7% and mostly attributed to multiorgan failure. Only 3% of the patients in this study were unable to have their pulmonary function stabilized, and after PECLA therapy was completed, the 30-day mortality was 13.6%.[38]

There are several case reports, retrospective analyses, and prospective studies that have validated the PECLA for use as a therapeutic measure for CO_2 removal. The

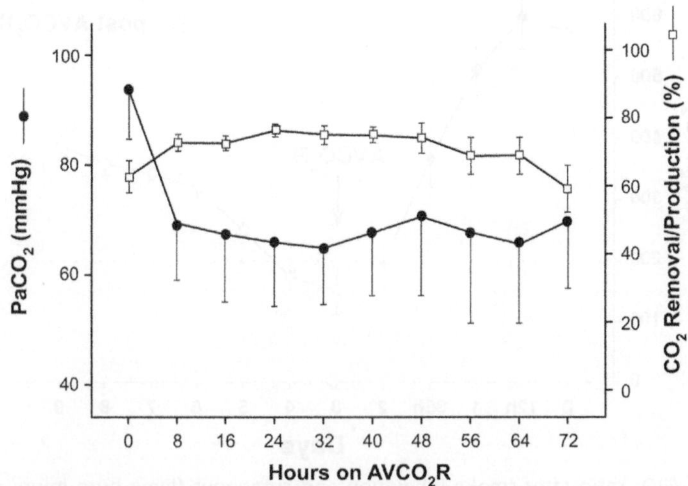

Fig. 2. At baseline, $PaCO_2$ was 93.6 ± 9.0 mm Hg and decreased to 69.0 ± 10.0 mm Hg on initiation of $AVCO_2R$. $AVCO_2R$ removed approximately 70% of total CO_2 production throughout the 72 hours of the study.

cases of respiratory failure in which Novalung has been reported efficacious include, but are not limited to, acute severe asthma[39]; support of influenza patients who require mechanical ventilation[40,41]; neurosurgery patients with repeated intracranial bleeds[42]; as an assist device for interhospital transfers of patients with severe, life-threatening acute respiratory failure[43,44]; as a bridge to lung transplant in patients with end-stage pulmonary hypertension or ventilator-refractory hypercapnia[45–48]; aiding in near-static ventilation in postpneumonectomy ARDS patients[49,50]; diffuse alveolar hemorrhage[51]; traumatic head injury patients[52]; an acute support measure in complex thoracic surgical procedures[53,54]; as a downgrade from ECMO to PECLA[55]; and for patients with ARDS.[56]

The most widely studied indication for the clinical use of Novalung is as a supportive therapy for patients with ARDS. In many studies, the PECLA system has proved superior to lung assist devices that require a pump because it significantly reduces the amount of mechanical blood trauma, bleeding, and hemolysis. The application of the Novalung facilitates the reversal of hypercapnia and stabilization of oxygenation. Due to its efficiency in removal of CO_2, the device allows maximized lung protection/rest and reduced incidence of ventilator-induced lung injury when combined with reduced tidal volumes ($\leq$4 mL/kg predicted body weight) and a high mean airway or positive end-expiratory pressure.

In all of these studies, the only reported complication to PECLA use is the chance for reversible distal limb ischemia.[56–69] A large cohort study, which included 96 patients with severe ARDS, evaluated the factors determining the efficacy of ILA and calculated its contributions to gas exchange by monitoring hemodynamic parameters, oxygen consumption, CO_2 production, and gas transfer through the device. Within 2 hours of Novalung therapy, Pao_2/FiO_2 ratio increased significantly, and a fast improvement in arterial CO_2 partial pressure and pH was observed in all patients. The PECLA removed 50% of the calculated total CO_2 production and rapidly normalized respiratory acidosis. As demonstrated in earlier studies, the patients who were on Novalung therapy were able to be ventilated with a protective lung strategy.[70]

Intravenacaval Oxygenation and CO_2 Removal with the Intravascular Oxygenator

The concept of an intravenacaval (intravascular) oxygenator and CO_2 removal device (IVOX) was originally conceived by Mortensen[71,72] as an intracorporeal gas exchange device in patients with ARDS. The IVOX consisted of multiple hollow fibers placed within the vena cava to provide blood oxygenation and CO_2 removal without the need for extracorporeal circulation or blood transfusion (**Fig. 3**). The fibers were joined together in a potted manifold that communicated with the dual-lumen gas conduit at both its proximal and distal ends. The fibers were silicone (Siloxone) coated and heparin bonded to create a thin true membrane on the previously porous hollow fibers.

The IVOX was first investigated in an ovine model that described the design features and delineated the experimental and potential clinical use. Implantation of the device did not adversely affect hemodynamic function nor was there evidence of significant hemolysis, thromboembolism, foaming in the blood, catheter migration, or venacaval intimal injury.[73–76] The significant reduction in foreign surface area as compared with ECMO resulted in fewer blood surface interactions, as evidenced by reduced pulmonary leukosequestration and complement activation.[77] In the initial design, IVOX was capable of removing up to 30% of CO_2 production in an ovine model (normal 150–180 mL/min) of severe smoke inhalation injury. The average CO_2 exchange was approximately 40 mL/min for size 7 IVOX and ranged from 30 mL/min to 55 mL/min.

The performance of the IVOX was limited in comparison to the natural lungs.[73] Our experience with the IVOX in animal and human studies demonstrated an average of 40

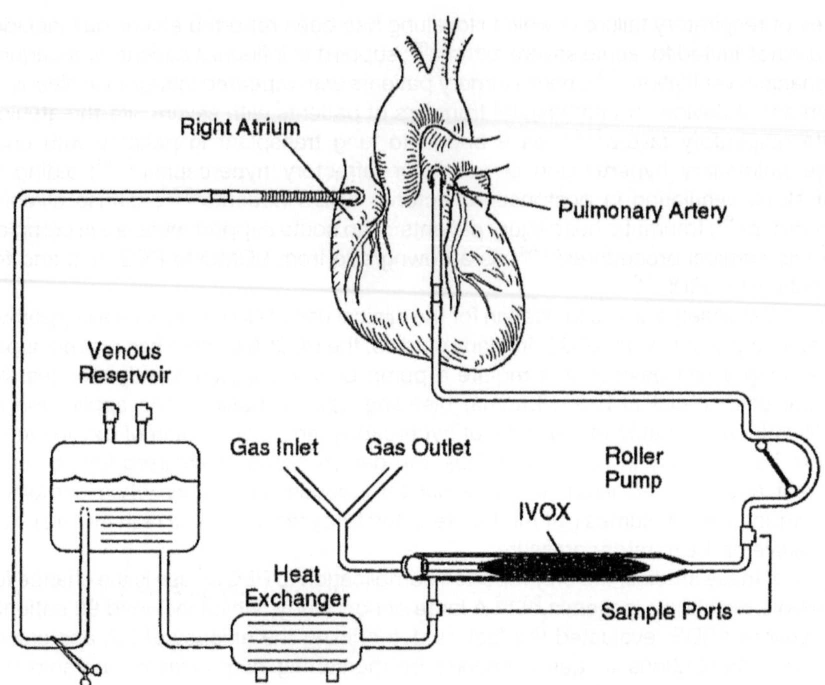

Fig. 3. Ivox circuit.

mL/min of CO_2 and O_2 exchange, approximately 25% to 30% of the metabolic demand of the patients implanted with the device.[74,75] Therefore, IVOX could not be used as a substitute for ECMO or provide total support for patients with acute respiratory failure.

An international, multicenter, phase I–II clinical trial of IVOX was conducted in major critical care centers in the United States and Europe. From February 1990 to May 1993, 164 IVOX devices were used in 160 patients as a means for temporary augmentation of gas exchange. These patients were considered to have developed severe, but potentially reversible, acute respiratory failure.[40]

Although overall survival of reported patients receiving IVOX was only 30%, survival was directly related to the severity of lung injury and patient selection. Unfortunately, there was no control arm to this study to evaluate improvement of survival with IVOX. Complications or adverse events associated with use of IVOX included mechanical and/or performance problems (29%), patient complications (bleeding, thrombosis, infection, venous occlusion, and arrhythmia), and user errors.

Based on the worldwide experience to date, IVOX demonstrated feasibility as a booster lung in patients with acute respiratory failure.[41–46] Gas exchange (usually 30% of the metabolic demands of the patients implanted with the device) can be achieved to allow a measurable reduction in ventilator settings. Improvements in design and engineering would be necessary for IVOX to become a more clinically applicable device.

The Intravascular Lung Assist Device

Vaslef and colleagues[77] developed an intravascular lung assist device (ILAD) by potting the membrane fibers into subunits of rosette-like layers, allowing the membrane surface area to increase up to 0.4 to 0.6 m^2 and blood flow perpendicular to the fibers without increasing the overall size for intravascular placement. Similar to IVOX, ILAD gas exchange efficiency increases with blood flow and gas pressure gradient across its membrane. In addition, it was shown that fibers arranged to allow cross-flow significantly increased gas exchange.

Although the device could achieve up to 100 mL/min of both O_2 and CO_2 exchange within the space of the vena cava in their in vitro studies, the blood pressure gradient needed to overcome the resistance of the device and achieve this gas exchange was high (23–105 mm Hg). Further attempts were made by the same group[78] to arrange the fibers in a helical or screw-like form. Unlike conventional devices, which depend on passive bulk blood flow around them, this pumping ILAD causes an active driving force for the blood when rotated.

The Hattler Respiratory Assist Catheter

Building on the lessons learned from the vitro testing of the IVOX, the Hattler catheter incorporates a small pulsating balloon into the middle of a hollow fiber bundle (**Fig. 4**). By testing a variety of balloon sizes and pulsation rates, it was determined that larger balloon volumes and higher pulsation rates increased both oxygen loading and CO_2 removal in a linear fashion in an in vitro model.[79]

Despite advances (described previously), the clinical translation of intravenous respiratory assist devices is still impeded by the insertion diameter of the catheter. The latest concepts in respiratory assist catheters that are being investigated are impeller percutaneous respiratory assist catheters, which incorporate rotating impellers within a stationary bundle of hollow fiber membranes (HFMs).

Decap

The latest device to enter the clinical arena is the Decap (Hemodec, Salerno, Italy). This system is essentially a modification of a continous VV hemodialysis machine (**Fig. 5**). Access is accomplished via a single double-lumen cannula inserted in the femoral vein. Blood flow is via a nonocclusive roller pump. Blood circulates through a membrane oxygenator then through a hemofilter. The ultrafiltrate from the hemofilter is recirculated into the pre–gas exchanger blood, increasing CO_2 removal.[80] This system's simplicity, although not allowing for total gas exchange, may allow for augmentation of CO_2 removal with a reduced need for high tidal volume ventilation. Only isolated case reports have been published; however, clinical trials are proposed.[48,80]

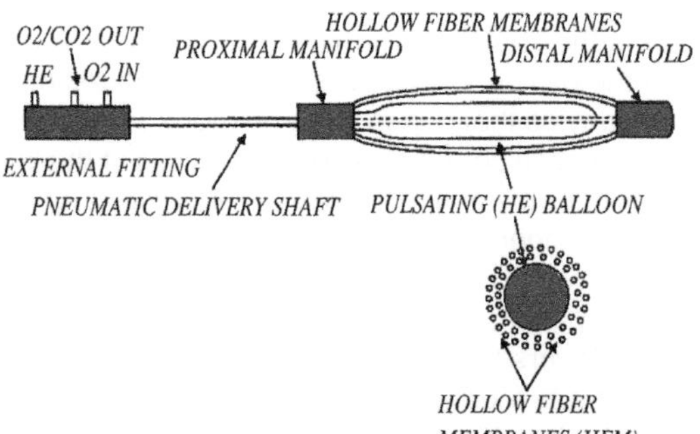

Fig. 4. Hattler catheter. Schematic of the Hattler catheter tested in the acute implants. HE, helium. (*From* Golob JF, Federspiel WJ, Merrill TL, et al. Acute in vivo testing of an intravascular respiratory support catheter. ASAIO J 2001;47:432–7; with permission.)

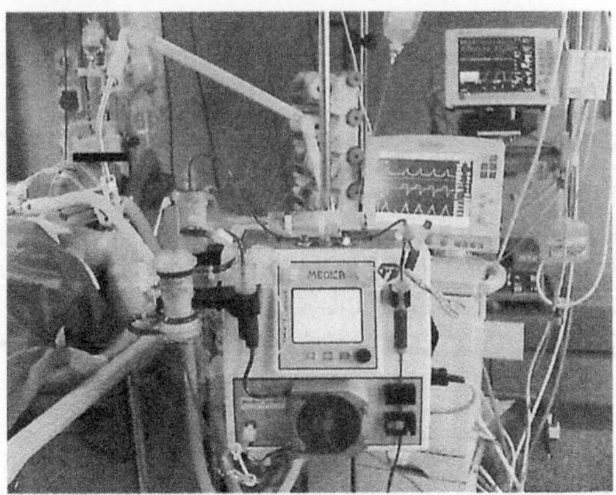

Fig. 5. $ECCO_2R$ device (Decap). The system consists of a standard continuous VV hemofiltration system equipped with a membrane lung with a total membrane surface of 0.33 m^2. (*From* Gramaticopolo S, Chronopoulos A, Piccinni P, et al. Extracorporeal CO_2 removal–a way to achieve ultraprotective mechanical ventilation and lung support: the missing piece of multiple organ support therapy. Contrib Nephrol 2010;165:174–84; with permission.)

Artificial Lungs

Long-term support for the failing lung has lagged behind that of the heart and kidney. Dialysis can provide years of support for those awaiting transplant, and modern ventricular assist devices have become an efficacious bridge to heart transplant or recovery, allowing for months of support. Although there are ECMO and extracorporeal lung assist devices ($AVCO_2R$ and PECLA) that have been applied to bridge lung transplant patients with some short-term success (approximately 1 month), no such long-term replacement device exists for the lungs. There is a need for a durable bridge to lung transplant because 30% of lung transplant candidates die while awaiting a suitable donor. Innovations in technologies with hemodynamic and hematologic compatibilities, such as prosthetic materials, pumps, membranes, and low-resistance oxygenators, must be achieved before the artificial lung can successfully move from the bench to the bedside.[81–88]

Controversy remains regarding the most effective configuration of an artificial lung. One current configuration being evaluated is pulmonary artery to left atrium (PA-LA). This configuration allows for partial support using a pumpless artificial lung. The pressure gradient between the mean pulmonary artery pressure and the left atrium provides flow through the device. Drawbacks to this configuration include unpredictability of flow through a device that depends on pulmonary vascular resistance, which can change dramatically over a short period of time; a loss of the lung vascular bed as a filter for clots; and, without the ability to create a shunt through the cannula, device malfunction or need for changeout involves considerable risk of systemic embolus or stroke.

In a hemodynamic study using a porcine model of the thoracic artificial lung (TAL) in parallel circulation (PA-LA) versus in-series pulmonary artery to pulmonary artery (PA-PA) to the natural lungs, it was found that the PA-LA configuration had lowered pulmonary system impedance, raised cardiac output, and provided the greatest TAL blood flow rate but reduced the natural lung blood flow rate, which could lead to serious cerebral embolic events in the long term.[89] In vivo sheep models have been used to study the effects of artificial lung compliance on right ventricular load, the durability of the PA-LA configuration of implantation, and the hemodynamic and functionality of the TAL in simulated pulmonary hypertension. A low-resistance but noncompliant artificial lung was found to increase pulmonary impedance and alter right ventricular function. The addition of a compliance chamber reduced pulse wave reflections and normalized ventricular function.[90] The TAL was discovered to be successfully implanted in the PA-LA configuration for 7 days, but improvements in the biocompatibility of the TAL are necessary to facilitate blood flow through the device for long periods of time.[91] In the pulmonary hypertension model, the TAL was found to not decrease cardiac output in rest or mild exercise, but it did not allow more vigorous exercise.[92]

Although the PA-LA configuration has not been approved for use in the United States, there are 2 case reports of its successful use in Europe. In the first case report, a PAL with PA-LA configuration was implanted in a 38-year-old woman with primary pulmonary hypertension. The patient was successfully supported for 62 days until an appropriate lung transplant was available.[93] The second patient had a pulmonary venoocculsive disease and was supported successfully for 18 days until he died from overwhelming sepsis.[94]

A PA-PA configuration uses the right heart as a pump. The device receives the total right ventricular output. This configuration was found to create an excessive amount of right heart strain resulting in a 50% incidence of right heart failure in early animal series.[81,95] To combat the right heart strain, an inflow compliance chamber was added to the low-resistance MC3 (Ann Arbor, MI, USA) prototype.[82] The addition of the compliance chamber caused the incidence of right heart failure to drop to 14% in the sheep model.[95] The ideal compliance of the chamber to maximize right heart function was found to be between 0.5 mL/mm Hg and 5 mL/mm Hg.[96] Technically, the modified compliance chamber achieved significant augmentation; however, the pulsatile third wave introduced into the delicate pulmonary artery caused severe hemorrhage. To try to diminish this effect, an optional active compliance chamber in a PA-PA PAL was studied in a sheep model. This device was unsuccessful due to the complexity in synchronizing the augmenting pulsations of the optional active compliance chamber with the cardiac cycle.[97] The PA-PA configuration would allow the artificial lung to be used in patients with elevated right heart pressures (pulmonary hypertension), but it would be a difficult surgery in humans. Sheep have long main pulmonary arteries (6 cm), which enables easy proximal and distal end-to-side anastomosis. The relatively short human pulmonary artery (2.5–3 cm) would require either dividing the main pulmonary artery with return of the blood postoxygenator to the transected main pulmonary artery or using a graft to the side of the main pulmonary artery and diverting all blood flow to the device and back to the right pulmonary artery. Unfortunately, either of these techniques requires CPB support and neither is an attractive long-term option.[82]

A third configuration being explored is the right atrium to pulmonary artery configuration. This configuration requires either integration or the coupling of the artificial lung to a pump. Functioning in a similar fashion to a right ventricular assist device, blood would flow from the right atrium to the device and be pumped into the main pulmonary artery. No CPB would be required for implant and removal, and temporary use of the native circulation would be possible to allow for device changeout. Two distinct approaches to this configuration have emerged. In one strategy, the pump and artificial lung are integrated. Through the use of centrifugal pumps with membrane fibers incorporated into the spinning disk, these all-in-one devices provide forward flow and gas exchange at the same time. Devices such as these have remained at the animal testing stage and have not received much interest in the past 5 years.

Another option for artificial lung configuration involves the use of a separate pump and oxygenator coupled together to power the device. Using a pulseless (axial or centrifugal) pump connected to an artificial lung, pump function and gas exchange function can be separated based on the needs of the patient. Drawbacks to this system include the increased complexity of 2 independent devices as well as the added bulk of a pump on the artificial lung. In vivo animal trials have been conducted to assess the safety and feasibility of obtaining total respiratory support using a pump-driven VV extracorporeal lung membrane attached through a single double-lumen cannula inserted in the femoral or jugular veins. In a pig study, the circuit successfully provided total respiratory support for 72 hours without inducing significant hemodynamic, coagulation, cellular, or inflammatory responses.[98]

Blood surface compatibility in the artificial lung provides a unique set of challenges. The blood contact with the prosthetic surfaces of artificial lungs causes extensive activation of molecular and cellular mediators of coagulation and inflammation that can lead to patient morbidity and mortality.[99,100] Methods tested to circumvent this issue include adhering endothelial cells to the microporous polypropylene HFMs[101] and modification of the HFM surface to promote endothelial cell attachment and growth.[102] Microfibricated biohybrid artificial lungs have also been created using poly(dimethylsiloxane) (PDMS) membranes. Successful seeding of endothelial cells on this membrane has provided a nonthrombogenic surface with adequate gas exchange properties.[103]

The fluid dynamics of a device also has a large impact on antithrombogenicity, gas exchange performance, and blood flow resistance. In recent years there have been many studies to elucidate the most effective flow configurations for artificial lungs. Areas of low flow were found to correlate with thrombus formation in animal studies, and microflow vectoral analysis could reliably predict problem areas for thrombus in artificial lung models.[104,105] The investigation in fluid dynamics of the artificial lung has now expanded to the development of microchannel technology, which has been used to design patterned PDMS membranes that allow adequate molecular diffusion and that are less prone to blockage.[106–109]

Palliation of end-stage lung disease patients with total or partial gas exchange devices remains a challenge. Short-term support can be accomplished currently with new generation hollow fiber oxygenation devices for up to weeks at a time. The length of time necessary for a device to be considered a bridge to transplant (6 months or longer) presents anticoagulation challenges that have not reached the stage of clinical trials. Also, many adverse events that must be dealt with will inevitably arise. Some of these include, but are not limited to, development of pulmonary hypertension from the constant barrage of small emboli to the lung bed and constant need for anticoagulation as well as low-level stimulation and complement activation. The goal of a bridge to transplant gas exchangers, although closer, remains mostly in animal testing phases. As materials and technologies continue to improve, the implantable artificial lung comes closer to a reality.

Ambulatory ECMO

Recent experiences have been described of patients ambulating on ECMO before lung transplantation.[110,111] Although this technique has not yet been applied to the ARDS patient population, the ability to perform total and near-total gas exchange through a simplified circuit should allow application to this population. The Avalon Elite cannula (Avalon Laboratories, Rancho Dominguez, CA, USA) is a highly efficient double-lumen ECMO cannula that allows for high blood flows with minimal recirculation and is placed under ultrasound guidance percutaneously at the bedside.[112] This

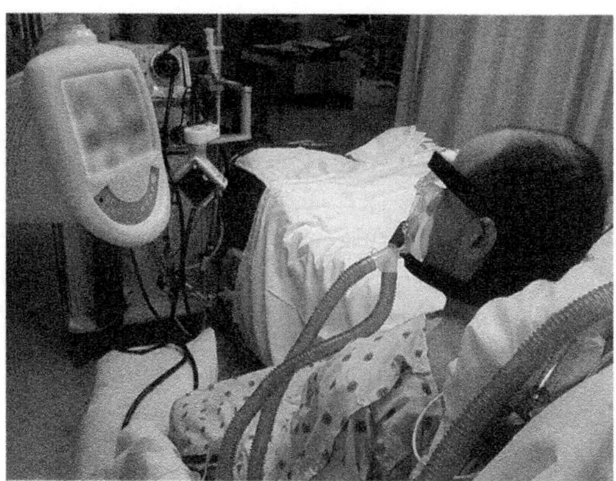

Fig. 6. Patient out of bed and awake with ECMO support. (*From* Mangi AA, Mason DP, Yun JJ, et al. Bridge to lung transplantation using short-term ambulatory extracorporeal membrane oxygenation. J Thorac Cardiovasc Surg 2010;140:713–5; with permission.)

single cannula approach to ECMO should allow even the sickest ARDS patient liberation from mechanical ventilation and the ability to ambulate (**Fig. 6**). Future studies are needed in this specific patient population.

SUMMARY

ARDS remains one of the most clinically vexing problems in critical care. As technology continues to evolve, it is likely that $ECCO_2R$ devices will become smaller, more efficient, and safer. As the risk of extracorporeal support decreases, their role for ARDS patients remains to be defined. Clinical trials assessing risk/benefit in this patient population are needed.

REFERENCES

1. Ventilation with lower tidal volumes as compared with traditional tidal volumes for acute lung injury and the acute respiratory distress syndrome. The Acute Respiratory Distress Syndrome Network. N Engl J Med 2000;342:1301–8.
2. Putensen C, Theuekaulf N, Zinserling J, et al. Meta-analysis: ventilation strategies and outcomes of the acute respiratory distress syndrome and acute lung injury. Ann Intern Med 2009;151:566–76.
3. Anderson H 3rd, Steimle C, Shapiro M, et al. Extracorporeal life support for adult cardiorespiratory failure. Surgery 1993;114(2):161–72 [discussion: 72–3].
4. Cornish JD, Heiss KF, Clark RH, et al. Efficacy of venovenous extracorporeal membrane oxygenation for neonates with respiratory and circulatory compromise. J Pediatr 1993;122(1):105–9.
5. Zwischenberger JB, Cox CS Jr, Minifee PK, et al. Pathophysiology of ovine smoke inhalation injury treated with extracorporeal membrane oxygenation. Chest 1993;103(5):1582–6.
6. Bartlett RH. Extracorporeal life support for cardiopulmonary failure. Curr Probl Surg 1990;27(10):621–705.
7. Amato MB, Barbas CS, Medeiros DM, et al. Effect of a protective-ventilation strategy on mortality in the acute respiratory distress syndrome. N Engl J Med 1998;338(6):347–54.

8. Bidani A, Tzouanakis AE, Cardenas VJ Jr, et al. Permissive hypercapnia in acute respiratory failure. JAMA 1994;272(12):957–62.
9. Hickling KG, Walsh J, Henderson S, et al. Low mortality rate in adult respiratory distress syndrome using low-volume, pressure-limited ventilation with permissive hypercapnia: a prospective study. Crit Care Med 1994;22(10):1568–78.
10. Milberg JA, Davis DR, Steinberg KP, et al. Improved survival of patients with acute respiratory distress syndrome (ARDS): 1983–1993. JAMA 1995;273(4):306–9.
11. Rappaport SH, Shpiner R, Yoshihara G, et al. Randomized, prospective trial of pressure-limited versus volume-controlled ventilation in severe respiratory failure. Crit Care Med 1994;22(1):22–32.
12. Willms D, Nield M, Gocka I. Adult respiratory distress syndrome: outcome in a community hospital. Am J Crit Care 1994;3(5):337–41.
13. Cardenas VJ Jr, Zwischenberger JB, Tao W, et al. Correction of blood pH attenuates changes in hemodynamics and organ blood flow during permissive hypercapnia. Crit Care Med 1996;24(5):827–34.
14. Gattinoni L, Kolobow T, Tomlinson T, et al. Low-frequency positive pressure ventilation with extracorporeal CO2 removal (LFPPV-ECCO2R): an experimental study. Anesth Analg 1978;57(4):470–7.
15. Gattinoni L, Kolobow T, Tomlinson T, et al. Control of intermittent positive pressure breathing (IPPB) by extracorporeal removal of CO2. Br J Anaesth 1978; 50(8):753–8.
16. Kolobow T, Gattinoni L, Tomlinson T, et al. An alternative to breathing. J Thorac Cardiovasc Surg 1978;75(2):261–6.
17. Brunet F, Belghith M, Mira JP, et al. Extracorporeal CO2 removal and low-frequency positive-pressure ventilation. Improvement in arterial oxygenation with reduction of risk of pulmonary barotrauma in patients with adult respiratory distress syndrome. Chest 1993;104(3):889–98.
18. Gattinoni L, Agostoni A, Pesenti A, et al. Treatment of acute respiratory failure with low-frequency positive-pressure ventilation and extracorporeal removal of CO2. Lancet 1980;2(8189):292–4.
19. Gattinoni L, Kolobow T, Agostoni A, et al. Clinical application of low frequency positive pressure ventilation with extracorporeal CO2 removal (LFPPV-ECCO2R) in treatment of adult respiratory distress syndrome (ARDS). Int J Artif Organs 1979;2(6):282–3.
20. Morris AH, Wallace CJ, Menlove RL, et al. Randomized clinical trial of pressure-controlled inverse ratio ventilation and extracorporeal CO2 removal for adult respiratory distress syndrome. Am J Respir Crit Care Med 1994;149(2 Pt 1): 295–305.
21. Tao W, Brunston RL Jr, Bidani A, et al. Significant reduction in minute ventilation and peak inspiratory pressures with arteriovenous CO2 removal during severe respiratory failure. Crit Care Med 1997;25(4):689–95.
22. Barthelemy R, Galletti PM, Trudell LA, et al. Total extracorporeal CO2 removal in a pumpless artery-to-vein shunt. Trans Am Soc Artif Intern Organs 1982;28: 354–8.
23. Awad JA, Deslauriers J, Major D, et al. Prolonged pumpless arteriovenous perfusion for CO2 extraction. Ann Thorac Surg 1991;51(4):534–40.
24. Young JD, Dorrington KL, Blake GJ, et al. Femoral arteriovenous extracorporeal CO2 elimination using low blood flow. Crit Care Med 1992;20(6):805–9.
25. Brunston RL Jr, Zwischenberger JB, Tao W, et al. Total arteriovenous CO2 removal: simplifying extracorporeal support for respiratory failure. Ann Thorac Surg 1997;64(6):1599–604 [discussion: 604–5].

26. Zwischenberger JB, Alpard SK, Conrad SA, et al. Arteriovenous CO2 removal: development and impact on ventilator management and survival during severe respiratory failure. Perfusion 1999;14(4):299–310.
27. Brunston RL Jr, Tao W, Bidani A, et al. Determination of low blood flow limits for arteriovenous CO2 removal. ASAIO J 1996;42(5):M845–9.
28. Brunston RL Jr, Tao W, Bidani A, et al. Organ blood flow during arteriovenous CO2 removal. ASAIO J 1997;43(5):M821–4.
29. Ronco JJ, Belzberg A, Phang PT, et al. No differences in hemodynamics, ventricular function, and oxygen delivery in septic and nonseptic patients with the adult respiratory distress syndrome. Crit Care Med 1994;22(5):777–82.
30. Brunston RL Jr, Tao W, Bidani A, et al. Prolonged hemodynamic stability during arteriovenous CO2 removal for severe respiratory failure. J Thorac Cardiovasc Surg 1997;114(6):1107–14.
31. Alpard SK, Zwischenberger JB, Tao W, et al. New clinically relevant sheep model of severe respiratory failure secondary to combined smoke inhalation/cutaneous flame burn injury. Crit Care Med 2000;28(5):1469–76.
32. Zwischenberger JB, Conrad SA, Alpard SK, et al. Percutaneous extracorporeal arteriovenous CO2 removal for severe respiratory failure. Ann Thorac Surg 1999;68(1):181–7.
33. Nielsen ND, Kjaergaard B, Koefoed-Nielsen J, et al. Apneic oxygenation combined with extracorporeal arteriovenous CO2 removal provides sufficient gas exchange in experimental lung injury. ASAIO J 2008;54(4):401–5.
34. Jungebluth P, Iglesias M, Go T, et al. Optimal positive end-expiratory pressure during pumpless extracorporeal lung membrane support. Artif Organs 2008;32(11):885–90.
35. Zick G, Schädler D, Elke G, et al. Effects of interventional lung assist on haemodynamics and gas exchange in cardiopulmonary resuscitation: a prospective experimental study on animals with acute respiratory distress syndrome. Crit Care 2009;13(1):R17.
36. Walles T. Clinical experience with the iLA Membrane Ventilator pumpless extracorporeal lung-assist device. Expert Rev Med Devices 2007;4(3):297–305.
37. Liebold A, Philipp A, Kaiser M, et al. Pumpless extracorporeal lung assist using an arterio-venous shunt. Applications and limitations. Minerva Anestesiol 2002;68(5):387–91.
38. Flörchinger B, Philipp A, Klose A, et al. Pumpless extracorporeal lung assist: a 10-year institutional experience. Ann Thorac Surg 2008;86(2):410–7 [discussion: 417].
39. Elliot SC, Paramasivam K, Oram J, et al. Pumpless extracorporeal CO2 removal for life-threatening asthma. Crit Care Med 2007;35(3):945–8.
40. Twigg S, Gibbon GJ, Perris T. The use of extracorporeal CO2 removal in the management of life-threatening bronchospasm due to influenza infection. Anaesth Intensive Care 2008;36(4):579–81.
41. Freed DH, Henzler D, White CW, et al. Extracorporeal lung support for patients who had severe respiratory failure secondary to influenza A (H1N1) 2009 infection in Canada. Can J Anaesth 2010;57(3):240–7.
42. Mallick A, Elliot S, McKinlay J, et al. Extracorporeal CO2 removal using the Novalung in a patient with intracranial bleeding. Anaesthesia 2007;62(1):72–4.
43. Zimmermann M, Bein T, Philipp A, et al. Interhospital transportation of patients with severe lung failure on pumpless extracorporeal lung assist. Br J Anaesth 2006;96(1):63–6.

44. Haneya A, Philipp A, Foltan M, et al. Extracorporeal circulatory systems in the interhospital transfer of critically ill patients: experience of a single institution. Ann Saudi Med 2009;29(2):110–4.
45. Fischer S, Simon AR, Welte T, et al. Bridge to lung transplantation with the novel pumpless interventional lung assist device NovaLung. J Thorac Cardiovasc Surg 2006;131(3):719–23.
46. Strueber M, Hoeper MM, Fischer S, et al. Bridge to thoracic organ transplantation in patients with pulmonary arterial hypertension using a pumpless lung assist device. Am J Transplant 2009;9(4):853–7.
47. Taylor K, Holtby H. Emergency interventional lung assist for pulmonary hypertension. Anesth Analg 2009;109(2):382–5.
48. Ricci D, Boffini M, Del Sorbo L, et al. The use of CO2 removal devices in patients awaiting lung transplantation: an initial experience. Transplant Proc 2010;42(4): 1255–8.
49. Iglesias M, Martinez E, Badia JR, et al. Extrapulmonary ventilation for unresponsive severe acute respiratory distress syndrome after pulmonary resection. Ann Thorac Surg 2008;85(1):237–44 [discussion: 244].
50. Iglesias M, Jungebluth P, Petit C, et al. Extracorporeal lung membrane provides better lung protection than conventional treatment for severe postpneumonectomy noncardiogenic acute respiratory distress syndrome. J Thorac Cardiovasc Surg 2008;135(6):1362–71.
51. Renner A, Neukam K, Rösner T, et al. Pumpless extracorporeal lung assist as supportive therapy in a patient with diffuse alveolar hemorrhage. Int J Artif Organs 2008;31(3):279–81.
52. McKinlay J, Chapman G, Elliot S, et al. Pre-emptive Novalung-assisted CO2 removal in a patient with chest, head and abdominal injury. Anaesthesia 2008; 63(7):767–70.
53. Meyer AL, Strueber M, Tomaszek S, et al. Temporary cardiac support with a mini-circuit system consisting of a centrifugal pump and a membrane ventilator. Interact Cardiovasc Thorac Surg 2009;9(5):780–3.
54. Wiebe K, Poeling J, Arlt M, et al. Thoracic surgical procedures supported by a pumpless interventional lung assist. Ann Thorac Surg 2010;89(6):1782–7 [discussion: 1788].
55. Floerchinger B, Philipp A, Foltan M, et al. Switch from venoarterial extracorporeal membrane oxygenation to arteriovenous pumpless extracorporeal lung assist. Ann Thorac Surg 2010;89(1):125–31.
56. Kopp R, Dembinski R, Kuhlen R. Role of extracorporeal lung assist in the treatment of acute respiratory failure. Minerva Anestesiol 2006;72(6):587–95.
57. Grubitzsch H, Beholz S, Wollert HG, et al. Pumpless arteriovenous extracorporeal lung assist: what is its role? Perfusion 2000;15(3):237–42.
58. Liebold A, Reng CM, Philipp A, et al. Pumpless extracorporeal lung assist—experience with the first 20 cases. Eur J Cardiothorac Surg 2000;17(5):608–13.
59. Reng M, Philipp A, Kaiser M, et al. Pumpless extracorporeal lung assist and adult respiratory distress syndrome. Lancet 2000;356(9225):219–20.
60. Bein T, Scherer MN, Philipp A, et al. Pumpless extracorporeal lung assist (pECLA) in patients with acute respiratory distress syndrome and severe brain injury. J Trauma 2005;58(6):1294–7.
61. Ruettimann U, Ummenhofer W, Rueter F, et al. Management of acute respiratory distress syndrome using pumpless extracorporeal lung assist. Can J Anaesth 2006;53(1):101–5.

62. von Mach MA, Kaes J, Omogbehin B, et al. An update on interventional lung assist devices and their role in acute respiratory distress syndrome. Lung 2006;184(3):169–75.
63. Zimmermann M, Philipp A, Schmid FX, et al. From Baghdad to Germany: use of a new pumpless extracorporeal lung assist system in two severely injured US soldiers. ASAIO J 2007;53(3):e4–6.
64. Muellenbach RM, Wunder C, Nuechter DC, et al. Early treatment with arteriovenous extracorporeal lung assist and high-frequency oscillatory ventilation in a case of severe acute respiratory distress syndrome. Acta Anaesthesiol Scand 2007;51(6):766–9.
65. Muellenbach RM, Kredel M, Wunder C, et al. Arteriovenous extracorporeal lung assist as integral part of a multimodal treatment concept: a retrospective analysis of 22 patients with ARDS refractory to standard care. Eur J Anaesthesiol 2008;25(11):897–904.
66. Hommel M, Deja M, von Dossow V, et al. Bronchial fistulae in ARDS patients: management with an extracorporeal lung assist device. Eur Respir J 2008; 32(6):1652–5.
67. Zimmermann M, Bein T, Arlt M, et al. Pumpless extracorporeal interventional lung assist in patients with acute respiratory distress syndrome: a prospective pilot study. Crit Care 2009;13(1):R10.
68. Bein T, Zimmermann M, Hergeth K, et al. Pumpless extracorporeal removal of CO2 combined with ventilation using low tidal volume and high positive end-expiratory pressure in a patient with severe acute respiratory distress syndrome. Anaesthesia 2009;64(2):195–8.
69. Weber-Carstens S, Bercker S, Hommel M, et al. Hypercapnia in late-phase ALI/ARDS: providing spontaneous breathing using pumpless extracorporeal lung assist. Intensive Care Med 2009;35(6):1100–5.
70. Müller T, Lubnow M, Philipp A, et al. Extracorporeal pumpless interventional lung assist in clinical practice: determinants of efficacy. Eur Respir J 2009;33(3): 551–8.
71. Mortensen JD. An intravenacaval blood gas exchange (IVCBGE) device. A preliminary report. ASAIO Trans 1987;33(3):570–3.
72. Mortensen JD, Berry G. Conceptual and design features of a practical, clinically effective intravenous mechanical blood oxygen/CO2 exchange device (IVOX). Int J Artif Organs 1989;12(6):384–9.
73. Cox CS Jr, Zwischenberger JB, Graves DF, et al. Intracorporeal CO2 removal and permissive hypercapnia to reduce airway pressure in acute respiratory failure. The theoretical basis for permissive hypercapnia with IVOX. ASAIO J 1993;39(2):97–102.
74. Cox CS Jr, Zwischenberger JB, Traber LD, et al. Use of an intravascular oxygenator/CO2 removal device in an ovine smoke inhalation injury model. ASAIO Trans 1991;37(3):M411–3.
75. Zwischenberger JB, Cox CS Jr. A new intravascular membrane oxygenator to augment blood gas transfer in patients with acute respiratory failure. Tex Med 1991;87(12):60–3.
76. Zwischenberger JB, Cox CS, Graves D, et al. Intravascular membrane oxygenation and CO2 removal–a new application for permissive hypercapnia? Thorac Cardiovasc Surg 1992;40(3):115–20.
77. Vaslef SN, Mockros LF, Anderson RW. Development of an intravascular lung assist device. ASAIO Trans 1989;35(3):660–4.

78. Makarewicz AJ, Mockros LF, Anderson RW. A pumping intravascular artificial lung with active mixing. ASAIO J 1993;39(3):M466–9.
79. Hattler BG, Lund LW, Golob J, et al. A respiratory gas exchange catheter: in vitro and in vivo tests in large animals. J Thorac Cardiovasc Surg 2002;124(3):520–30.
80. Ruberto F, Pugliese F, D'Alio A, et al. Extracorporeal removal of CO2 using a venovenous, low-flow system (Decapsmart) in a lung transplanted patient: a case report. Transplant Proc 2009;41:1412–4.
81. Zwischenberger JB, Anderson CM, Cook KE, et al. Development of an implantable artificial lung: challenges and progress. ASAIO J 2001;47(4):316–20.
82. Lick SD, Zwischenberger JB. Artificial lung: bench toward bedside. ASAIO J 2004;50(1):2–5.
83. Matheis G. New technologies for respiratory assist. Perfusion 2003;18(4):245–51.
84. Kolobow T. The artificial lung: the past. A personal retrospective. ASAIO J 2004; 50(6):xliii–xlviii.
85. Zwischenberger JB. Future of artificial lungs. ASAIO J 2004;50(6):xlix–xlli.
86. Lick SD, Zwischenberger JB, Wang D, et al. Improved right heart function with a compliant inflow artificial lung in series with the pulmonary circulation. Ann Thorac Surg 2001;72(3):899–904.
87. Go T, Macchiarini P. Artificial lung: current perspectives. Minerva Chir 2008; 63(5):363–72.
88. Ota K. Advances in artificial lungs. J Artif Organs 2010;13(1):13–6.
89. Perlman CE, Cook KE, Seipelt JR, et al. In vivo hemodynamic responses to thoracic artificial lung attachment. ASAIO J 2005;51(4):412–25.
90. Haft JW, Alnajjar O, Bull JL, et al. Effect of artificial lung compliance on right ventricular load. ASAIO J 2005;51(6):769–72.
91. Sato H, Griffith GW, Hall CM, et al. Seven-day artificial lung testing in an in-parallel configuration. Ann Thorac Surg 2007;84(3):988–94.
92. Akay B, Reoma JL, Camboni D, et al. In-parallel artificial lung attachment at high flows in normal and pulmonary hypertension models. Ann Thorac Surg 2010; 90(1):259–65.
93. Schmid C, Philipp A, Hilker M, et al. Bridge to lung transplantation through a pulmonary artery to left atrial oxygenator circuit. Ann Thorac Surg 2008;85(4):1202–5.
94. Camboni D, Philipp A, Arlt M, et al. First experience with a paracorporeal artificial lung in humans. ASAIO J 2009;55(3):304–6.
95. Lick SD, Deyo DJ, Wang D, et al. Paracorporeal artificial lung: perioperative management for survival study in sheep. J Invest Surg 2003;16(3):177–84.
96. Sato H, McGillicuddy JW, Griffith GW, et al. Effect of artificial lung compliance on in vivo pulmonary system hemodynamics. ASAIO J 2006;52(3):248–56.
97. Alpard SK, Wang D, Deyo DJ, et al. Optional active compliance chamber performance in a pulmonary artery-pulmonary artery configured paracorporeal artificial lung. Perfusion 2007;22(2):81–6.
98. Sanchez-Lorente D, Go T, Jungebluth P, et al. Single double-lumen venous-venous pump-driven extracorporeal lung membrane support. J Thorac Cardiovasc Surg 2010;140(3):558–63, 563,e1–2.
99. Cook KE, Maxhimer J, Leonard DJ, et al. Platelet and leukocyte activation and design consequences for thoracic artificial lungs. ASAIO J 2002;48(6):620–30.
100. Schmalstieg FC, Zwischenberger JB. The artificial lung/inflammatory interface: a refocus of the problem. ASAIO J 2004;50(1):6–8.
101. Takagi M, Shiwaku K, Inoue T, et al. Hydrodynamically stable adhesion of endothelial cells onto a polypropylene hollow fiber membrane by modification with adhesive protein. J Artif Organs 2003;6(3):222–6.

102. Polk AA, Maul TM, McKeel DT, et al. A biohybrid artificial lung prototype with active mixing of endothelialized microporous hollow fibers. Biotechnol Bioeng 2010;106(3):490–500.
103. Burgess KA, Hu HH, Wagner WR, et al. Towards microfabricated biohybrid artificial lung modules for chronic respiratory support. Biomed Microdevices 2009; 11(1):117–27.
104. Fritsche CS, Simsch O, Weinberg EJ, et al. Pulmonary tissue engineering using dual-compartment polymer scaffolds with integrated vascular tree. Int J Artif Organs 2009;32(10):701–10.
105. Funakubo A, Taga I, McGillicuddy JW, et al. Flow vectorial analysis in an artificial implantable lung. ASAIO J 2003;49(4):383–7.
106. Taga I, Funakubo A, Fukui Y. Design and development of an artificial implantable lung using multiobjective genetic algorithm: evaluation of gas exchange performance. ASAIO J 2005;51(1):92–102.
107. Lee JK, Kung HH, Mockros LF. Microchannel technologies for artificial lungs: (1) theory. ASAIO J 2008;54(4):372–82.
108. Kung MC, Lee JK, Kung HH, et al. Microchannel technologies for artificial lungs: (2) screen-filled wide rectangular channels. ASAIO J 2008;54(4):383–9.
109. Lee JK, Kung MC, Kung HH, et al. Microchannel technologies for artificial lungs: (3) open rectangular channels. ASAIO J 2008;54(4):390–5.
110. Garcia JF, Iacono A, Kon ZN, et al. Ambulatory extracorporeal membrane oxygenation: a new approach for bridge-to-lung transplantation. J Thorac Cardiovasc Surg 2010;139:e137–8.
111. Mangi AA, Mason DP, Yun JJ, et al. Bridge to lung transplantation using short-term ambulatory extracorporeal membrane oxygenation. J Thorac Cardiovasc Surg 2010;140:713–5.
112. Javidfar J, Wang D, Zwischenberger JB, et al. Insertion of a bicaval dual lumen extracorporeal membrane oxygenation catheter with image guidance. ASAIO J 2011;57(3):203–5.

Extracorporeal Membrane Oxygenation in Adult Acute Respiratory Distress Syndrome

Pauline K. Park, MD, FCCM*, Lena M. Napolitano, MD, Robert H. Bartlett, MD, FCCM

KEYWORDS

- Extracorporeal membrane oxygenation
- Extracorporeal life support
- Acute respiratory distress syndrome • Respiratory failure

The role of extracorporeal membrane oxygenation (ECMO) in supporting refractory respiratory failure in adults continues to evolve. Interest in ECMO surged after reports of severe acute respiratory distress syndrome (ARDS) associated with the 2009 H1N1 pandemic viral infection.[1] As physicians struggled to treat young, previously healthy patients failing conventional therapy,[2] heightened media and Internet coverage drove the discussion of rescue measures into the public forum. Published systematic review[3] and pooled analyses[4,5] point out that high-quality experimental evidence available for guidance is limited. While the results of further randomized controlled trials are awaited,[6] considerable new experience with adult ECMO continues to accrue.

ECMO is supportive care and is not intended as a primary ARDS treatment; an artificial membrane lung and blood pump (a modified cardiopulmonary bypass circuit) provides gas exchange and ensures systemic perfusion to sustain the life of the patient when native heart and lung function cannot.[7] Continuous cardiopulmonary support stabilizes critical derangements of oxygenation and ventilation and allows additional time to continue to diagnose, treat, and allow recovery from the underlying cause of respiratory failure. During this period, typically days to weeks, further iatrogenic ventilator-induced lung injury can be avoided.

At its heart, ECMO is an invasive, complex, resource-intensive form of support. Safe delivery requires considerable institutional and caregiver commitment. Because of

Division of Acute Care Surgery, Department of Surgery, University of Michigan Health System, 1500 East Medical Center Drive, 1C340A-UH, SPC 5033, Ann Arbor, MI 48109-5033, USA
* Corresponding author.
E-mail address: parkpk@umich.edu

Crit Care Clin 27 (2011) 627–646
doi:10.1016/j.ccc.2011.05.009 criticalcare.theclinics.com
0749-0704/11/$ – see front matter

this, its use is advocated only in those patients believed to be at substantial risk of death. Nevertheless, as cardiac surgery and destination support of heart failure have become more commonplace, the personnel and devices required to provide prolonged support are now routinely deployed in many intensive care units (ICUs). The availability of simpler, compact support devices, combined with improved clinical management, has lowered the barriers to broader adoption of ECMO as a rescue therapy for refractory respiratory failure. This article reviews the current evidence supporting the use of extracorporeal support in refractory respiratory failure and discusses contemporary management of adult patients receiving ECMO.

REVIEW OF SUPPORTING EVIDENCE

In a recently published systematic review,[3] Mitchell and colleagues identified only 3 randomized controlled trials[8–10] and 3 cohort studies[11–13] evaluating ECMO in patients with acute respiratory failure. Meta-analysis of the randomized controlled trials revealed significant heterogeneity in risk of mortality, with the summary risk ratio 0.93 (95% confidence interval, 0.71–1.22); however, it was noted that the most recent trial showed a reduction in mortality and severe disability in patients randomized to receive ECMO. These trials are reviewed in the following sections, followed by discussion of additional available data.

Randomized Controlled Trials of ECMO Versus Conventional Ventilation

Interest in ECMO support of adult respiratory failure was stimulated after its successful use in a trauma patient.[14] By 1974, there were 20 case reports in adults and children. In response, the US National Institutes of Health sponsored a multicenter randomized trial comparing venoarterial (VA) ECMO with conventional mechanical ventilation in adult patients with severe acute respiratory failure.[8] At that time, the standard ECMO circuit was based on a servoregulated roller pump coupled to a high-resistance, thrombogenic membrane lung that required full anticoagulation, technology that is no longer in use. Patients were drawn from a larger cohort of 686 hypoxemic patients; 90 patients who met prespecified criteria for severity of illness (ECMO entry criteria, fast-entry: PaO_2 <50 mm Hg for >2 hours at inspired oxygen fraction [FiO_2] of 1.0 and positive end-expiratory pressure [PEEP] $\geq$5 cm H_2O; or slow-entry: after 48 hours of maximal medical therapy, PaO_2 <50 mm Hg for >12 hours at FiO_2 1.0 and PEEP $\geq$5 cm H_2O and Q_s/Q_T >30% of cardiac output) were enrolled. Overall survival of the larger group of patients was 34%[15]; the high-risk patients randomized to receive VA ECMO plus conventional ventilation and those receiving conventional ventilation alone had dismal survival rates of 8.7% and 9.5%.

In 1994, Morris and colleagues[9] reported a second single-center, randomized, controlled trial. Based on Gattinoni and colleagues[16] initial experience with extracorporeal CO_2 removal ($ECCO_2R$), 40 patients meeting the ECMO entry criteria were randomized to receive either $ECCO_2R$ with venovenous (VV) ECMO or pressure-controlled inverse ratio ventilation. No survival difference was noted between the 2 study arms (33% vs 42%); however, overall ARDS survival at that institution was significantly higher than in the previous decade.[17] Based on the negative results from these 2 trials, use of ECMO support for adult respiratory failure was largely restricted to a few centers.

Most recently, a pragmatic randomized controlled trial was conducted in the United Kingdom, following the design used in the previous UK study of ECMO in neonatal respiratory failure.[18] The Conventional Ventilation or ECMO for Severe Adult Respiratory Failure (CESAR) trial[10] used different entry criteria (severe, but potentially reversible, ARDS with Murray lung injury score >3 or pH <7.20) and specific exclusion criteria (high pressure or high FiO_2 ventilation for more than 7 days, signs of intracranial bleeding, contraindications to limited heparinization, or contraindication to continuation of active treatment). Patients were randomized to either conventional care at 1 of 68 tertiary care centers or to a single center using a treatment protocol that included ECMO. The trial was stopped for efficacy after 180 patients. Survival without severe disability at 6 months was 47% for those treated at tertiary care centers and 63% at 6 months for patients referred to the ECMO center. The trial has been criticized for lack of standardized mechanical ventilation protocols in the conventional care group and because the intention-to-treat analysis included patients who did not go on to receive ECMO; nevertheless, CESAR did show that protocolized care including ECMO in an expert ARDS center led to improved outcomes.[19]

Cohort Studies of ECMO with Comparison Groups

Lewandowski and colleagues[12] conducted a single-center, prospective trial evaluating a criteria-based treatment algorithm in 122 consecutive patients. Patients received either advanced ventilation or advanced ventilation plus ECMO, based on their clinical status. As specified by the treatment protocol, baseline measures of acuity (APACHE II, Murray scores, duration of mechanical ventilation before admission and PaO_2/FiO_2 ratio) differed between groups. Survival was 89% in the group without ECMO and 55% in the ECMO group. The investigators concluded that high survival rates could be achieved using their ARDS algorithm.

Mols and colleagues[11] reported a cohort of 245 patients with ARDS, of whom approximately one-quarter received ECMO. Overall survival in the non-ECMO patients was 61% and 55% in the ECMO group. The investigators concluded that ECMO should be used in selected patients with severe ARDS.[11]

Beiderlinden and colleagues[13] conducted a single-center, prospective observational study of 150 patients with severe ARDS. Of the group 78.7% were treated conservatively; 32 patients received ECMO. Survival was higher in the conservative group, but there was significant survival in the ECMO group as well (71% vs 53%, $P = .059$). Again, patients in the ECMO group presented with baseline higher Murray and simplified acute physiology scores. Predictors of mortality included age, mean pulmonary artery pressure, sequential organ failure assessment score, and duration of mechanical ventilation before referral, but not allocation to receive ECMO.

Observational Series of ECMO in Adult ARDS

In addition to multiple institutional and national case series[5,20–23] and individual case reports,[24–26] 2 large observational studies of adult respiratory ECMO have recently been reported: the Extracorporeal Life Support Organization (ELSO) registry review and the Australia and New Zealand (ANZ) ECMO H1N1 experience.

Brogan and colleagues[27] conducted a retrospective review of the ELSO registry and identified 1473 adult patients who received ECMO for severe respiratory failure between 1986 and 2006. Patients were not randomized to specific ventilator protocols, and registry reporting was on a voluntary basis. The median patient age was 34 years; the median time on ECMO was 154 hours. In this series, VV ECMO was associated with increased survival compared with VA ECMO. Approximately 9% of patients sustained radiographic evidence of cerebral infarction, hemorrhage, or brain death. Overall survival to hospital discharge was 50%.

The ANZ-ECMO Influenza Investigators[28] reported their experience treating 201 patients in ICUs with confirmed or suspected 2009 influenza A (H1N1) infection

Table 1
ELSO patient outcomes: neonatal, pediatric, and adult, by indication, as of July, 2010

	Total	Survive ECLS (n, %)		Survive to Discharge (n, %)	
Neonatal					
Respiratory	24,017	20,346	85	18,044	75
Cardiac	4103	2,474	60	1603	39
ECPR	586	373	64	224	38
Pediatric					
Respiratory	4635	3002	65	2575	56
Cardiac	5026	3179	63	2386	47
ECPR	1128	594	53	442	39
Adult					
Respiratory	2121	1319	62	1124	53
Cardiac	1238	598	48	424	34
ECPR	476	179	38	137	29
Total	43,330	32,064	74	26,959	62

Abbreviation: ECPR, extracorporeal cardiopulmonary resuscitation.

between June 1 and August 31, 2009. During this period, most cases receiving ECMO support were adults, with a median age of 34 years. Sixty-eight patients received ECMO after failing to improve on conventional treatment; 72% were transported to a tertiary care center on ECMO. Before commencing ECMO, the patients were quite ill, with median Murray score 3.8, PaO_2/FiO_2 ratio of 56, lowest pH 7.20, PEEP 18 cm H_2O, and peak airway pressure 36 cm H_2O. The median time on ventilator before initiating ECMO was 2 days and median duration of ECMO support was 10 days. Final survival to hospital discharge in this series was 75%.[29]

Complementary data exist in the pediatric critical care literature,[18] in which ECMO has been the accepted standard of care in neonatal respiratory failure from a variety of causes. The use of ECMO has been related to a reduced neonatal mortality at the population level in the state of Michigan.[30] A meta-analysis of pediatric cases showed favorable survival outcome with ECMO.[31]

In summary, randomized data available to address the question of efficacy of extracorporeal support in adult ARDS are limited to 3 trials, only one of which was conducted within the past decade. Considerable observational and anecdotal data exist to support use of ECMO once conventional measures have failed, including successful experience during the recent H1N1 epidemic. Current ELSO summary statistics for 2010 are presented in **Table 1** and **Fig. 1**; preliminary subset analysis of more than 175 adult H1N1 cases shows an overall survival to discharge of 67% (ELSO, unpublished data, 2011).

CANDIDATES FOR ECMO SUPPORT

ECMO support should be considered only in patients with respiratory failure refractory to conventional therapy. Ideally, the risks of initiating ECMO therapy should be balanced against the risk of subsequent mortality; much of the controversy regarding ECMO hinges on our ability to accurately risk-stratify ARDS mortality. Identification of early predictors of adverse outcome would allow optimization of the referral criteria.

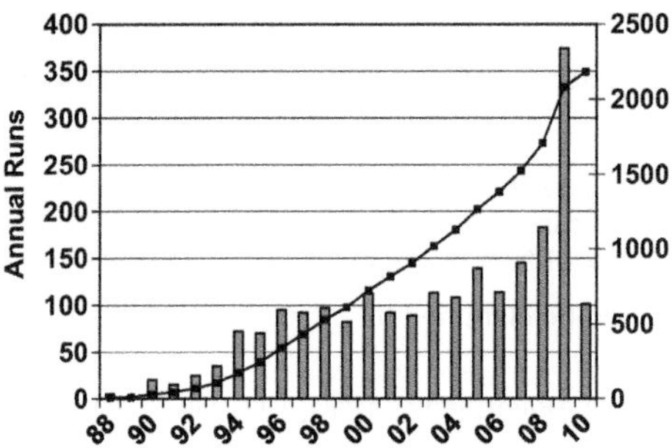

Fig. 1. ELSO, adult respiratory failure cases, 1988 to 2010, annual and cumulative.

Given the available data, it would be reasonable to use the CESAR trial entry criteria (adult patients 18–65 years old, with Murray score >3 or uncompensated hypercarbia with pH <7.20, duration of mechanical ventilation <7 days) to trigger early referral to a center with ECMO capability. The Murray score[32] uses the average score of 4 elements graded on a 0 to 4 scale to establish ARDS severity. For convenience, the following Web site contains a calculator to assist in the computation: http://www.lshtm.ac.uk/msu/trials/cesar/murrayscorecalculator.htm.

The CESAR Trial Criteria[10] and the ELSO guidelines for referral for ECMO for adult respiratory failure[33] are reproduced in **Boxes 1** and **2**.

METHODS OF ECMO SUPPORT

Detailed discussion of ECMO indications, management, complications, and outcome beyond the scope of this article may be found on the Extracorporeal Life Support Organization Web site: http://www.elso.med.umich.edu/.

Box 1
Selection of patients with respiratory failure for ECMO CESAR trial enrollment criteria

1. Inclusion Criteria
   a. Adult patients (18–65 years)
   b. Severe, but potentially reversible, respiratory failure
   c. Murray score >3.0, or uncompensated hypercapnia with a pH <7.20
2. Exclusion Criteria
   a. Duration of high pressure and/or high FiO_2 ventilation >7 days
   b. Intracranial bleeding
   c. Any other contraindication to limited heparinization
   d. Patients who are moribund and have any contraindication to continuation of active treatment

Data from Peek GJ, Mugford M, Tiruvoipati R, et al. Efficacy and economic assessment of conventional ventilatory support versus extracorporeal membrane oxygenation for severe adult respiratory failure (CESAR): a multicentre randomised controlled trial. Lancet 2009; 374(9698):1351–63.

Box 2
ELSO general guidelines: Selection of adult patients with respiratory failure for ECMO

A. Indications

1. In hypoxic respiratory failure from any cause (primary or secondary) extracorporeal life support (ECLS) should be considered when the risk of mortality is 50% or greater, and is indicated when the risk of 80% or greater.
   a. 50% mortality risk can be identified by a PaO_2/FiO_2 <150 on FiO_2 >90% and/or Murray score 2–3
   b. 80% mortality risk can be identified by a PaO_2/FiO_2 <80 on FiO_2 >90% and Murray score 3–4
2. CO_2 retention caused by asthma or permissive hypercapnia with a $PaCO_2$ >80 or inability to achieve safe inflation pressures (P-plat $\leq$30 cm H_2O) is an indication for ECLS.
3. Severe air leak syndromes

B. Contraindications

There are no absolute contraindications to ECLS, because each patient is considered individually with respect to risks and benefits. However, there are conditions that are known to be associated with a poor outcome despite ECLS, and can be considered relative contraindications.

1. Mechanical ventilation at high settings (FiO_2 >.9, P-plat >30) for 7 days or more
2. Major pharmacologic immunosuppression (absolute neutrophil count <400/mL^3
3. Central nervous system hemorrhage that is recent or expanding

C. Specific patient considerations

1. Age: no specific age contraindication but consider increasing risk with increasing age
2. Weight: more than 125 kg can be associated with technical difficulty in cannulation, and the risk of not being able to achieve an adequate blood flow based on patient size
3. Nonfatal comorbidities may be a relative indication based on the individual case (ie, diabetes and renal transplant and retinopathy and pulmonary venoocclusive disease complicated by severe pneumonia)
4. Bridging to lung transplant: generally bridging to lung transplant is impractical because of limited donors. Using an implanted membrane lung (in a paracorporeal position) with extubation and ambulation is being evaluated in some transplant centers

Abbreviation: P-plat, plateau pressure.
Data from ELSO. Extracorporeal Life Support Organization patient specific guidelines. A supplement to the ELSO General Guidelines (April 2009) Version 1.1.2011. Available at: http://www.elso.med.umich.edu/Guidelines.html.

COMPONENTS

Over the past decade, technical advances have led to improvements in all major components used in extracorporeal support. The ECMO circuit consists of the cannulae used to provide vascular access to the patient's native circulation, a pump to propel blood through the circuit, and the artificial membrane lung oxygenator. In addition, smaller integrated devices with prepackaged components offering off-the-shelf circuit availability have recently received approval from the US Food and Drug Administration for marketing in the United States.[33,34]

Cannulation in adults is now primarily performed percutaneously via the Seldinger technique, using either 2 separate cannulae, one for drainage and one for return, or a single bicaval cannula with drainage from the retrohepatic vena cava and return directly into the right atrium.[35] For many years, the standard ECMO circuit used a servoregulated roller pump with passive drainage. Current centrifugal pump design has evolved to minimize hemolysis related to stagnation, heating, and thrombosis.[36,37] These features have been successfully incorporated in ECMO circuits, with improved circuit durability and reduced hemolysis.[38] Priming times and plasma leak have been reduced as oxygenator design has moved from early, high-resistance designs[39] to low-resistance, hollow-fiber poly-(4-methyl-1-pentene).[40–42] In many institutions, heparin-bonded or surface-treated[43] tubing is used to complete the circuit, with conflicting data reporting reduced[44,45] or unchanged[46] thrombogenicity secondary to decreased blood-prosthetic interaction.

Reports of current adult practice are primarily anecdotal; the CESAR trial used roller pump and polymethylpentene oxygenators and the ANZ-ECMO experience used centrifugal pump and polymethylpentene oxygenators.[28] Direct comparison with pediatric experience is hampered by differences in component availability for neonatal patients. A 2008 ELSO survey of 80 of 103 (78%) North American neonatal ECMO centers indicated that 82.5% routinely used roller pumps for neonatal ECMO, whereas the remaining 17.5% used centrifugal pumps; 67% used silicone membrane oxygenators, 14% used polymethylpentene hollow-fiber oxygenators, and a surface coating was used by 44% of the centers on all their neonatal patients receiving ECMO. Compared with a 2002 survey, this finding represented a decrease in silicone membrane use and increase in the use of centrifugal blood pumps and coated ECMO circuits.[47]

CIRCUIT CONFIGURATIONS

ECMO support is configured as VV or VA with drainage and blood return based on site of vascular access. In VV ECMO, the oxygenator is placed in series with the native pulmonary circulation; in VA ECMO, it is placed in parallel. Overall blood flow rates for full ECMO support are 50 to 100 mL/kg/min.

VV ECMO

VV ECMO is the most commonly used means of supporting adult patients with respiratory failure and stable hemodynamics. In VV ECMO, venous blood is withdrawn through a large-bore venous cannula (21–25 Fr) and passes through the membrane lung, and newly oxygenated blood is returned to the venous circulation close to the right atrium. Venous cannulation reduces the risks of cannula-related arterial ischemia and systemic emboli. The location of the oxygenator between 2 venous limbs also functions to prevent venous air emboli. Access for VV ECMO can be obtained through either 2 single-lumen catheters, typically placed via the right internal jugular and femoral veins, or 1 bicaval dual-lumen catheter (27–31 Fr) placed via the right internal jugular vein, with the drainage port situated in the retrohepatic cava and the return port within the right atrium (**Fig. 2**). Placement of the dual-lumen catheter is facilitated by digital bedside radiology, fluoroscopic or ultrasound guidance; misplacement can occur, with resultant inadequate flow or even cardiac perforation.[48]

VA ECMO

VA ECMO provides additional cardiac as well as respiratory support. Blood is withdrawn from the venous circulation, passed through the oxygenator, and returned to the arterial circulation. Femoral venous and femoral arterial cannulation is preferred in adult patients (**Fig. 3**). Ischemic complications (ischemia of the distal extremity or other organs) may accompany arterial cannulation; the incidence may be reduced by using ultrasound evaluation to permit size-matching the cannula and the target

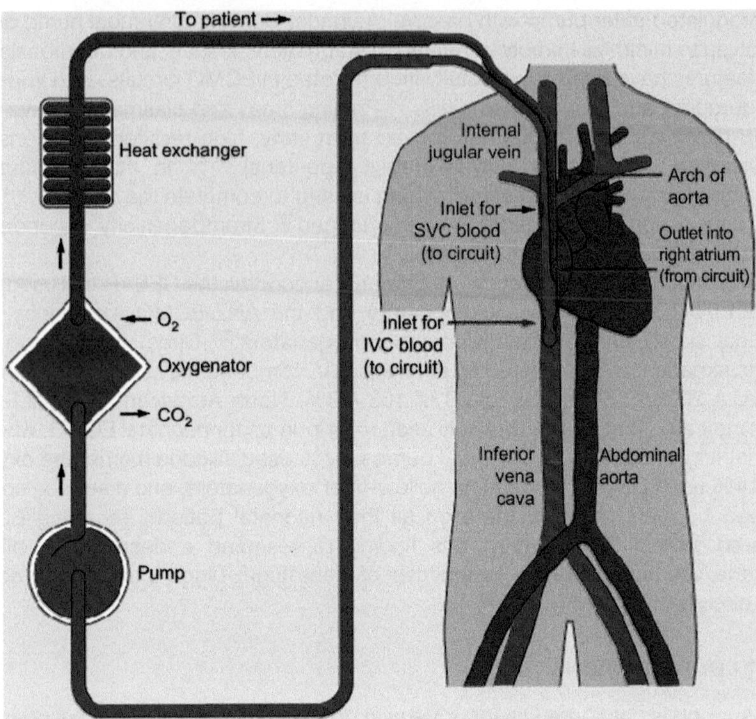

Fig. 2. Dual-lumen cannula VV extracorporeal circuit configuration. (*Reproduced from* Gaffney AM, Wildhirt SM, Griffin MJ, et al. Extracorporeal life support. BMJ 2010;341:983; with permission.)

vessel or by using a separate reperfusion cannula to separately perfuse the distal limb. In addition, because VA ECMO returns oxygenated blood retrograde through the aorta, flow dynamics must be monitored closely to ensure that adequate oxygen is reaching the proximal cerebral circulation. With direct arterial access, thromboemboli or air emboli may enter the systemic circulation.

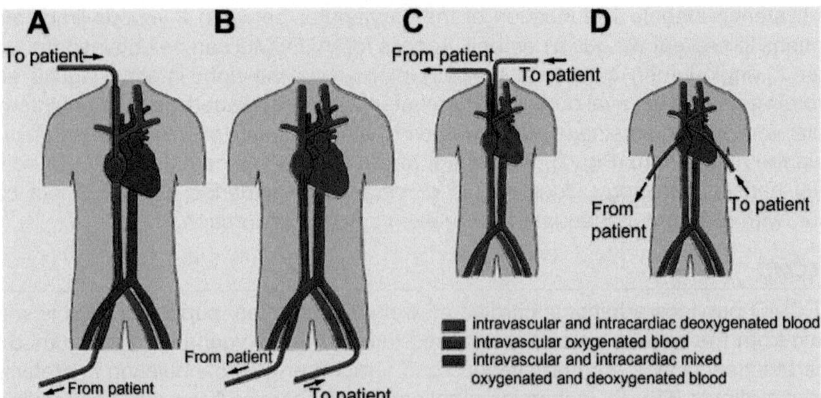

Fig. 3. Alternative cannulation configurations. (*Reproduced from* Gaffney AM, Wildhirt SM, Griffin MJ, et al. Extracorporeal life support. BMJ 2010;341:985; with permission.)

Pumpless Arteriovenous ECMO/ECCO$_2$R

Arteriovenous (AV) ECMO[49,50] depends on the native cardiac output to propel blood through the oxygenator and thus has the advantage of simplifying circuit configuration. Access is most frequently obtained through the femoral artery and femoral vein. AV ECMO is limited by the lower total flow volume through the oxygenator and, by itself, may not provide sufficient oxygenation, particularly in the face of shock or heart failure. Nevertheless, flow is sufficient to allow carbon dioxide exchange, and its use as an adjunct to mechanical ventilation has been piloted in patients with ARDS.[51]

A variation on this technique, ECCO$_2$R, replaces the arterial inflow with a second venous cannula and adds back a small roller pump to achieve VV blood flow (10 – 15 mL/kg/min) sufficient to clear CO_2.[52] This technique has the advantage of avoiding arterial complications, taking advantage of the ability to use small-bore cannulae and minimizing extracorporeal blood volume. Because CO_2 removal and pH are managed by the circuit, ventilator settings can be reduced to lung protective levels, or simple oxygen insufflation may be sufficient to ensure oxygenation.[53,54]

ECMO TRANSPORT

For patients considered too tenuous for conventional transport, ECMO has been used to facilitate safe transfer from outlying hospitals to referral centers. Cannulation is performed on site, either by the referring team or by the retrieving team, and the patient is stabilized before transport. The process requires a specialized team and resources dedicated to retrieval; availability in the United States is limited.

A handful of centers have reported their experience with ECMO-based retrieval and transport over the past 2 decades. The University of Arkansas,[55] the Karolinska Institute,[56] Wilford Hall,[57] and the University of Michigan[21] have all reported transporting critically ill patients on ECMO, safely traveling several hours and in some cases hundreds or thousands of kilometers. These series report no mortalities during transport, and transported patients had overall survivals similar to patients who were in-house or transferred without ECMO support.

Similarly, Forrest and colleagues[58] reported the experience in the state of New South Wales, Australia. New South Wales represents a large catchment area of more than 800,000 km^2, with ECMO support limited to 2 hospitals in Sydney. A state-wide, mobile ECMO support service was established with the goal of providing equitable access for patients with severe lung failure whose condition physicians felt precluded safe conventional transport. Using a prespecified protocol for ECMO referral, teams were mobilized to transport patients with severe respiratory failure. Forty patients, with a median age of 34 years, were transported on ECMO over the past 3 years (42% for H1N1-related respiratory failure). Ten percent were accomplished by helicopter, 25% by jet, and 65% traveled by road; the median distance for transport was 250 km, with a mean travel time of 4.8 hours. Median time from acceptance of referral to establishment of ECMO was 6.5 hours. Two patients died at the referral hospital before cannulation. Complications, primarily hypothermia, occurred in 42% of patients during transport, but pump failure, hypotension, and arrhythmia were also noted. No significant short-term patient morbidity was noted. Survival to hospital discharge was 85%. The investigators concluded that the program enhanced the ability of the state to respond to increased demand for ECMO support during the H1N1 influenza outbreak.

In the military setting, the simplified pumpless AV CO_2 removal (AVCO$_2$R) circuit, in tandem with conventional ventilation, has been used to facilitate interhospital transport of critically ill patients.[59–61] In-theater casualties requiring definitive ICU care and requiring evacuation to Landstuhl Regional Medical Center, Germany were successfully transferred using $AVCO_2R$. Most recently a US combat casualty with severe penetrating thoracic trauma wounded in Afghanistan required initiation of VV ECMO for stabilization before transport to Germany.[62] A specialized acute lung rescue team (ALRT), equipped with advanced ventilator and ECLS capability, has been developed to assist in transport of soldiers with severe lung injury.[63]

MANAGEMENT ON ECMO

After initiation of ECMO, the patient often stabilizes rapidly, with improved hemodynamics and weaning of vasopressors. Over the next 24 hours, ongoing, continuous blood exposure to the nonbiologic extracorporeal circuit provokes an inflammatory response with associated fluid shifts, consumption, and activation of procoagulant and anticoagulant blood components.[64,65] Full-blown systemic inflammatory response syndrome may develop, with characteristic cytokine level increase, leukocyte activation, and multisystem organ dysfunction. This process is believed to be related to mobilization of preformed cytokine stores rather than de novo synthesis.[66]

Supportive ICU therapy is continued, with attention to appropriate treatment of sepsis and de-escalation of ventilator settings as ECMO support permits. Positive-pressure ventilation should be reduced to lung protective settings. Chest radiographs initially worsen; however, if ventilator pressures are significantly decreased once extracorporeal support is established, derecruitment may occur, and radiographic changes may not necessarily reflect increasing pulmonary edema. Oxygen delivery is primarily related to blood flow rate through the oxygenator and is titrated to the SaO_2; because CO_2 is more readily diffusible across the membrane lung, ventilation is managed by titrating the sweep gas flow rate to remove carbon dioxide.

Oximetric assessment of the return circuit limb may be used as a surrogate SvO_2 to trend adequacy of ECMO support. This measure may be falsely increased in the presence of significant recirculation (blood traversing from the inflow cannula through the vena cava directly into the return circuit limb, rather than entering the right heart circulation). If this situation occurs, it may be addressed by cannula repositioning. In hyperdynamic states, native cardiac output may greatly exceed circuit pump flow, resulting in significant venous admixture and lowering arterial oxygen saturations. As such, ECMO traditionally is conducted using a high-hematocrit target to ensure adequate oxygen delivery in the face of relative hypoxemia.

Systemic anticoagulation is initiated to prevent circuit clotting. Platelet consumption at the oxygenator interface may necessitate regular platelet transfusion. The adult patient requires substantially larger platelet and red blood cell transfusion volumes than a neonate; whereas a pediatric ECMO program may create minimal burden on the transfusion service,[67] an adult ECMO program has a greater impact on blood bank resources. Data from the recent H1N1 experience suggest that at 1 center, despite long ECMO runs, blood product use was 45% less than historical reports, suggesting improved circuit biocompatibility and transfusion practice.[68,69]

Neuromuscular blockade should be discontinued as soon as feasible and oversedation avoided. In some centers, clinical management is moving toward maintaining the patient awake and spontaneously breathing, similar to the experience with ECMO patients receiving bridge-to-lung transplant.

PHARMACOTHERAPY ON ECMO

ECMO creates additional challenges for drug dosing because of drug binding to circuit components and thrombus, increases in the overall volume of distribution, and asymmetric laminar flow distributions.[70] Pharmacokinetics may be further complicated by the presence of renal failure or continuous renal replacement therapy.

Ex vivo work suggests that concentrations of commonly used ICU drugs (including fentanyl, morphine, aminoglycosides, vancomycin, phenytoin) decrease over time, with significant drug sequestration in the circuit varying by the age of the circuit.[71] Increased circuit drug absorption is correlated with increased drug lipophilicity.[72] Centrifugal pump circuits with hollow-fiber oxygenators had lower drug absorption than other configurations.[72]

In neonates, in vivo fentanyl requirements were noted to be increased[73] and morphine half-life prolonged.[74] Midazolam kinetics show large interpatient variability, and close titration of continuous infusions is required.[75] Metabolite accumulation during ECMO increases over time, and substantial dose increases may be required after 5 days. Despite this variability, daily sedation holidays were feasible in a neonatal population.[76]

When available, regular monitoring of drug levels is mandatory to ensure adequate dosing and avoid toxicity. Vancomycin and gentamicin elimination half-life is prolonged[77,78] on ECMO. Ahsman and colleagues[79] showed that cefotaxime dosing was unchanged in neonates on ECMO. Oseltamivir dosing does not seem to be affected by the ECMO circuit[80]; however, adjustments are necessary if concomitant continuous venovenous hemodialysis is administered.[81,82]

ECMO PROVIDER MODELS IN THE ICU

ECMO requires a collaborative multidisciplinary team approach to achieve the best outcome.[83] A 2008 survey of North American neonatal ECMO centers showed that registered nurses, respiratory therapists and perfusionists participated at 70%, 46% and 54% of centers, respectively. In the United States, many centers favor stationing a dedicated ECMO team member at the bedside to supervise the circuit, with the bedside nurse also providing direct patient care. In other countries, a single caregiver supervises the circuit as part of routine care, a model that is used in US cardiac units for patients with implanted ventricular assist devices, but may be unsuitable for critically ill patients with ARDS and multisystem failure. Dedicated ECMO specialists continue to serve in a consultative role. As ECMO circuits continue to become simpler and easier to manage, the bedside care model will likely continue to evolve, and careful attention must be paid to workload and safety considerations.

COMPLICATIONS ON ECMO

Complications on ECMO occur frequently and are associated with increased overall mortality.[27]

Hemorrhage

The most frequent complication during ECMO is hemorrhage. Bleeding is managed by decreasing or temporarily stopping anticoagulation and transfusing platelets and blood products, and occasional use of antifibrinolytics. Concerns that use of a prophylactic or therapeutic bleeding protocol reduces circuit lifespan may be unfounded.[84] Cannula sites and airway are frequent sites. Airway hemorrhage may require multiple bronchoscopies for pulmonary toilet.

Invasive procedures should be deferred when possible. For any invasive procedures, such as tracheostomy, careful hemostasis with electrocautery is mandatory. Tube thoracostomy while on ECMO should be avoided if there is no hemodynamic compromise, because this may precipitate massive intrathoracic hemorrhage. Thoracotomy on ECMO can lead to significant morbidity.[85]

Intracerebral hemorrhage or infarction on ECMO is a devastating and often fatal complication, occurring in approximately 10% to 15% of patients with ARDS on ECMO. Forty-three percent of the deaths in the ANZ-ECMO series were related to intracranial hemorrhage (ICH).[28] In a retrospective review of 74 adults receiving VA ECMO at a single center, the ICH rate was 18.9%. Increased risk of ICH was correlated with female gender (odds ratio [OR] 6.5), use of heparin (OR 8.5), renal failure (OR 6.5), need for dialysis (OR 4.3), and, most strongly, with thrombocytopenia (OR 18.3). Mortality was 92.3% in patients with ICH versus 61% in those without.[86]

Cannula complications are primarily vascular. Vascular access should be performed under direct ultrasound visualization. Limb ischemia can occur with arterial cannulation; perfusion of the distal extremity with retrograde posterior tibial catheters or antegrade percutaneous femoral catheters[87] may allow limb salvage. Fatal vascular perforation of the arterial or venous system can occur during cannula insertion.[48]

Systemic anticoagulation is required to avoid circuit clotting. Bedside monitoring can be performed based on activated clotting times (ACT), thromboelastography (TEG), activated partial thromboplastin time, or laboratory testing of coagulation factor levels. The ideal goal and the best method of anticoagulation monitoring are not known. In 12 infants receiving VA ECMO support, Nankervis and colleagues[88] found poor correlation between ACT and dose of unfractionated heparin (UFH), but strong correlation between anti-Xa levels and dose of UFH. Anti-Xa levels increased during time on ECMO, suggesting that UFH may collect in the circuit over time. Baird and colleagues[89] reported modest correlation of the ACT with UFH and ACT. TEG may be useful in functionally evaluating coagulation status; however, the technique is not always readily available on an ongoing basis.

As circuit components have become less thrombogenic, anticoagulation goals are being reduced in an attempt to reduce hemorrhagic complications. In some centers, fixed low-dose heparin is administered empirically. A multicenter placebo-controlled trial of prophylactic antifibrinolytic therapy[90] failed to confirm the results of an earlier cohort study[91] and showed no statistically significant reduction in the incidence of ICH. A study evaluating regional circuit anticoagulation using citrate was suspended pending further animal data.[92]

Hemolysis

Hemolysis does not occur during ECMO unless there is a problem in the circuit or with the patient. Plasma-free hemoglobin in serum should be checked daily; values more than 10 mg/dL require further investigation in identifying and repairing the cause. Circuit-related hemolysis is caused by cavitation, which occurs when blood is exposed to negative pressure in excess of −650 mm Hg.[36] This situation can occur at even less-negative levels in the presence of a blood-air interface. The presence of venous line chatter, which results from a transient drop in venous line pressure associated with interrupted flow, can also result in hemolysis. This situation can be minimized by maintaining safe rotor speed (3000–3500 rpm). If flow needs are greater, the adequacy of blood volume should be assessed and adding additional venous drainage by placement of an additional venous cannula or cannula repositioning should be considered before depending solely on increasing pump revolutions per minute.

Circuit Infection in Sepsis

In patients with active sepsis who are receiving ECMO, routine surveillance was not of additional value and hence routine cultures are not recommended.[93] The main risk factor for component infection seems to be the duration of the ECMO run,[94] and awareness of the circuit as a potential source of occult sepsis has been recommended.[95] Bacterial contamination of oxygenator biofilm may be responsible. Muller and colleagues[96] reported a case of unexplained bleeding diathesis associated with negative peripheral blood cultures, but a single positive bacterial culture was obtained from the oxygenator biofilm; the question that infection may have contributed to the clinical course was raised.

OUTCOMES IN ECMO

Mortality

Several factors have been associated with mortality on ECMO. The ELSO review[27] identified advanced patient age, pre-ECMO arterial blood pH less than 7.18, increased duration of pre-ECMO ventilation, decreasing patient weight, underlying cause of respiratory failure, and complications on ECMO to be associated with increased mortality. Hemmila and colleagues[21] derived a logistic equation to predict mortality that included similar variables: age, pre-ECLS ventilator days, initial PaO_2/FiO_2 ratio, pre-ECMO pH, and gender. In both of these series, the only non-fixed patient variable was the duration of pre-ECMO ventilation, and this has been incorporated into many recommendations for ECMO referral.

Cost

The initial cost of ECMO, in terms of circuit components, intensive care time, and personnel time is considerable. In the ANZ-ECMO series, significant resource allocation was required, with 828 patient days of ECMO support used for the 68 patients. Compared with the 133 patients who improved with conventional care, patients treated with ECMO had higher median days of mechanical ventilation; ICU length of stay was longer, despite a higher ICU mortality.

Follow-up from the UK neonatal ECMO study suggested that the incremental cost per disability-free life year gained was well below willingness-to-pay levels, and the probability that ECMO was cost-effective at 7 years was calculated to be 0.98.[97] The CESAR trial economic analysis concluded that the average cost per patient for ECMO referral was more than double the cost of treatment with conventional management. Nevertheless, the lifetime predicted cost-usefulness was approximately $31,000 per quality-adjusted life year, and the investigators concluded that "referral for ECMO is likely to prove more efficient than conventional management."[10]

Long-term Follow-up

Recovery from ARDS has been found to be associated with pulmonary and nonpulmonary functional deficits that may persist for years after ICU discharge.[98] Specific long-term follow-up in patients with ARDS who additionally undergo ECMO is limited. Post-discharge follow-up of pediatric ECMO survivors showed that most required at least 1 readmission to the hospital, one-third of them for respiratory diagnoses.[99] Linden and colleagues[100] evaluated 21 patients with severe ARDS treated with ECMO. On high-resolution thoracic computed tomography, residual changes consisting of areas of fibrosis were identified that correlated with the duration of ECMO support. Although many patients had persistent reduction in the health-related quality of life, they had less respiratory symptoms than reported by conventionally treated patients with ARDS in previous studies, and 76% of patients were able to return to their former occupations.

SUMMARY

In adult patients with respiratory failure refractory to conventional treatment, ECMO represents a potentially life-saving option. Although debate continues regarding the appropriate interpretation of limited randomized clinical trial data,[19,101–105] a significant and growing body of observational data supports the use of ECMO in severe adult respiratory failure. The issues of selection bias and survivor bias in unselected case series should not be ignored. The series reporting little[106] or no[107] ECMO use and excellent survival should also be carefully considered. It is also likely that at least some of the patients receiving ECMO after conventional measures fail represent sicker patients than those typically enrolled in clinical trials.[103]

A French prospective, randomized multicenter trial (EOLIA) (Extracorporeal Membrane Oxygenation to Rescue Lung Injury in ARDS) has opened and will enroll patients to test the efficacy of early VV ECMO in ARDS. In an effort to address some of the criticism of the CESAR trial, the protocol includes explicitly specified ventilator management and early ECMO transport from referral centers without cannulation capability.[6]

As we await the results of further randomized trials, several questions still remain to be considered. Which patients are the best candidates for ECMO? Should ECMO be initiated early in the course of ARDS or only in the cases of late failure? How can we minimize the ECMO-associated inflammatory response? What is optimal "lung rest" strategy in the face of cardiopulmonary bypass? What are the long-term functional outcomes of patients undergoing ECMO, and can intervention in the ICU improve their recovery? What is the safest and most effective ECMO team composition? What competencies and resources are necessary to deliver care safely? Would treatment outcomes be further improved by regionalization? The critical care community needs to consider these questions as we move forward in advancing ARDS care.

RESOURCES

The ELSO Web site contains a member list with contacts, management guidelines,[108] references, and training/education materials. http://www.elso.med.umich.edu/.

REFERENCES

1. Dominguez-Cherit G, Lapinsky SE, Macias AE, et al. Critically ill patients with 2009 influenza A(H1N1) in Mexico. JAMA 2009;302(17):1880–7.
2. Carrell S. Pregnant woman with swine flu airlifted to Sweden. London (UK): The Guardian; 2009. Accessed April 30, 2011.
3. Mitchell MD, Mikkelsen ME, Umscheid CA, et al. A systematic review to inform institutional decisions about the use of extracorporeal membrane oxygenation during the H1N1 influenza pandemic. Crit Care Med 2010;38(6):1398–404.
4. Chalwin RP, Moran JL, Graham PL. The role of extracorporeal membrane oxygenation for treatment of the adult respiratory distress syndrome: review and quantitative analysis. Anaesth Intensive Care 2008;36(2):152–61.
5. Allen S, Holena D, McCunn M, et al. A review of the fundamental principles and evidence base in the use of extracorporeal membrane oxygenation (ECMO) in critically ill adult patients. J Intensive Care Med 2011;26(1):13–26.
6. Combes A. EOLIA (Extracorporeal membrane oxygenation (ECMO) to rescue Lung Injury in severe ARDS). 2011. Available at: http://reaweb.org/gb/etudes.php#e2. Accessed May 2, 2011.

7. van Muers K, Lally K, Peek G, et al. ECMO. Extracorporeal cardiopulmonary support in critical care. 3rd edition. Ann Arbor (MI): Extracorporeal Life Support Organization (ELSO); 2005.
8. Zapol WM, Snider MT, Hill JD, et al. Extracorporeal membrane oxygenation in severe acute respiratory failure. A randomized prospective study. JAMA 1979; 242(20):2193–6.
9. Morris AH, Wallace CJ, Menlove RL, et al. Randomized clinical trial of pressure-controlled inverse ratio ventilation and extracorporeal CO2 removal for adult respiratory distress syndrome. Am J Respir Crit Care Med 1994;149(2 Pt 1): 295–305.
10. Peek GJ, Mugford M, Tiruvoipati R, et al. Efficacy and economic assessment of conventional ventilatory support versus extracorporeal membrane oxygenation for severe adult respiratory failure (CESAR): a multicentre randomised controlled trial. Lancet 2009;374(9698):1351–63.
11. Mols G, Loop T, Geiger K, et al. Extracorporeal membrane oxygenation: a ten-year experience. Am J Surg 2000;180(2):144–54.
12. Lewandowski K, Rossaint R, Pappert D, et al. High survival rate in 122 ARDS patients managed according to a clinical algorithm including extracorporeal membrane oxygenation. Intensive Care Med 1997;23(8):819–35.
13. Beiderlinden M, Eikermann M, Boes T, et al. Treatment of severe acute respiratory distress syndrome: role of extracorporeal gas exchange. Intensive Care Med 2006;32(10):1627–31.
14. Hill JD, De Leval MR, Fallat RJ, et al. Acute respiratory insufficiency. Treatment with prolonged extracorporeal oxygenation. J Thorac Cardiovasc Surg 1972; 64(4):551–62.
15. Bartlett RH, Morris AH, Fairley HB, et al. A prospective study of acute hypoxic respiratory failure. Chest 1986;89(5):684–9.
16. Gattinoni L, Pesenti A, Mascheroni D, et al. Low-frequency positive-pressure ventilation with extracorporeal CO2 removal in severe acute respiratory failure. JAMA 1986;256(7):881–6.
17. Suchyta MR, Clemmer TP, Orme JF Jr, et al. Increased survival of ARDS patients with severe hypoxemia (ECMO criteria). Chest 1991;99(4):951–5.
18. UK collaborative randomised trial of neonatal extracorporeal membrane oxygenation. UK Collaborative ECMO Trail Group. Lancet 1996;348(9020): 75–82.
19. Zwischenberger JB, Lynch JE. Will CESAR answer the adult ECMO debate? Lancet 2009;374(9698):1307–8.
20. Nehra D, Goldstein AM, Doody DP, et al. Extracorporeal membrane oxygenation for nonneonatal acute respiratory failure: the Massachusetts General Hospital experience from 1990 to 2008. Arch Surg 2009;144(5):427–32 [discussion: 432].
21. Hemmila MR, Rowe SA, Boules TN, et al. Extracorporeal life support for severe acute respiratory distress syndrome in adults. Ann Surg 2004;240(4):595–605 [discussion: 605–7].
22. Buckley E, Sidebotham D, McGeorge A, et al. Extracorporeal membrane oxygenation for cardiorespiratory failure in four patients with pandemic H1N1 2009 influenza virus and secondary bacterial infection. Br J Anaesth 2010; 104(3):326–9.
23. Freed DH, Henzler D, White CW, et al. Extracorporeal lung support for patients who had severe respiratory failure secondary to influenza A (H1N1) 2009 infection in Canada. Can J Anaesth 2010;57(3):240–7.

24. Grasselli G, Foti G, Patroniti N, et al. A case of ARDS associated with influenza A - H1N1 infection treated with extracorporeal respiratory support. Minerva Anestesiol 2009;75(12):741–5.
25. Liong T, Lee KL, Poon YS, et al. The first novel influenza A (H1N1) fatality despite antiviral treatment and extracorporeal membrane oxygenation in Hong Kong. Hong Kong Med J 2009;15(5):381–4.
26. Kao TM, Wang CH, Chen YC, et al. The first case of severe novel H1N1 influenza successfully rescued by extracorporeal membrane oxygenation in Taiwan. J Formos Med Assoc 2009;108(11):894–8.
27. Brogan TV, Thiagarajan RR, Rycus PT, et al. Extracorporeal membrane oxygenation in adults with severe respiratory failure: a multi-center database. Intensive Care Med 2009;35(12):2105–14.
28. Davies A, Jones D, Bailey M, et al. Extracorporeal membrane oxygenation for 2009 influenza A(H1N1) acute respiratory distress syndrome. JAMA 2009; 302(17):1888–95.
29. Davies A, Jones D, Gattas D, et al; for the ANZ-ECMO Investigators. Extracorporeal membrane oxygenation for ARDS due to 2009 influenza A (H1N1) [reply]. JAMA 2010;303(10):942.
30. Campbell BT, Braun TM, Schumacher RE, et al. Impact of ECMO on neonatal mortality in Michigan (1980–1999). J Pediatr Surg 2003;38(3):290–5 [discussion: 290–5].
31. Green TP, Timmons OD, Fackler JC, et al. The impact of extracorporeal membrane oxygenation on survival in pediatric patients with acute respiratory failure. Pediatric Critical Care Study Group. Crit Care Med 1996;24(2):323–9.
32. Murray JF, Matthay MA, Luce JM, et al. An expanded definition of the adult respiratory distress syndrome. Am Rev Respir Dis 1988;138(3):720–3.
33. Arlt M, Philipp A, Voelkel S, et al. Hand-held minimised extracorporeal membrane oxygenation: a new bridge to recovery in patients with out-of-centre cardiogenic shock. Eur J Cardiothorac Surg 2011. [Epub ahead of print].
34. Philipp A, Arlt M, Amann M, et al. First experience with the ultra compact mobile extracorporeal membrane oxygenation system Cardiohelp in interhospital transport. Interact Cardiovasc Thorac Surg 2011. [Epub ahead of print].
35. Wang D, Zhou X, Liu X, et al. Wang-Zwische double lumen cannula-toward a percutaneous and ambulatory paracorporeal artificial lung. ASAIO J 2008; 54(6):606–11.
36. Toomasian JM, Bartlett RH. Hemolysis and ECMO pumps in the 21st century. Perfusion 2011;26(1):5–6.
37. Zhang J, Gellman B, Koert A, et al. Computational and experimental evaluation of the fluid dynamics and hemocompatibility of the CentriMag blood pump. Artif Organs 2006;30(3):168–77.
38. Thiara AP, Hoel TN, Kristiansen F, et al. Evaluation of oxygenators and centrifugal pumps for long-term pediatric extracorporeal membrane oxygenation. Perfusion 2007;22(5):323–6.
39. Kolobow T, Zapol W, Pierce JE, et al. Partial extracorporeal gas exchange in alert newborn lambs with a membrane artificial lung perfused via an A-V shunt for periods up to 96 hours. Trans Am Soc Artif Intern Organs 1968;14:328–34.
40. Lehle K, Philipp A, Gleich O, et al. Efficiency in extracorporeal membrane oxygenation-cellular deposits on polymethylpentene membranes increase resistance to blood flow and reduce gas exchange capacity. ASAIO J 2008;54(6):612–7.
41. Peek GJ, Killer HM, Reeves R, et al. Early experience with a polymethyl pentene oxygenator for adult extracorporeal life support. ASAIO J 2002;48(5):480–2.

42. Horton S, Thuys C, Bennett M, et al. Experience with the Jostra Rotaflow and QuadroxD oxygenator for ECMO. Perfusion 2004;19(1):17–23.
43. Bindslev L. Adult ECMO performed with surface-heparinized equipment. ASAIO Trans 1988;34(4):1009–13.
44. Moen O, Hogasen K, Fosse E, et al. Attenuation of changes in leukocyte surface markers and complement activation with heparin-coated cardiopulmonary bypass. Ann Thorac Surg 1997;63(1):105–11.
45. Fosse E, Moen O, Johnson E, et al. Reduced complement and granulocyte activation with heparin-coated cardiopulmonary bypass. Ann Thorac Surg 1994; 58(2):472–7.
46. Meinhardt JP, Annich GM, Miskulin J, et al. Thrombogenicity is not reduced when heparin and phospholipid bonded circuits are used in a rabbit model of extracorporeal circulation. ASAIO J 2003;49(4):395–400.
47. Lawson DS, Lawson AF, Walczak R, et al. North American neonatal extracorporeal membrane oxygenation (ECMO) devices and team roles: 2008 survey results of Extracorporeal Life Support Organization (ELSO) centers. J Extra Corpor Technol 2008;40(3):166–74.
48. Bare JB, Abramowsky CR, Denton TD, et al. Perforation of the superior vena cava during ECMO catheterization in two neonates with congenital diaphragmatic hernia: a cause of accidental death. Am J Forensic Med Pathol 2008; 29(3):271–3.
49. Ruettimann U, Ummenhofer W, Rueter F, et al. Management of acute respiratory distress syndrome using pumpless extracorporeal lung assist. Can J Anaesth 2006;53(1):101–5.
50. Reng M, Philipp A, Kaiser M, et al. Pumpless extracorporeal lung assist and adult respiratory distress syndrome. Lancet 2000;356(9225):219–20.
51. Zimmermann M, Bein T, Arlt M, et al. Pumpless extracorporeal interventional lung assist in patients with acute respiratory distress syndrome: a prospective pilot study. Crit Care 2009;13(1):R10.
52. Habashi NM, Borg UR, Reynolds HN. Low blood flow extracorporeal carbon dioxide removal (ECCO2R): a review of the concept and a case report. Intensive Care Med 1995;21(7):594–7.
53. Terragni PP, Del Sorbo L, Mascia L, et al. Tidal volume lower than 6 ml/kg enhances lung protection: role of extracorporeal carbon dioxide removal. Anesthesiology 2009;111(4):826–35.
54. Terragni PP, Birocco A, Faggiano C, et al. Extracorporeal CO2 removal. Contrib Nephrol 2010;165:185–96.
55. Clement KC, Fiser RT, Fiser WP, et al. Single-institution experience with interhospital extracorporeal membrane oxygenation transport: a descriptive study. Pediatr Crit Care Med 2010;11(4):509–13.
56. Linden V, Palmer K, Reinhard J, et al. Inter-hospital transportation of patients with severe acute respiratory failure on extracorporeal membrane oxygenation–national and international experience. Intensive Care Med 2001;27(10): 1643–8.
57. Coppola CP, Tyree M, Larry K, et al. A 22-year experience in global transport extracorporeal membrane oxygenation. J Pediatr Surg 2008;43(1):46–52 [discussion: 52].
58. Forrest P, Ratchford J, Burns B, et al. Retrieval of critically ill adults using extracorporeal membrane oxygenation: an Australian experience. Intensive Care Med 2011;37(5):824–30.

59. Zimmermann M, Bein T, Philipp A, et al. Interhospital transportation of patients with severe lung failure on pumpless extracorporeal lung assist. Br J Anaesth 2006;96(1):63–6.
60. Zimmermann M, Philipp A, Schmid FX, et al. From Baghdad to Germany: use of a new pumpless extracorporeal lung assist system in two severely injured US soldiers. ASAIO J 2007;53(3):e4–6.
61. Bein T, Osborn E, Hofmann HS, et al. Successful treatment of a severely injured soldier from Afghanistan with pumpless extracorporeal lung assist and neurally adjusted ventilatory support. Int J Emerg Med 2010;3(3):177–9.
62. Robbins S. A breath of life: U.S. medical team uses new method to save soldier's life. Washington, DC: Stars and Stripes; 2010.
63. Dorlac GR, Fang R, Pruitt VM, et al. Air transport of patients with severe lung injury: development and utilization of the acute lung rescue team. J Trauma 2009;66(Suppl 4):S164–71.
64. Underwood MJ, Pearson JA, Waggoner J, et al. Changes in "inflammatory" mediators and total body water during extra-corporeal membrane oxygenation (ECMO). A preliminary study. Int J Artif Organs 1995;18(10):627–32.
65. Halter J, Steinberg J, Fink G, et al. Evidence of systemic cytokine release in patients undergoing cardiopulmonary bypass. J Extra Corpor Technol 2005; 37(3):272–7.
66. McILwain RB, Timpa JG, Kurundkar AR, et al. Plasma concentrations of inflammatory cytokines rise rapidly during ECMO-related SIRS due to the release of preformed stores in the intestine. Lab Invest 2010;90(1):128–39.
67. McCoy-Pardington D, Judd WJ, Knafl P, et al. Blood use during extracorporeal membrane oxygenation. Transfusion 1990;30(4):307–9.
68. Butch SH, Knafl P, Oberman HA, et al. Blood utilization in adult patients undergoing extracorporeal membrane oxygenated therapy. Transfusion 1996;36(1): 61–3.
69. Cooling L, Park PK, Napolitano L. Blood transfusion support in critically ill H1N1 patients. Transfusion 2010;50S:27–28A.
70. Noerr B. ECMO and pharmacotherapy. Neonatal Netw 1996;15(6):23–31.
71. Dagan O, Klein J, Gruenwald C, et al. Preliminary studies of the effects of extracorporeal membrane oxygenator on the disposition of common pediatric drugs. Ther Drug Monit 1993;15(4):263–6.
72. Wildschut ED, Ahsman MJ, Allegaert K, et al. Determinants of drug absorption in different ECMO circuits. Intensive Care Med 2010;36(12):2109–16.
73. Arnold JH, Truog RD, Orav EJ, et al. Tolerance and dependence in neonates sedated with fentanyl during extracorporeal membrane oxygenation. Anesthesiology 1990;73(6):1136–40.
74. Dagan O, Klein J, Bohn D, et al. Effects of extracorporeal membrane oxygenation on morphine pharmacokinetics in infants. Crit Care Med 1994;22(7):1099–101.
75. Ahsman MJ, Hanekamp M, Wildschut ED, et al. Population pharmacokinetics of midazolam and its metabolites during venoarterial extracorporeal membrane oxygenation in neonates. Clin Pharmacokinet 2010;49(6):407–19.
76. Wildschut ED, Hanekamp MN, Vet NJ, et al. Feasibility of sedation and analgesia interruption following cannulation in neonates on extracorporeal membrane oxygenation. Intensive Care Med 2010;36(9):1587–91.
77. Bhatt-Mehta V, Johnson CE, Schumacher RE. Gentamicin pharmacokinetics in term neonates receiving extracorporeal membrane oxygenation. Pharmacotherapy 1992;12(1):28–32.

78. Buck ML. Pharmacokinetic changes during extracorporeal membrane oxygenation: implications for drug therapy of neonates. Clin Pharmacokinet 2003;42(5):403–17.
79. Ahsman MJ, Wildschut ED, Tibboel D, et al. Pharmacokinetics of cefotaxime and desacetylcefotaxime in infants during extracorporeal membrane oxygenation. Antimicrob Agents Chemother 2010;54(5):1734–41.
80. Wildschut ED, de Hoog M, Ahsman MJ, et al. Plasma concentrations of oseltamivir and oseltamivir carboxylate in critically ill children on extracorporeal membrane oxygenation support. PLoS One 2010;5(6):e10938.
81. Eyler RF, Pleva M, Sowinski KM, et al. Oseltamivir & oseltamivir carboxylate pharmacokinetics in critically ill patients receiving continuous venovenous hemodialysis (CVVHD). Paper presented at: 50th Interscience Conference on Antimicrobial Agents and Chemotherapy. Boston, September 15, 2011.
82. Ariano RE, Sitar DS, Zelenitsky SA, et al. Enteric absorption and pharmacokinetics of oseltamivir in critically ill patients with pandemic (H1N1) influenza. CMAJ 2010;182(4):357–63.
83. Oliver WC. Anticoagulation and coagulation management for ECMO. Semin Cardiothorac Vasc Anesth 2009;13(3):154–75.
84. Muensterer OJ, Laney D, Georgeson KE. Survival time of ECMO circuits on and off bleeding protocol: is there a higher risk of circuit clotting? Eur J Pediatr Surg 2011;21(1):30–2.
85. Marasco SF, Preovolos A, Lim K, et al. Thoracotomy in adults while on ECMO is associated with uncontrollable bleeding. Perfusion 2007;22(1):23–6.
86. Kasirajan V, Smedira NG, McCarthy JF, et al. Risk factors for intracranial hemorrhage in adults on extracorporeal membrane oxygenation. Eur J Cardiothorac Surg 1999;15(4):508–14.
87. Rao AS, Pellegrini RV, Speziali G, et al. A novel percutaneous solution to limb ischemia due to arterial occlusion from a femoral artery ECMO cannula. J Endovasc Ther 2010;17(1):51–4.
88. Nankervis CA, Preston TJ, Dysart KC, et al. Assessing heparin dosing in neonates on venoarterial extracorporeal membrane oxygenation. ASAIO J 2007;53(1):111–4.
89. Baird CW, Zurakowski D, Robinson B, et al. Anticoagulation and pediatric extracorporeal membrane oxygenation: impact of activated clotting time and heparin dose on survival. Ann Thorac Surg 2007;83(3):912–9 [discussion: 919–20].
90. Horwitz JR, Cofer BR, Warner BW, et al. A multicenter trial of 6-aminocaproic acid (Amicar) in the prevention of bleeding in infants on ECMO. J Pediatr Surg 1998;33(11):1610–3.
91. Wilson JM, Bower LK, Fackler JC, et al. Aminocaproic acid decreases the incidence of intracranial hemorrhage and other hemorrhagic complications of ECMO. J Pediatr Surg 1993;28(4):536–40 [discussion: 540–1].
92. Clinical Trials.gov. Available at: http://clinicaltrials.gov/ct2/show/NCT00968565. Accessed May 1, 2011.
93. Elerian LF, Sparks JW, Meyer TA, et al. Usefulness of surveillance cultures in neonatal extracorporeal membrane oxygenation. ASAIO J 2001;47(3):220–3.
94. Steiner CK, Stewart DL, Bond SJ, et al. Predictors of acquiring a nosocomial bloodstream infection on extracorporeal membrane oxygenation. J Pediatr Surg 2001;36(3):487–92.
95. Burket JS, Bartlett RH, Vander Hyde K, et al. Nosocomial infections in adult patients undergoing extracorporeal membrane oxygenation. Clin Infect Dis 1999;28(4):828–33.

96. Muller T, Lubnow M, Phillipp A, et al. Risk of circuit infection in septic patients on extracorporeal membrane oxygenation: a preliminary study. Artif Organs 2011; 35(4):E84–90.
97. Petrou S, Bischof M, Bennett C, et al. Cost-effectiveness of neonatal extracorporeal membrane oxygenation based on 7-year results from the United Kingdom Collaborative ECMO Trial. Pediatrics 2006;117(5):1640–9.
98. Herridge MS, Tansey CM, Matte A, et al. Functional disability 5 years after acute respiratory distress syndrome. N Engl J Med 2011;364(14):1293–304.
99. Jen HC, Shew SB. Hospital readmissions and survival after nonneonatal pediatric ECMO. Pediatrics 2010;125(6):1217–23.
100. Linden VB, Lidegran MK, Frisen G, et al. ECMO in ARDS: a long-term follow-up study regarding pulmonary morphology and function and health-related quality of life. Acta Anaesthesiol Scand 2009;53(4):489–95.
101. Morris AH, Hirshberg E, Miller RR, et al. Efficacy of ECMO in H1N1 influenza: sufficient evidence? Chest 2010;138(4):778–81.
102. Park PK, Dalton HJ, Bartlett RH. Point: efficacy of extracorporeal membrane oxygenation in 2009 influenza A(H1N1): sufficient evidence? Chest 2010; 138(4):776–8.
103. White DB, Angus DC. Preparing for the sickest patients with 2009 influenza A(H1N1). JAMA 2009;302(17):1905–6.
104. Dalton HJ, MacLaren G. Extracorporeal membrane oxygenation in pandemic flu: insufficient evidence or worth the effort? Crit Care Med 2010;38(6):1484–5.
105. Finney SJ, Cordingley JJ, Griffiths MJ, et al. ECMO in adults for severe respiratory failure finally comes of age: just in time? Thorax 2010;65(3):194–5.
106. Kumar A, Zarychanski R, Pinto R, et al. Critically ill patients with 2009 influenza A(H1N1) infection in Canada. JAMA 2009;302(17):1872–9.
107. Miller RR, Markewitz BA, Rolfs RT, et al. Clinical findings and demographic factors associated with ICU admission in Utah due to novel 2009 influenza A(H1N1) infection. Chest 2010;137(4):752–8.
108. ELSO. Extracorporeal Life Support Organization Patient Specific Guidelines. A supplement to the ELSO General Guidelines (April 2009) Version 1.1. 2011. Available at: http://www.elso.med.umich.edu/Guidelines.html. Accessed May 1, 2011.

Nutrition Therapy for ALI and ARDS

Anna Krzak, RD[a], Melissa Pleva, PharmD[b], Lena M. Napolitano, MD[c,*]

KEYWORDS

- Nutrition therapy • Enteral nutrition
- Acute respiratory distress syndrome • Acute lung injury

The importance of nutrition support in critically ill patients with acute lung injury (ALI) and acute respiratory distress syndrome (ARDS) cannot be overstated. ALI and ARDS are characterized by a proinflammatory response associated with hypercatabolism that could lead to significant nutrition deficits. Nutrition support is necessary to prevent cumulative caloric deficits, malnutrition, loss of lean body mass, and deterioration of respiratory muscle strength.[1–3] Furthermore, early delivery of enteral nutrition (EN) has been associated with modulation of stress and the systemic immune response as well as attenuation of disease severity.[1] Such factors make the delivery of EN in critically ill patients, particularly in high-risk patients, such as those with ALI and ARDS, a vital component of quality care and management.

NUTRITION REQUIREMENTS AND SUBSTRATE USE

Although the importance of nutrition in this patient population is widely accepted, determining nutrition requirements and designing a nutrition support regimen is challenging. Secondary diagnoses in patients with ALI and ARDS, such as sepsis, trauma, major surgery, and multisystem organ failure, significantly alter metabolism.[4,5] Various comorbidities, sedation, and neuromuscular blockade use further complicate comprehensive assessment of energy expenditure and implementation of a safe and appropriate nutrition support regimen.[5]

Determining Energy Requirements

The many metabolic and nutrition-related manifestations associated with ALI, ARDS, and common secondary diagnoses make standard equations for determining energy expenditure highly inaccurate.[4] Indirect calorimetry (IC) is considered the gold standard

Conflicts of interests: none.

[a] Nutrition Services, University of Michigan Health System, Ann Arbor, MI, USA
[b] Department of Pharmacy Services, University of Michigan Health System, Ann Arbor, MI, USA
[c] Division of Acute Care Surgery, Department of Surgery, University of Michigan Health System, 1500 East Medical Center Drive, 1C340A-UH, SPC 5033, Ann Arbor, MI 48109–5033, USA
* Corresponding author.
E-mail address: lenan@med.umich.edu

Crit Care Clin 27 (2011) 647–659
doi:10.1016/j.ccc.2011.05.004
0749-0704/11/$ – see front matter

for assessing energy requirements.[1] Unfortunately, because of cost and lack of trained personnel, IC is frequently unavailable. Even when available, technical factors, such as FiO_2 greater than or equal to 60%, positive end expiratory pressure greater than 12 cm H_2O, and hyperventilation/hypoventilation (acute changes altering body CO_2 stores), prohibit accurate study measurement.[4,5] When available, IC captures shifts in metabolism during critical illness, allowing clinicians to design safe and appropriate nutrition support regimens while minimizing complications of underfeeding or overfeeding.[4,5] Although traditionally respiratory quotient was thought to represent substrate use, it is now more often used to confirm the validity of the study.[4] Ideally, the aim is to obtain IC at baseline and repeat when the patient clinical status changes in an effort to provide the safest and most appropriate nutrition therapy.[4,5]

Hypercapnia and Substrate Use

Previously, high carbohydrate provision was considered most detrimental in terms of hypercapnia associated with overfeeding. However, Talpers and colleagues[6] demonstrated that increasing caloric provision rather than excessive carbohydrate substrate correlated more closely with CO_2 production (**Fig. 1**). When the carbohydrate-to-fat-calorie ratio was constant, increasing total calorie intake resulted in a statistically significant increase in VCO_2 production.[6]

Before the Talpers and colleagues study in 1992, a study (n = 20) reported a reduction in duration of mechanical ventilation with the use of a high-fat, low-carbohydrate formula compared with a standard formula.[1,7,8] Additional review of other pertinent literature on this subject demonstrates no improvement in CO_2 production or improved outcomes correlated with use of high-fat, low-carbohydrate formulas.[1,7,8] Moreover, the American Society for Parenteral and Enteral Nutrition (ASPEN)/Society of Critical Care Medicine (SCCM) consensus guidelines for nutrition support therapy in adult, critically ill patients published in 2009, state that, "Specialty high-lipid low-carbohydrate formulations designed to manipulate the respiratory quotient and reduce CO_2 production are not recommended for routine use in [intensive care unit] ICU patients with acute respiratory failure."[1]

Because of a high risk of CO_2 retention, patients with ALI and ARDS on nutrition support should be frequently monitored for signs of underfeeding or overfeeding. Attention should be paid to unanticipated acid/base changes or difficulty weaning from mechanical ventilation.[5] Nutrition requirements for these patients should be

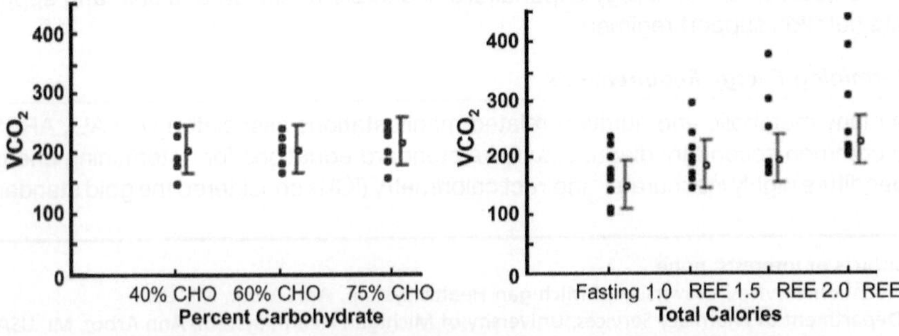

Fig. 1. Effect of carbohydrate versus total calories on CO_2 production. Increasing caloric provision rather than excessive carbohydrate substrate correlated more closely with CO_2 production. When carbohydrate-to-fat-calorie ratio was constant, increasing total calorie intake resulted in a statistically significant increase in VCO_2 production. *Abbreviations*: CHO, carbohydrate; REE, resting energy expenditure. (*Adapted from* Talpers SS, Romberger DJ, Bunce SB, et al. Nutritionally associated increased carbon dioxide production. Excess total calories vs high proportion of carbohydrate calories. Chest 1992;102:551–5; with permission.)

reevaluated and the nutrition support regimen adjusted frequently as indicated by the patients' clinical status.

Complications of Underfeeding and Overfeeding

The fundamental goal of providing adequate nutrition support therapy to critically ill patients is to avoid gross underfeeding or overfeeding. The metabolic implications characteristic of ALI and ARDS place these patients at higher risk for complications related to underfeeding or overfeeding (**Table 1**). Deleterious effects of underfeeding in patients with ALI and ARDS, such as a reduction in respiratory muscle strength and ventilatory drive, could lead to failure to wean from mechanical ventilation.[9] Underfeeding is also associated with immunosuppression, poor wound healing, and increased risk of nosocomial infections.[9] The effects of inadequate nutrition in critically ill patients are more frequently highlighted, but it should be recognized that overfeeding may also lead to undesirable outcomes. Similar to the consequences of underfeeding, hypercapnia resulting from overfeeding may delay ventilator weaning.[9] Stress hyperglycemia, which is common in critically ill patients, is exacerbated by overfeeding and may also prolong wound healing and increase risk of infection.[9]

TIMING OF THERAPY: EARLY ENTERAL NUTRITION

Early initiation of enteral nutrition in critical illness is important to achieve clinical benefit. See **Box 1** for a summary of the clinical benefits of early enteral nutrition. Once patients are fluid resuscitated and hemodynamically stable, enteral nutrition should be initiated within 24 to 48 hours and advanced to goal over the next 48 to 72 hours.[1,10,11] Feeding initiated within 24 to 72 hours of ICU admission, compared with feeding started later, is associated with reduced gastrointestinal permeability; reduced activation and release of inflammatory cytokines; and decreased infectious morbidity, mortality, and hospital length of stay.[1,10,11]

ROUTE OF DELIVERY (GASTRIC VS SMALL-BOWEL FEEDS)

The most appropriate route of delivery of enteral nutrition is an area of intense debate. Although small-bowel feeding may decrease the incidence of gastroesophageal reflux, meta-analyses evaluating gastric and small-bowel feeding reported no

Table 1
Complications of underfeeding and overfeeding

Underfeeding	Overfeeding
Decreased ventilatory drive	Hypercapnia
Depressed respiratory muscle strength	Azotemia
Failure to wean from mechanical ventilation	Failure to wean from mechanical ventilation
Immunosuppression	Electrolyte imbalances
Poor wound healing	Hyperglycemia
Infections	Infections
	Poor wound healing
	Immunosuppression
	Hepatic steatosis

Data from Refs.[3,6,9]

Box 1
Benefits of early enteral nutrition

Attenuation of hypercatabolism

Decreased gastrointestinal permeability

Improved hepatic and visceral blood flow

Reduced activation and release of inflammatory cytokines

Decreased infectious morbidity

Decreased mortality

Shorter hospital length of stay

Data from Refs.[1,10,11]

significant difference in pneumonia, ICU length of stay, or mortality.[12–15] Some of the benefits of gastric feeding include ease of tube placement and earlier feeding initiation.[13] In fact, ASPEN/SCCM guidelines recognize that gastric feeding is appropriate for many critically ill patients.[1] However, at the height of critical illness, patients are prone to gastrointestinal dysfunction, gastroparesis, and potential feeding intolerance.[1] Therefore, small-bowel feeding tube placement should be considered for high-risk patients, particularly those with a history of aspiration or intolerance to gastric feeding.[1,5] Frequent withholding of EN because of elevated gastric residual volumes also warrants evaluation for small-bowel feeding.[1]

SPECIAL CONSIDERATIONS FOR NUTRITION SUPPORT IN ALI AND ARDS

ALI and ARDS are characterized by a persistent production of oxygen free radicals and arachidonic acid (AA)-derived inflammatory mediators.[16–20] These mediators result in lung inflammation, edema, and diffuse alveolar damage. A key aim in treating patients with ALI and ARDS is to modulate pulmonary inflammation and permeability characteristic of the disease, thereby improving oxygenation.[16] A diet enriched with eicosapentaenoic acid (EPA) and γ-linolenic acid (GLA) has been shown to modify the availability of AA in tissue and cell phospholipids as well as stimulate proinflammatory eicosanoid production from AA.[16–20] Additionally, EPA shifts production of cytokines from the highly proinflammatory 4-series leukotrienes and dienoic prostaglandins to the less-inflammatory 5-series leukotrienes and trienoic prostaglandins. Through a series of pathways, GLA is metabolized to prostaglandin E1, a potent vasodilator of pulmonary and systemic circulation. Consequently, a combination of EPA and GLA may favorably reduce the pulmonary inflammatory response and support vasodilation and oxygenation (**Fig. 2**).[16–20]

CLINICAL TRIALS WITH IMMUNE-MODULATING NUTRITION IN ALI/ARDS

Several studies in patients with ALI or ARDS have shown that the use of omega-3 fatty acids, specifically EPA and GLA, and antioxidants may prevent oxidative cellular injury, modify the metabolic response caused by stress, and modulate immunity and inflammation.[16–20] This specialized nutrition support therapy was associated with improved outcomes, including improved ventilation and oxygenation, shorter ICU length of stay, and decreased morbidity and mortality.[21–23]

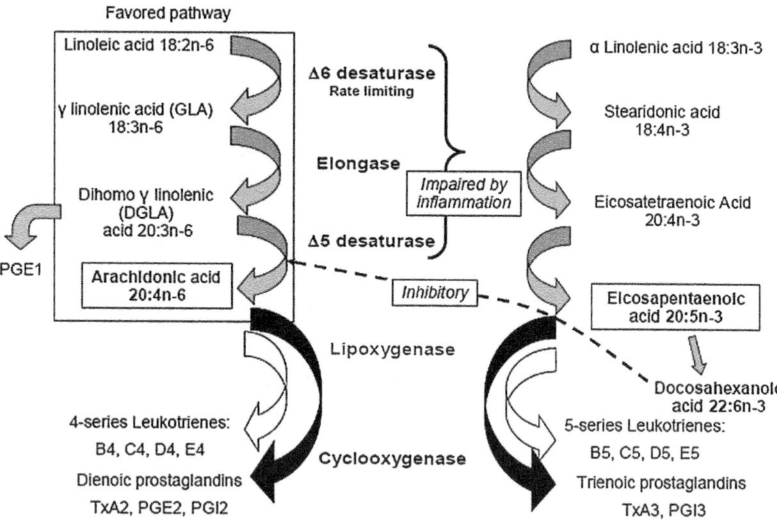

Fig. 2. Pathophysiology: metabolism of omega-6 fatty acids and omega-3 fatty acids. The major product of omega-6 fatty acid metabolism is arachidonic acid. Cyclooxygenase and lipoxygenase enzymes use arachidonic acid to form prostaglandins of the 2 series and leukotrienes of the 4 series. These compounds are known to be proinflammatory. The metabolites of omega-3 fatty acids (primarily EPA and docosahexaenoic acid) compete with arachidonic acid for use of the same enzymes. As a result, more omega-3 fatty acids lead to both an increase in antiinflammatory mediators and a decrease in proinflammatory mediators. (Created by Todd W. Rice, MD, MSc and Arthur P. Wheeler, MD and Presented at A.S.P.E.N. Clinical Nutrition Week 2011; with permission.)

Three prospective, randomized clinical trials highlighted the use of omega-3 fatty acids and antioxidants in patients with ALI and ARDS. Two of these studies were single-center studies and one study was completed at 5 sites in the United States. The sample size in each study ranged from 100 to 165 patients. All three trials followed a similar study design comparing a diet enriched with EPA, GLA, and antioxidants (Oxepa; Abbott Nutrition, Abbott Laboratories, Columbus, OH, USA) with an isocaloric and isonitrogenous control diet (Pulmocare; Abbott Nutrition, Abbott Laboratories).[4,5,9,16]

In a meta-analysis of these 3 trials, the diet enriched with EPA, GLA, and antioxidants was associated with the following outcomes: (1) a 60% reduction in 28-day, in-hospital, all-cause mortality (odds ratio [OR] 0.404; 95% confidence interval [CI] 0.241–0.678; P = .001); (2) a mean increase of 4.9 ventilator-free days; (3) a mean increase of 4.3 ICU-free days; (4) an 83% reduction in the risk of developing new organ failures, (The study reported by Singer and colleagues was excluded because it did not assess the development of new organ failures); and (5) improvement in oxygenation status (**Figs. 3** and **4**).[16,21–23]

However, a recent study reported different findings. The ARDSNet EDEN-Omega study was entitled "Early Versus Delayed Enteral Feeding and Omega-3 Fatty Acid/Antioxidant Supplementation for Treating People With Acute Lung Injury or Acute Respiratory Distress Syndrome."[24] This phase III clinical trial was a prospective, randomized trial of initial trophic enteral feeding followed by advancement to full-calorie enteral feeding versus early advancement to full-calorie enteral feeding. This trial was run simultaneously with a trial of omega-3 fatty acid, GLA, and antioxidant

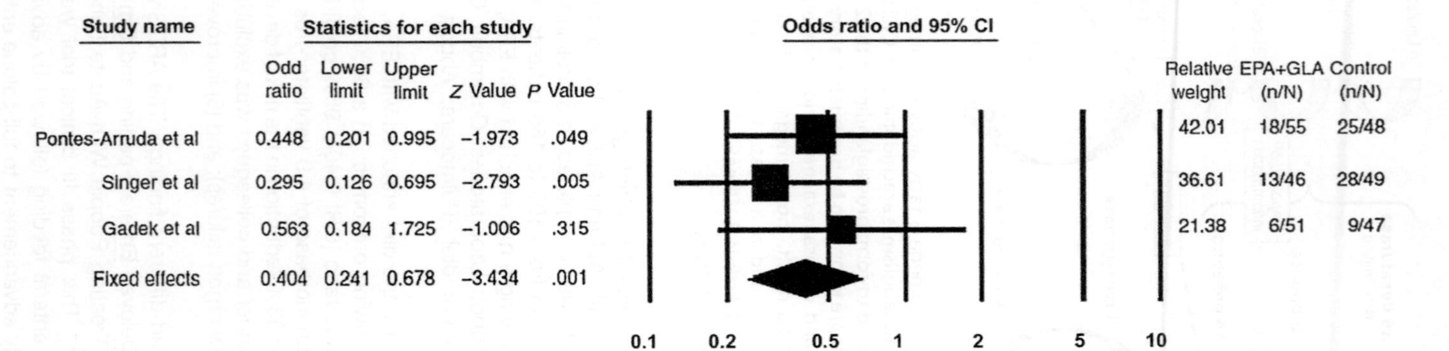

Fig. 3. Effect of inflammation-modulating diet on mortality in ALI/ARDS. Effect of the EPA and GLA diet when compared with the control diet on 28-day, in-hospital, all-cause mortality. Data are presented as OR for each study (*boxes*), 95% CI (*horizontal lines*), and summary as OR with 95% CI (*diamond*). (*Adapted from* Pontes-Arruda A, Demichele S, Seth A, et al. The use of an inflammation-modulating diet in patients with acute lung injury or acute respiratory distress syndrome: a meta-analysis of outcome data. JPEN J Parenter Enteral Nutr 2008;32:596; with permission.)

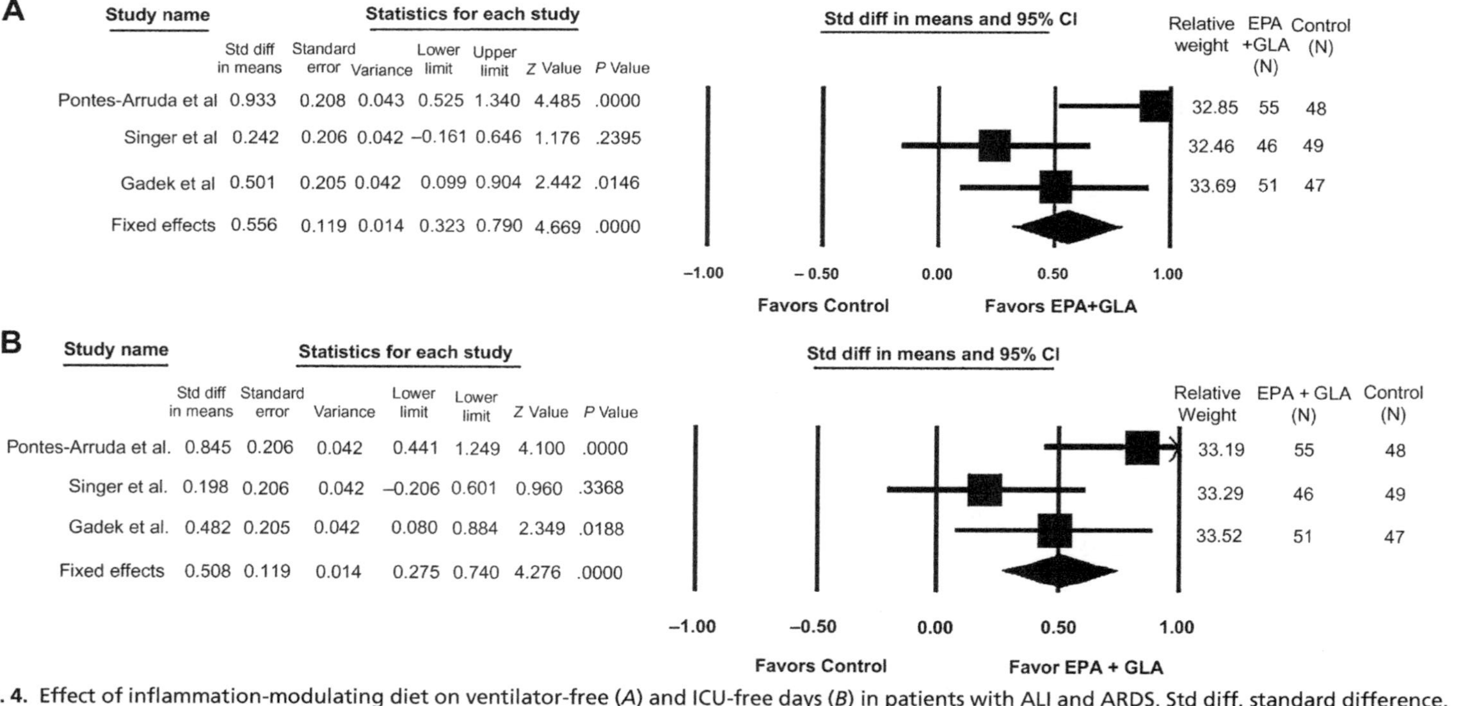

A
Study name
Statistics for each study
Std diff in means
Standard error
Variance
Lower limit
Upper limit
Z Value
P Value
Pontes-Arruda et al 0.933 0.208 0.043 0.525 1.340 4.485 .0000
Singer et al 0.242 0.206 0.042 –0.161 0.646 1.176 .2395
Gadek et al 0.501 0.205 0.042 0.099 0.904 2.442 .0146
Fixed effects 0.556 0.119 0.014 0.323 0.790 4.669 .0000
Std diff in means and 95% CI
–1.00
– 0.50
0.00
0.50
1.00
Favors Control
Favors EPA+GLA
Relative weight
EPA +GLA (N)
Control (N)
32.85 55 48
32.46 46 49
33.69 51 47
B
Study name
Statistics for each study
Std diff in means
Standard error
Variance
Lower limit
Lower limit
Z Value
P Value
Pontes-Arruda et al. 0.845 0.206 0.042 0.441 1.249 4.100 .0000
Singer et al. 0.198 0.206 0.042 –0.206 0.601 0.960 .3368
Gadek et al. 0.482 0.205 0.042 0.080 0.884 2.349 .0188
Fixed effects 0.508 0.119 0.014 0.275 0.740 4.276 .0000
Std diff in means and 95% CI
–1.00
–0.50
0.00
0.50
1.00
Favors Control
Favor EPA + GLA
Relative Weight
EPA + GLA (N)
Control (N)
33.19 55 48
33.29 46 49
33.52 51 47

Fig. 4. Effect of inflammation-modulating diet on ventilator-free (*A*) and ICU-free days (*B*) in patients with ALI and ARDS. Std diff, standard difference. (*Adapted from* Pontes-Arruda A, Demichele S, Seth A, et al. The use of an inflammation-modulating diet in patients with acute lung injury or acute respiratory distress syndrome: a meta-analysis of outcome data. JPEN J Parenter Enteral Nutr 2008;32:596; with permission.)

supplementation versus comparator enteral solution. The primary outcome measures were number of ventilator-free days and mortality before hospital discharge with unassisted breathing. This trial added an omega-3 fatty acid and antioxidant supplement to usual feeding (did not use a commercially available product). This difference is important in this trial design from prior studies in that it separated the immune-modulating nutrients from the continuous delivery of EN.

Participants assigned to initial minimal enteral feedings received feedings at 10 mL/h and continued at this rate for 144 hours, provided that the participant remained on mechanical ventilation. After 144 hours, the feeding rate was advanced to the full-calorie target rate. Participants assigned to initial full-calorie enteral feedings received feedings at 25 mL/h, and the feeding rate was increased by 25 mL increments every 6 hours until the goal rate was reached. Omega-3 fatty acid, antioxidant, and placebo supplements were administered with a syringe into the participant's feeding tube every 12 hours until day 21 or discontinuation of the ventilator.

The Data Safety and Monitoring Board performed an interim analysis and examined the data of the EDEN-Omega study. The study was terminated early for futility. In a brief report in *Surgery News*,[25] the preliminary data was reviewed. The mortality rate at 60 days was significantly lower at 16.3% in the control group versus 26.6% in the experimental cohort ($P = .05$). In addition, patients randomized to the omega-3 fatty acid–supplement group had significantly fewer ventilator-free days within 28 days (14.6 days, compared with 17.4 days for the control group, $P = .03$) and significantly fewer ICU-free days within 28 days (13.9 days, compared with 16.8 days for the control group, $P = .02$; **Tables 2** and **3**). Further review of the data from this prospective clinical trial awaits peer-reviewed publication.

CONTROVERSIES WITH IMMUNE-MODULATING NUTRITION IN ALI/ARDS

Despite several reports regarding the positive effects of omega-3 fatty acids on the inflammatory response in patients with ALI and ARDS, there are still areas of uncertainty and controversy.

First, in the original 3 trials on omega-3 fatty acids, the medical management of the patients is not consistently controlled or reported. The recent ARDSNet EDEN-Omega study was the first to report important components of medical management, such as fluid therapy and tidal volume.[5,16,24]

Second, many studies on the use of enteral omega-3 fatty acids used a comparator formula (Pulmocare) that was high in fat and low in carbohydrate. The fat source in this comparator formula is primarily omega-6 fatty acids.[16] Omega-6 fatty acids have been associated with proinflammatory characteristics in critically ill patients.[1,26–28] It could be presumed that the results reported in studies using this high-fat, low-carbohydrate formula as the control were distorted because of the potential proinflammatory characteristics of omega-6 fatty acids.

Third, timing of initiation of therapy, optimal dose, and duration of therapy remain uncertain. As previously mentioned, early delivery of EN is pivotal to obtain clinical benefit.[1,10,11] The same is true when using immune-modulating, specialized nutrition support. Studies suggest that delivery of more than 50% to 65% of goal calories is more closely associated with positive outcomes of EN, when compared with lower calorie provision.[1] The period of time needed from delivery to clinical effect may vary based on the dose and the route of delivery. See **Table 3** for more information regarding the dosing ranges of EPA, docosahexaenoic acid, and GLA in important trials. Additional studies are needed to come to a definitive conclusion.

Table 2
Antiinflammatory immune-modulating enteral nutrition versus standard enteral nutrition in ALI, ARDS, and sepsis

Study	Population	Study Groups	Mortality	LOS Days, Mean ± SD	Ventilator Days, Mean ± SD	New Organ Dysfunction
Gadek et al,[21] 1999	ARDS (n = 146)	EPA/GLA/AO	11/70 (16%)	11.0 ± 0.9 ICU[a]	9.6 ± 0.9[a]	7/70 (10%)[a]
		Control EN	19/76 (25%)	14.8 ± 1.3 ICU	13.2 ± 1.4	19/76 (25%)
		EPA/GLA/AO	ICU mortality	27.9 ± 2.1 Hospital		
		Control EN		31.1 ± 2.4 Hospital		
Singer et al,[22] 2006	ARDS and ALI (n = 100)	EPA/GLA/AO	14/46 (30%)[a]	13.5 ± 11.8 ICU	12.1 ± 11.3	NR
		Control EN	26/49 (53%) 28d mortality	15.6 ± 11.8 ICU	14.7 ± 12.0	
Pontes-Arruda et al,[23] 2006	Severe sepsis (n = 165)	EPA/GLA/AO	26/83 (31%)[a]	17.2 ± 4.9 ICU[a]	14.6 ± 4.3[a]	32/83 (39%)[a]
		Control EN	38/82 (46%) 28d mortality	23.4 ± 3.5 ICU	22.2 ± 5.1	66/82 (80%)

Abbreviations: AO, antioxidants; EN, enteral nutrition; EPA, eicosapentaenoic acid; GLA, γ-linolenic acid; LOS, length of stay; NR, not reported; SD, standard deviation.

[a] $P \leq 05$.

Data from McClave SA, Martindale RG, Vanek VW, et al; A.S.P.E.N. Board of Directors; American College of Critical Care Medicine; Society of Critical Care Medicine. Guidelines for the provision and assessment of nutrition support therapy in the adult critically ill patient: Society of Critical Care Medicine (SCCM) and American Society for Parenteral and Enteral Nutrition (A.S.P.E.N.). JPEN J Parenter Enteral Nutr 2009;33(3):277–316.

Table 3
Summary of clinical studies

	Gadek et al[21]	Singer et al[22]	Pontes-Arruda et al[23]	ARDSNet EDEN-Omega[24]
Design	P, R, C, DB Full feeds	P, R, C Full feeds	P, R, C, DB Full feeds	P, R, C Full feeds/ trophic feeds
Setting	Multicenter	Single center	Single center	Multicenter
Patients	146 ARDS	100 ALI	165 severe sepsis/ septic shock	272 ALI/ARDS
Interventions	Omega-3 FA + AO	Omega-3 FA + AO	Omega-3 FA + AO	Omega-3 FA + AO
Mean fatty-acid intake				
EPA (g/d)	6.9	5.4	4.9	6.8
DHA (g/d)	2.9	2.5	2.2	3.4
GLA (g/d)	5.8	5.1	4.6	5.9
Omega-3 delivery	Continuous	Continuous	Continuous	Bolus BID
Control formula	High fat (omega-6, 9)	High fat (omega-6, 9)	High fat (omega-6, 9)	High carbohydrate
Tidal volume	Uncontrolled	Uncontrolled	Uncontrolled	6 mL/kg PBW
Fluid therapy	Uncontrolled	Uncontrolled	Uncontrolled	Conservative
Outcomes[a]				
Improved oxygenation	X	X	X	—
Reduced vent days	X	X	X	X
Reduced ICU length of stay	X	X	X	X
Reduced new organ failure	X	Not assessed	X	—
Reduced 28-day mortality	—	X	X	—

Abbreviations: AO, antioxidants; C, controlled; CD, control diet; DB, double blind; DHA, docosahexaenoic acid; EPA, eicosapentaenoic acid; FA, fatty acid; GLA, γ-linolenic acid; P, prospective; PBW, predicted body weight; R, randomized.

[a] X: statistically significant ($P<.05$) for EPA + GLA versus control diet.

Data from Pontes-Arruda A, Demichele S, Seth A, et al. The Use of an inflammation-modulating diet in patients with acute lung injury or acute respiratory distress syndrome: a meta-analysis of outcome data. JPEN J Parenter Enteral Nutr 2008;32:596.

RECOMMENDATIONS FOR NUTRITION SUPPORT IN CRITICALLY ILL PATIENTS WITH ALI AND ARDS

General

- EN is preferred when the gastrointestinal tract is functional.
- Initiate early EN after patients are resuscitated.
  - Initiate within 24 to 48 hours and advance to the goal over the next 48 to 72 hours.
- Withhold EN if patients are hypotensive or on increasing doses of vasopressors.
- Polymeric formula is preferred.

- Either gastric or small-bowel feeds are acceptable.
  - Consider small-bowel feeding tube placement in high-risk patients with history of aspiration or intolerance to gastric feeding.
- Consider prokinetics in patients with feeding intolerance.
- Provide antioxidants and trace minerals.
- Fluid-restricted formulas should be considered in patients with respiratory failure.
- Aggressively replace phosphorus in patients with normal renal function.

Evidence-based consensus guidelines on nutrition support in adult, critically ill patients endorse the following:

ASPEN/SCCM Guidelines

The ASPEN/SCCM Guidelines for the Provision and Assessment of Nutrition Support Therapy in the Adult Critically Ill Patient published in 2009[1,2] recommend the following:

> *Patients with ARDS and severe ALI should be placed on an enteral formulation characterized by an anti-inflammatory lipid profile (ie, omega-3 fish oils, borage oil) and antioxidants.*

Canadian Clinical Practice Guidelines

The "Canadian Clinical Practice Guidelines for Nutrition Support in Mechanically Ventilated, Critically Ill Adult Patients," published in the January 2009 update, recommends the following:[10]

> *"Based on one level 1 study and four level 2 studies, we recommend the use of an enteral formula with fish oils, borage oils and antioxidants in patients with ALI and ARDS."*

SUMMARY

Nutrition support is a critical component of care in patients with ALI/ARDS. Early EN support is recommended, using either gastric or small-bowel feeding dependent on patient tolerance. Indirect calorimetry is the ideal method for determination of caloric requirements in patients with ALI/ARDS. Specialized nutrition support, with an enteral diet enriched with omega-3 fatty acid, GLA, and antioxidant supplementation, should be considered in patients with ALI and ARDS based on the available clinical trial data. However, results from the recent ARDSNet EDEN-Omega study are not yet published. The optimal dosage, composition of fatty acids, and the ratio of individual immune-modulating nutrients in specialized enteral formulations remain controversial.

REFERENCES

1. McClave SA, Martindale RG, Vanek VW, et al, A.S.P.E.N. Board of Directors, American College of Critical Care Medicine, Society of Critical Care Medicine. Guidelines for the provision and assessment of nutrition support therapy in the adult critically ill patient: Society of Critical Care Medicine (SCCM) and American Society for Parenteral and Enteral Nutrition (A.S.P.E.N.). JPEN J Parenter Enteral Nutr 2009;33(3):277–316.
2. Martindale RG, McClave SA, Vanek VW, et al, American College of Critical Care Medicine, A.S.P.E.N. Board of Directors. Guidelines for the provision and assessment of nutrition support therapy in the adult critically ill patient: Society of Critical

Care Medicine and American Society for Parenteral and Enteral Nutrition: executive summary. Crit Care Med 2009;37(5):1757–61.
3. Fraser IM. Effects of refeeding on respiration and skeletal muscle function. Clin Chest Med 1986;7:131–9.
4. Wooley JA, Sax HC. Indirect calorimetry: applications to practice. Nutr Clin Pract 2003;18(5):434–9.
5. Turner KL, Moore FA, Martindale RG. Nutrition support for the acute lung injury/adult respiratory distress syndrome patient: a review. Nutr Clin Pract 2011;26:14.
6. Talpers SS, Romberger DJ, Bunce SB, et al. Nutritionally associated increased carbon dioxide production. Excess total calories vs high proportion of carbohydrate calories. Chest 1992;102:551–5.
7. al-Saady NM, Blackmore CM, Bennett ED. High fat, low carbohydrate, enteral feeding lowers PaCO2 and reduces the period of ventilation in artificially ventilated patients. Intensive Care Med 1989;15:290–5.
8. Barale F, Verdy S, Boillot A, et al. Calorimetric study of enteral low-carbohydrate diet in patients with respiratory insufficiency and decompensation. Agressologie 1990;31:77–9.
9. McClave SA. The consequences of overfeeding and underfeeding. J Respir Care Pract 1997;10:57–64.
10. Heyland DK, Dhaliwal R, Drover JW, et al, Canadian Critical Care Clinical Practice Guidelines Committee. Canadian clinical practice guidelines for nutrition support in mechanically ventilated, critically ill adult patients. JPEN J Parenter Enteral Nutr 2003;27(5):355–73. Update January 2009. Available at: http://www.criticalcarenutrition.com/docs/cpg/srrev.pdf. Accessed April 24, 2011.
11. Marik PE, Zaloga GP. Early enteral nutrition in acutely ill patients: a systematic review. Crit Care Med 2001;29:2264–70.
12. Heyland DK, Drover JW, MacDonald S, et al. Effect of postpyloric feeding on gastroesophageal regurgitation and pulmonary microaspiration: results of a randomized controlled trial. Crit Care Med 2001;29:1495–501.
13. Ho KM, Dobb GJ, Webb SA. A comparison of early gastric and post-pyloric feeding in critically ill patients: a meta-analysis. Intensive Care Med 2006;32:639–49.
14. Marik PE, Zaloga GP. Gastric versus post-pyloric feeding: a systematic review. Crit Care 2003;7:R46–51.
15. Heyland DK, Drover JW, Dhaliwal R, et al. Optimizing the benefits and minimizing the risks of enteral nutrition in the critically ill: role of small bowel feeding. JPEN J Parenter Enteral Nutr 2002;26(Suppl 6):S51–5.
16. Pontes-Arruda A, Demichele S, Seth A, et al. The use of an inflammation-modulating diet in patients with acute lung injury or acute respiratory distress syndrome: a meta-analysis of outcome data. JPEN J Parenter Enteral Nutr 2008;32:596.
17. DeMichele SJ, Wood SM, Wennberg AK. A nutritional strategy to improve oxygenation and decrease morbidity in patients who have acute respiratory distress syndrome. Respir Care Clin N Am 2006;12:547–66.
18. Mizock BA. Nutritional support in acute lung injury and acute respiratory distress syndrome. Nutr Clin Pract 2001;16:319–28.
19. Mizock BA, DeMichele SJ. The acute respiratory distress syndrome: role of nutritional modulation through dietary lipids. Nutr Clin Pract 2004;19:563–74.
20. Nelson JL, DeMichele SJ, Pacht E, et al, Enteral Nutrition in ARDS Study Group. Effect of enteral feeding with eicosapentaenoic acid, gamma-linolenic acid, and antioxidants on antioxidant status in patients with acute respiratory distress syndrome. JPEN J Parenter Enteral Nutr 2003;27:98–104.

21. Gadek JE, DeMichele SJ, Karlstad MD, et al. Effect of enteral feeding with eicosapentaenoic acid, gamma-linolenic acid, and antioxidants in patients with acute respiratory distress syndrome. Crit Care Med 1999;27:1409–20.
22. Singer P, Theilla M, Fisher H, et al. Benefit of an enteral diet enriched with eicosapentaenoic acid and gamma-linolenic acid in ventilated patients with acute lung injury. Crit Care Med 2006;34:1033–8.
23. Pontes-Arruda A, Aragao AM, Albuquerque JD. Effects of enteral feeding with eicosapentaenoic acid, gamma-linolenic acid, and antioxidants in mechanically ventilated patients with severe sepsis and septic shock. Crit Care Med 2006; 34:2325–33.
24. Early versus delayed enteral feeding and omega-3 fatty acid/antioxidant supplementation for treating people with acute lung injury or acute respiratory distress syndrome (The EDEN-Omega Study). Available at: http://clinicaltrials.gov/ct2/show/NCT00609180. Accessed April 24, 2011.
25. Available at: http://www.facs.org/surgerynews/1209.pdf. Accessed April 24, 2011.
26. Battistella FD, Widergren JT, Anderson JT, et al. A prospective, randomized trial of intravenous fat emulsion administration in trauma victims requiring total parenteral nutrition. J Trauma 1997;43:52–8.
27. Mayer K, Kiessling A, Ott J, et al. Acute lung injury is reduced in fat-1 mice endogenously synthesizing n-3 fatty acids. Am J Respir Crit Care Med 2009; 179:474–83.
28. Pluess T, Hayoz D, Berger MM, et al. Intravenous fish oil blunts the physiological response to endotoxin in healthy subjects. Intensive Care Med 2007;33:789–97.

Biomarkers in Acute Lung Injury—Marking Forward Progress

Nicolas Barnett, MB ChB, Lorraine B. Ware, MD*

KEYWORDS

• Biomarkers • Clinical predictors • ALI • ARDS

An invited commentary in the *Lancet* in 1997 noted, "despite two decades of intense effort, there is still no means of predicting reliably whether an individual patient will develop the acute respiratory distress syndrome (ARDS)".[1] Shortly thereafter, the National Institutes of Health National Heart, Lung, and Blood Institute ARDS Clinical Network (ARDSNet) trial of lower tidal volume ventilation,[2] with an unprecedented 21% relative risk reduction in mortality, led to renewed optimism in the field of acute lung injury (ALI). In addition to guiding clinical management, this and subsequent ARDSNet studies have served as valuable sources of biologic samples for large-scale validation of multiple biomarkers.[3]

This article reviews the state of the art regarding biomarkers for prediction, diagnosis, prognosis, and surrogate endpoints in ALI, drawing on data from ARDSNet studies as well as other well-characterized patient populations. In addition to candidate biomarker studies, contributions from the omics revolution, with its many subgenres—genomics, proteomics, metabolomics, and others—are discussed. Given the significant progress in the past decade, there is optimism that the next decade will be marked by continued advancements in the ability to apply biomarkers to the diagnosis, treatment, and prognostication in the clinical syndrome of ALI.

BIOMARKER RESEARCH IN ALI: DEFINITIONS AND GOALS

A widely cited definition for a biomarker came from the 1998 National Institutes of Health Biomarker Definitions Working Group: "a characteristic that is objectively measured and evaluated as an indicator of normal biological processes, pathogenic processes, or pharmacologic responses to a therapeutic intervention".[4] This definition

This work was supported by HL 103836 and HL 088263 from the National Institutes of Health and an American Heart Association Established Investigator Award.

Division of Allergy, Pulmonary and Critical Care Medicine, Department of Medicine, Vanderbilt University, Nashville, TN, USA

* Corresponding author. Division of Allergy, Pulmonary and Critical Care Medicine, Vanderbilt University, T1218 MCN, 1161 21st Avenue South, Nashville, TN 37232-2650.

E-mail address: Lorraine.ware@vanderbilt.edu

Crit Care Clin 27 (2011) 661–683
doi:10.1016/j.ccc.2011.04.001

0749-0704/11/$ – see front matter

makes no supposition about the material nature of the characteristic in question. Reflecting this, the World Health Organization suggests that a biomarker is “any substance, structure or process that can be measured in the body or its products and influence or predict the incidence or outcome of disease”.[5] More broadly, the World Health Organization proposed that a biomarker is “almost any measurement reflecting an interaction between a biological system and a potential hazard, which may be chemical, physical or biological. The response may be functional and physiological, biochemical at the cellular level, or a molecular interaction.”[6] This definition provides a mechanistic framework for conceptualizing biomarkers in ALI and serves as a reminder that clinical signs, such as pulse and blood pressure, can also be biomarkers. The fundamental goal of biomarker research is to determine the relationship between a given biomarker and relevant clinical endpoints.[7]

Several relevant clinical endpoints have been the focus of biomarker research in ALI. The most clinically important outcome is mortality,[8] and prediction of hospital or short-term mortality has been the predominant focus of biomarker research in the past decade.[9] Another clinical endpoint of import is that of diagnosis—can a biomarker that is specific to lung injury facilitate the diagnosis in high-risk patients or distinguish between the high permeability pulmonary edema of ALI and cardiogenic edema? Related to diagnosis is the prediction of ALI in at-risk patients. More accurate identification of patients likely to develop ALI would facilitate trials of novel agents or quality-improvement initiatives for prevention of ALI. Similarly, identification of subgroups of patients either at risk of or with established ALI who may have a differential response to treatment could facilitate enrollment of more homogenous populations into clinical trials and represents an additional clinical endpoint of interest.

A further potential role for biomarkers of ALI is as surrogate endpoints in clinical trials.[7] A biomarker response to treatment might substitute for a hierarchically more important clinical endpoint, such as mortality in early-phase clinical trials, that are not powered for mortality.[10] The use of surrogate endpoints, however, can be problematic in critical care. Improvements in surrogate endpoints, such as oxygenation and organ failures, have not consistently been associated with mortality reductions in sepsis or ALI studies.[2] Conversely, an absence of signal in a surrogate endpoint does not necessarily imply a failure to improve mortality outcomes.[11] In summary, there are many potential roles for biomarkers in clinical ALI and these roles coalesce around predicting progression from the at-risk state, to diagnosis, to response to treatment, to risk stratification and to prognosis.

Biomarkers—Illuminating Biologic Pathways

Another important goal of biomarker research is to shed light on the relative contribution of biologic pathways to ALI pathogenesis. Assays of candidate biomarkers that reflect various aspects of ALI pathogenesis derived from experimental models can provide confirmation that these pathways are important in the pathophysiology of human disease. Furthermore, modeling candidate biomarkers in a head-to-head comparison has emerged as a powerful tool to determine the best performing biomarkers, an approach that can also provide important glimpses into pathogenesis.[12]

The apparent association of cytokines, biologic pathways, and clinical outcomes in ALI must be tempered, however, by the knowledge that biomarkers, such as cytokines, are members of complex cascades and networks. Assessing levels of an individual cytokine dissociated from the levels of its antagonists or natural inhibitors may lead to the erroneous impression that an altered cytokine level reflects derangements in a biologic pathway.[13] In addition, immune-reactive assays that measure the presence of a protein may provide qualitatively different information from bioactivity assays that measure the functional, downstream signaling activity of the protein.[14]

Biomarker Performance and Validity

Assessment of biomarker performance is a function of sensitivity (the probability of a positive test given the presence of disease) and specificity (the probability of a negative test given the absence of disease). The ratio of sensitivity to 1-specificity (the false-positive rate) yields a likelihood ratio. When the likelihood ratio exceeds 1, then the odds of the disease based on the test under examination is increased and the test has greater discriminatory value.[10] The likelihood ratio is particularly useful because it can be examined at incremental values of the diagnostic test. Values for the sensitivity and 1-specificifity depicted graphically result in a receiver operating characteristic (ROC) curve (**Fig. 1**). The area under the curve (AUC) is a measure of performance. ROC curve analysis is particularly indicated to assess the diagnostic accuracy of a biomarker but newer statistical models suggest a role in disease prediction.[15] A related term often used in the literature is accuracy. Accuracy is an aggregate (rather than a multiplicative) of sensitivity and specificity modified by the underlying prevalence of the disease.[16]

Validity is an overarching term that incorporates aspects of precision, performance, and reproducibility. Validity can be assessed at multiple levels. First is measurement validity: Is the biomarker measurable with precision and reproducibility? Second is internal validity: For a given study and clinical outcome, how well does the biomarker under scrutiny perform. Third is external validity: What is the predictive power of the biomarker beyond its initial evaluation and its capacity for surrogacy—can the biomarker be used to stratify patient groups based on risk for ALI or responsiveness to therapy?[7] A valid biomarker may be considered to have high effectiveness if it meets all aspects of validity.

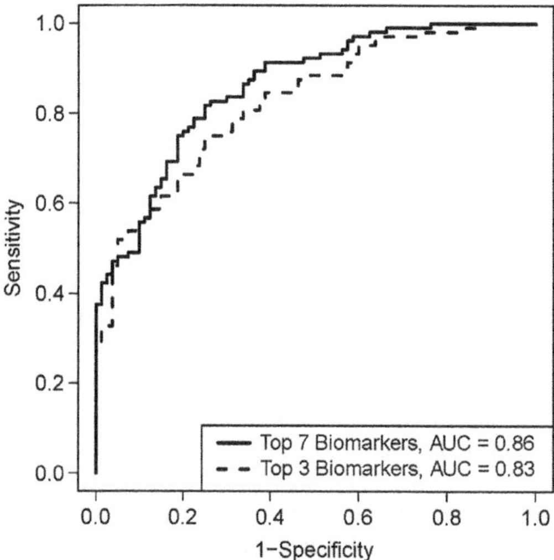

Fig. 1. ROC curve analysis for the 7 best performing biomarkers from a 21-biomarker panel for the diagnosis of trauma-induced ALI. The 3 most discriminatory biomarkers were RAGE, brain natriuretic peptide, and PCP III, with an AUC of 0.83. (*From* Fremont RD, Koyama T, Calfee CS, et al. Acute lung injury in patients with traumatic injuries: utility of a panel of biomarkers for diagnosis and pathogenesis. J Trauma 2010;68:1124; with permission.)

Characteristics of the Ideal Biomarker—the SMART Biomarker

The SMART criteria and mnemonic, a transplant from the business world, has been suggested for assessment of the disparate elements of quality control (performance and accuracy) and quality assurance (process measures, such as reproducibility, accessibility, ease of use, and internal validity). Shehabi and Seppelt[17] suggested that a SMART biomarker is *S*ensitive (and *S*pecific), *M*easurable (with a high degree of precision), *A*vailable (*A*ffordable and safely *A*ttainable), and *R*esponsive (and *R*eproducible) in a *T*imely fashion (to expedite clinical decision making). Two additional words making the comparative SMARTER[18]—*E*valuate (validate) and *R*e-evaluate (revalidate) emphasize that biomarker research needs to be in a continuous cycle of appraisal and reappraisal.

THE BIOMARKER AND ALI INTERFACE

ALI and ARDS are complex, inflammatory syndromes of noncardiogenic pulmonary edema. Nonpulmonary sepsis and pneumonia are the most common causes followed by major trauma, shock, and aspiration of gastric contents.[19] Injury to and permeabilization of endothelial and alveolar epithelial membranes, by a variety of injurious stimuli, leads to flooding of the alveolar compartment with protein-rich edema fluid, neutrophils, cellular debris, and inflammatory mediators. Multiple overlapping biologic pathways and cell and tissue types are deranged or injured, reflecting both the local (site-specific) and systemic (site-independent) perturbations that arise in ALI. This complex pathophysiology and heterogeneity of cause yields a large number of potential biomarkers.[20]

BIOMARKERS OF ACUTE LUNG INJURY—A RATIONAL CLASSIFICATION

Biomarkers of ALI can be classified according to clinical, molecular biologic, or pathophysiologic dimensions. A clinical classification should take into consideration the underlying cause of lung injury, the phase of disease (early exudative or late fibroproliferative), and the site of sampling. Biomarkers of ALI may be measured in exhaled breath condensate, undiluted pulmonary edema fluid, saline-diluted bronchoalveolar lavage (BAL), plasma, serum, whole blood for gene expression analysis, and urine. Additional considerations include the direction of change in the biomarker, the clinical outcome under investigation, the grade of evidence, and the performance characteristics for the outcome of interest.

A molecular biologic classification categorizes biomarkers by their place in the central dogma of molecular biology, namely the genome, transcriptome, proteome, and metabolome. Most currently described biomarkers of ALI belong to the proteome and include proteins, such as enzymes, receptors, polypeptides, lipoproteins, and glycoproteins.[21–24] It is likely that as understanding of the genetics of ALI deepens, the focus may shift to genetic markers for identification of individuals or populations at risk.[25]

Mechanistically, biomarkers can be classified by their role in the pathophysiology of ALI, which involves alveolar-capillary membrane injury, inflammation, activation of coagulation, and increased permeability pulmonary edema.[26,27] For example, biomarkers reflecting local injury to the alveolar-capillary membrane can be organized by compartment of origin (alveolar vs vascular) and further organized according to the cell or tissue of origin (epithelial, endothelial, or extracellular matrix) from which they are released. Surfactant proteins (SPs), for example, are released from alveolar epithelial cells and are considered markers of alveolar epithelial cell injury.[3] Biomarkers mediating inflammation can be linked to their cell of origin (neutrophil, alveolar macrophage, or platelets) or to their mode of action (cytokine, chemokine, protease, antiprotease, or lipid signaling molecule). Biomarkers of coagulation can reflect activation of coagulation, endogenous anticoagulant systems, or impaired fibrinolysis. Finally, increased pulmonary permeability results in a high ratio of protein in the pulmonary edema compared with plasma. This ratio in and of itself can be a useful biomarker for diagnosis of ALI.[28] Alternatively, biomarkers may track the repair and resolution pathways that mitigate or prolong the high-permeability edema state.

Although these classification systems create an orderly framework for consideration of ALI biomarkers, they may create artificial distinctions between overlapping pathways. The more integrated systems biology approach considers all these elements and classifications as interlinked, weaving together structural (molecular and cellular) and dynamic (pathophysiological) features into a unified whole.[29] For example, epithelial repair mechanisms are instances of an anatomic or structural defect in the epithelium with clear pathogenic (dynamic) consequences. Potential biomarkers of ALI are summarized in **Fig. 2** according to pathophysiology and/or tissue of origin.

PROTEIN BIOMARKERS FOR PREDICTION OF ALI IN AT-RISK PATIENTS

Inflammation and Cytokines

ALI is characterized by intra-alveolar inflammation mediated in part by proinflammatory cytokines. Differing cytokine profiles are characteristic of the early stages of ALI (termed *early response cytokines*) compared with the later fibroproliferative phase. Rising levels of inflammatory cytokines might be expected to precede the development of ALI in the at-risk patient population. Cytokines that have been identified in ALI include the interleukins (ILs), IL-2, IL-6, IL-8, IL-10, and IL-1β and its receptor antagonist, IL-1ra; tumor necrosis factor (TNF)-α; and the soluble TNF-1 (sTNFR-1) and TNF-2 receptors—not strictly cytokines but an integral part of the downstream cytokine cascade.[30,31] Remarkably for such central mediators, neither proinflammatory nor anti-inflammatory plasma cytokines have proved particularly useful in predicting ALI development.

Parsons and colleagues[32] measured plasma levels of the anti-inflammatory cytokines, IL-10 and IL-1ra, both anti-inflammatory cytokines, and found no association with disease prediction. Similarly, Bouros and colleagues[33] failed to show a strong positive predictive value of either plasma or BAL IL-6 or IL-8 for development of ARDS in patients at risk. TNF-α, a pleiotropic and early-phase cytokine, has also repeatedly failed to predict ALI development[34,35] although issues with both the sensitivity and the internal validity of TNF-α assays (immunoassay vs bioassay) are well documented.[34] In contrast, Takala and colleagues[36] found elevated serum IL-8, IL-6, and soluble IL-2 receptor concentrations in at-risk patients who went on to develop ALI, although none of the markers was able to discriminate between ARDS and non-ARDS patients. Donnelly and colleagues[37] measured plasma and BAL IL-8 in 29 consecutively enrolled at-risk patients. They showed significantly elevated BAL (but not plasma) IL-8 in the at-risk cohort who went on to develop ALI.

High-mobility group box 1 protein (HMGB1) is a DNA-binding protein and inflammatory cytokine. HMGB1 is a ligand for and mediates part of its inflammatory effects through the receptor for advanced glycation end products (RAGE), a marker of epithelial injury. Cohen and colleagues[38] showed that HMBG1 was released early (within 30 minutes) into the circulation of patients admitted to an emergency department after trauma and correlated with the development of acute organ dysfunction, including ALI.

Overall, the evidence to date indicates that cytokine levels are characteristic of but only weakly predictive for ALI. Causal heterogeneity, lack of statistical power, and the

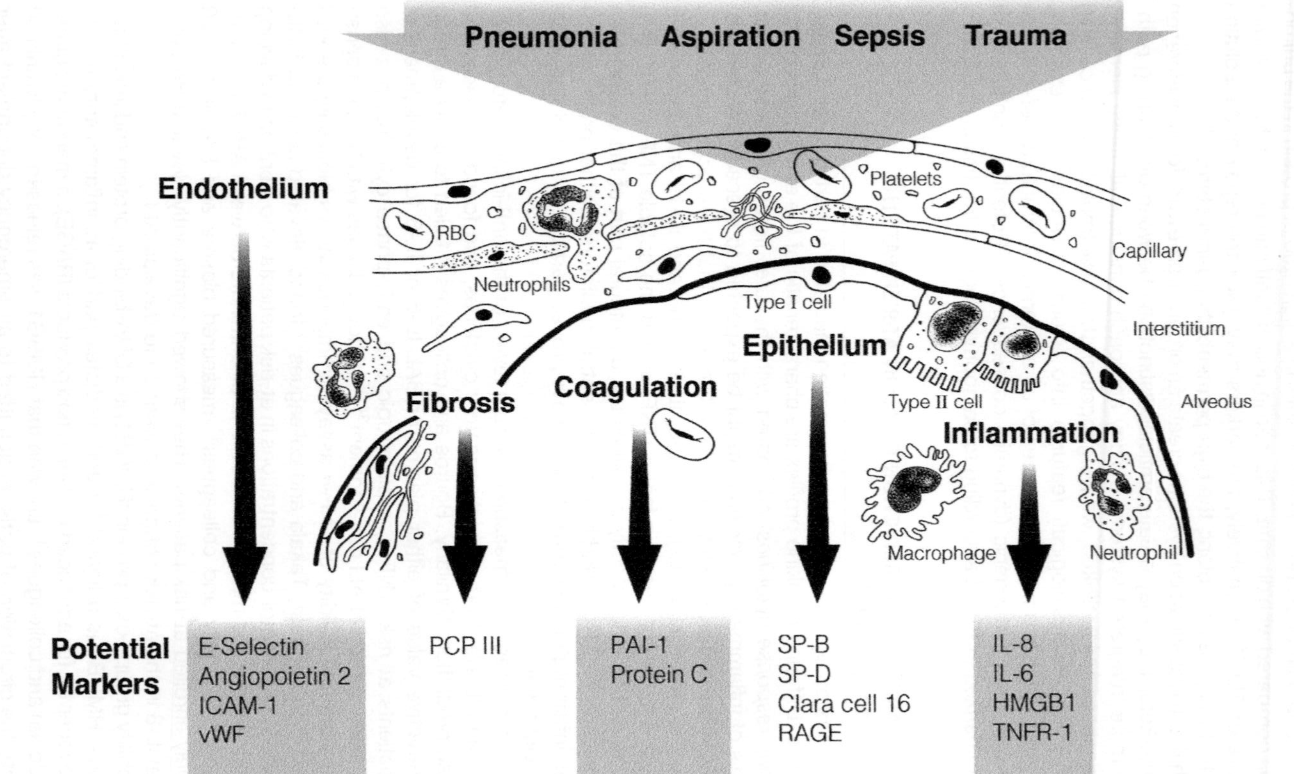

Fig. 2. Schematic representation of an alveolus and the alveolar-capillary interface demonstrating causes, pathophysiology, and important potential biomarkers for prediction, diagnosis, and prognosis in ALI. RBC, red blood cell.

observational nature of the studies undertaken suggest that there could still be some scope in determining the role of selected cytokine biomarkers (eg, HMGB1) in ALI prediction.

Markers of Endothelial Injury

Lung endothelial injury and activation lead to the increase in vascular permeability and influx of protein-rich edema fluid in ALI. Endothelial activation can be viewed as a 3-fold process. Neutrophils are mobilized from the circulation to the alveolar space by bridging molecules that support neutrophil margination and adhesion (selectins and intercellular adhesion molecules [ICAMs]).[39] This process is abetted by the secretion of angiopoietin-2 from endothelial cells, which further destabilizes and permeabilizes the endothelial membrane—a process that is believed essential to allow endothelial cell migration and new vessel formation.[40] Simultaneously, the injured endothelium releases proteins, such as von Willebrand factor, that encourage vascular hemostasis.[41] Endothelial activation and injury is thus an essential mechanism of non-cardiogenic pulmonary edema, and biomarkers that reflect this process are promising in identifying at-risk critically ill patients who progress to ALI.

Angiopoietin-2

The angiopoietins are potent regulators of vascular permeability in critical illness, pulmonary diseases, and beyond.[40] Four ligands (Ang 1–4) have been identified but Ang-1 and Ang-2 are the best characterized.[42] Both Ang-1 and Ang-2 bind to a common receptor, termed *Tie* 2, a tyrosine kinase receptor present on the endothelial cell surface. Ang-1 is constitutively expressed in all vessels under quiescent conditions to maintain vessel wall stability and homeostasis. Injury to the vessel wall tilts the balance towards Ang-2 expression, which counteracts Ang-1 via Tie 2 inhibition.[41] Ang-2 activates Rho kinase, causing disaggregation of cell-cell junctions and potentiation of the inflammatory nuclear factor (NF)-κB pathway while silencing protective phosphoinositide-3 kinase/Akt signaling vital to cell survival. The net result is capillary leak, neutrophil transmigration, and angiogenesis.[40]

Clinical measurements of circulating Ang-2 have provided interesting results. Gallagher and colleagues[43] in 63 at-risk surgical ICU patients showed higher median levels of Ang-2 in the patients who developed ALI compared with those who did not (10.1 ng/mL vs 3.7 ng/mL) and significantly higher median levels (19.8 ng/mL vs 5.3 ng/mL, $P = 0.004$) in ALI patients who did not survive in samples obtained on the day of meeting ALI criteria.

Of particular interest are data linking polymorphisms in the Ang-2 gene (ANGPT2) to susceptibility to trauma-induced ALI.[44,45] Using a large-scale candidate gene platform, the two single nucleotide polymorphisms most strongly associated with ALI were present in the Ang-2 gene. These findings were validated in 2 separate populations across two ethnicities. One of the ANGPT2 polymorphisms was associated with higher levels of a variant Ang-2 isoform in plasma.[46]

Vascular endothelial growth factor

Vascular endothelial growth factor (VEGF) is another novel mediator of vascular permeability and angiogenesis functionally related to the angiopoeitins with an adjuvant role in repair after lung injury.[47] The inter-relation of VEGF and Ang-2 is complex. VEGF up-regulates Ang-2[48] but also seems to induce shedding of Tie 2 to its soluble form, thereby mitigating its effect on downstream signal transduction.[49] In contrast to Ang-2, however, recent studies of VEGF have not corroborated earlier positive data and either showed no differences in plasma or edema fluid levels[50] or a weak but nonsignificant signal for ALI or prediction of ALI.[51]

von Willebrand factor antigen

von Willebrand factor antigen (vWF) is a large multimeric glycoprotein involved in hemostasis. vWF performs the dual functions of coupling platelets to the endothelium via its platelet-binding domain and as a transport protein for factor VIII. It is synthesized principally in endothelial cells (where it resides within Weibel-Palade bodies) and to a lesser extent in platelets. Although it is constitutively expressed, release is greatly augmented by a wide variety of injurious stimuli.[52] In a small cohort of 45 patients with nonpulmonary sepsis at risk for ALI, a level above 450% of control had a positive predictive value of 80% for ALI.[53] Bajaj and Tricomi[54] and Moss and colleagues[55] in broader study populations comprising both septic and nonseptic patients could not replicate those findings, although the study populations may have differed in relation to chest x-ray findings. In the study by Rubin,[53] the patients all had normal chest radiographs at enrollment whereas some of the patients in the other 2 studies already had chest x-ray abnormalities and thus may have had a subclinical stage of ALI.

Selectins

Selectins are cell-surface adhesion molecules involved in the early phase of neutrophil rolling and homing to a site of inflammation. There are 3 types: endothelial (E), leucocyte (L), and platelets (P).[56] E-selectin is selectively synthesized under conditions of cellular stress such as hypotension or organ hypoperfusion.[57] Okajima and colleagues[24] measured E-selectin by a rapid laboratory assay in 50 unselected patients with *systemic inflammatory response syndrome* (SIRS) admitted to an emergency department. Higher levels of E-selectin had a positive predictive value of 68% and negative predictive value of 86% for the development of ALI. The assay was also predictive for other organ failures. Donnelly and colleagues[58] measured all 3 selectins in plasma in 82 at-risk patients with trauma, pancreatitis, or perforated bowel. Cleaved, soluble L-selectin (sL-selectin) was significantly lower in those patients who progressed to ARDS than those who did not. Unlike Okajima and colleagues, they found no differences in plasma E-selectin or P-selectin. The biologic rationale for lower sL-selectin is as follows: cleaved L-selectin is required for normal leukocyte migration but the investigators speculated that sL-selectin may become bound to a ligand present on the endothelium, reducing circulating levels.

Markers of Epithelial Injury

Epithelial injury is a pivotal step that contributes to inflammation and the influx of pulmonary edema fluid in ALI. Injury to the epithelium also compromises alveolar fluid clearance and surfactant production (from type II cells), facilitates bacterial transmigration into the systemic circulation, and impairs alveolar repair mechanisms.[59] Evidence of epithelial injury through release of an intracellular or cell-surface biomarker into the alveolar space and circulation represents a powerful potential tool for prediction of at-risk patients.[60,61]

Surfactant proteins

Surfactant is a matrix of amphipathic lipoproteins and phospholipids whose major property is to lower surface tension at end-expiration preventing alveolar collapse. Four SPs have been identified, lettered SP-A through SP-D. SP-A and SP-D are high-molecular-weight hydrophilic molecules with marked roles in innate immunity[62] whereas SP-B and SP-C are low-molecular-weight hydrophobic species essential for alveolar epithelial membrane integrity.[63]

BAL SP-A levels were low in 1 study of patients at risk for ALI with a negative predictive value of 100% for ALI[64] when the levels remained above a cutoff of 1.2 μg/mL. The same investigators found elevated plasma SP-A levels in an at-risk cohort who developed ARDS secondary to sepsis and aspiration but not trauma.[65] These findings suggest that alveolar-capillary membrane permeability leading to leak of SP-A from the airspace into the plasma is a marker of lung epithelial injury.

In a single-center study of 54 patients at risk for ALI, Bersten and colleagues generated ROC curves for plasma SP-B with an AUC of 0.77 for all-cause prediction of ALI increasing to 0.87 for ALI from direct lung injury.[66] In contrast to the above study,[65] plasma SP-A was not predictive for ALI with an AUC 0.61.[66]

No further research on SP-B has ensued as a biomarker for detection of at-risk patients, perhaps due to the difficulty of measuring this hydrophobic protein in the circulation. In addition, plasma SP-D has emerged in subsequent well-powered publications as a diagnostic and prognostic (but not predictive) biomarker in ALI (discussed later).[3]

Clara cell protein

Clara cell protein (CC-16) is a small 16-kDa anti-inflammatory protein secreted almost exclusively by Clara cells of the terminal bronchial epithelium.[67] It is postulated to exert its actions through blockade of the phospholipase A2 second messenger system. Results from studies of CC-16 as a biomarker for prediction of ALI have been somewhat discordant. In a small study of 22 patients with ventilator-associated pneumonia at risk for ALI/ARDS, an acute elevation in plasma CC-16 occurred prior to the diagnosis of the clinical syndrome of ALI.[68] Sustained elevation of 30% or more yielded a diagnostic AUC of 0.91. Kropski and colleagues[69] found that plasma and pulmonary edema fluid CC-16 levels were lower in patients with ALI/ARDS than control patients with cardiogenic pulmonary edema. Prospective validation in larger-scale trials of this interesting biomarker is still required.

PROTEIN BIOMARKERS FOR DIAGNOSIS OF ALI

Distinct from prediction of ALI in at-risk patients is the use of biomarkers to confirm the diagnosis of ALI similar to the use of cardiac troponins for myocardial infarction.[70] Ideally a biomarker would function and perform under all clinical conditions (ie, be universal). For biomarker characterization, however, it is useful to specify the control group (patients with cardiogenic pulmonary edema, patients in an ICU with clear chest radiographs, normal controls, or patients at risk) against which cases are compared as well the phenotypic subtype (sepsis-induced, trauma-induced ALI, or ventilator-induced lung injury) being evaluated. In addition, the North American–European Consensus Committee definitions of ALI and ARDS that are applied as the gold standard for assessment of diagnostic biomarkers have limitations in the area of specificity.[71,72]

Many individual biomarkers from diverse biologic ontologies have been tested that reflect the heterogeneity of ALI. Some of the most promising markers with the strongest associations across important clinical endpoints are discussed. First the most straightforward method is discussed—measurement of total protein ratios.

Endothelial and Epithelial Injury—Edema Fluid to Plasma Protein Ratios and Plasma Protein Levels

Protein-rich pulmonary edema due to increased permeability of the alveolar-capillary membrane is a pathophysiologic feature of ALI. Measurement of the pulmonary edema fluid to plasma protein ratio is an intuitive, easy-to-perform, and rapid way to distinguish between high and low permeability pulmonary edema. Ware and colleagues[28] used a predefined edema fluid to plasma protein ratio of greater than or equal to 0.65 and compared its performance by ROC analysis with expert clinical diagnosis as the gold standard in a large cohort of 390 patients. The AUC for discriminating ALI from cardiogenic edema was 0.81, increasing to 0.85 for measurements taken within 3 hours of endotracheal intubation. This technique is limited by the need to perform measurements early after intubation because fluid resorption mechanisms (if intact) tend to concentrate protein levels in the alveolar space over time, potentially confounding results.

Using a related approach, Aman and colleagues[60,73] showed that low plasma levels of albumin and/or transferrin were predictive of a pulmonary leak index greater than 30×10^{-3}/min with an AUC of 0.85 for albumin. The pulmonary leak index, however, is only a surrogate marker of extravascular lung water and pulmonary edema and is not currently part of the consensus criteria for ARDS.

Epithelial Markers

Receptor for advanced glycation end products

RAGE is a transmembrane protein of the immunoglobulin superfamily and multiligand receptor that binds modified glycoproteins, including HMGB-1, transmitting a proinflammatory downstream intracellular signal via NF-κB.[74] Although it is ubiquitously expressed, expression levels are highest in the lung; RAGE is a specific marker of lung epithelial damage because it is anchored on the basolateral membrane of the alveolar type I cell. RAGE levels are increased in the plasma and pulmonary edema fluid of patients with ALI compared with patients with hydrostatic pulmonary edema.[75] In a study of patients with severe trauma at high risk for ALI, RAGE was the best performing biomarker out of a panel of 21 biomarkers for distinguishing patients with ALI from those without ALI.[76] In a larger study of 676 patients from the ARDSNet trial of low tidal volume ventilation, Calfee and colleagues[60] showed that after adjusting for potential confounders, RAGE was also a marker of worse clinical outcomes (including mortality) only in patients in the higher tidal volume arm of the study. The overall impression is that RAGE is associated with alveolar epithelial injury and has diagnostic abilities both for ALI and worsening of ALI by ventilator-induced lung injury.

Laminin-5

Laminin-5, a polymorphic, polyfunctional epithelial cell adhesion molecule, has recently been identified as a potential marker of early ALI. Laminins play an important role in cell adhesion, growth, and differentiation.[77] Katayama and colleagues[78] showed that a degradation product of laminin-5, G2F, the terminal active portion of its γ2-chain, was significantly increased in the plasma of ALI patients as compared with patients with cardiogenic pulmonary edema. High levels were maintained in nonsurviving patients.

Endothelial Markers–Intercellular Adhesion Molecule-1

As the name suggests, ICAM-1 mediates intercellular adhesion of leukocytes to the endothelium and epithelium where it colocates to the cell membrane of all 3 cell types. ICAM-1 is up-regulated in inflammatory states and facilitates movement of neutrophils across endothelial barriers to sites of inflammation.[79] In a small pilot study, ICAM-1 was elevated in both the plasma and edema fluid of patients with ALI as compared with patients with cardiogenic pulmonary edema.[80] Earlier studies found similar results but the elevation was confined to edema fluid only prompting the suggestion that this was a dual endothelial-epithelial membrane marker.[81]

Markers of Coagulation and Fibrinolysis–Plasminogen Activator Inhibitor-1

Plasminogen activator inhibitor-1 (PAI-1) is an antiprotease inhibitor of fibrinolysis that promotes fibrin deposition, one of the pathologic hallmarks of the ARDS.[19] Prakhakaran and colleagues[82] reported increases in plasma and pulmonary edema fluid of patients with early ALI compared with patients with severe hydrostatic pulmonary edema.

Extracellular Matrix–Procollagen Peptide Type III

Procollagen peptide type III (PCP III) is a marker of collagen synthesis. Two small studies[83,84] have suggested an association of higher edema fluid levels of PCP III with ALI. In the trauma study (discussed previously),[76] among a panel of 21 plasma biomarkers PCP III was the second-best performing biomarker for distinguishing patients with ALI from severely injured controls without ALI. In another larger study, plasma and BAL PCP III levels decreased with steroid treatment,[85] suggesting that PCP III levels potentially mirror disease activity.

Inflammation–Lipopolysaccharide-Binding Protein

Lipopolysaccharide (LPS)-binding protein (LBP) produced by alveolar epithelial type II cells is an acute-phase reactant that mediates transduction of a proinflammatory response to LPS by binding of LPS from gram-negative bacteria or lipotechoic acid from gram-positive organisms.[86] Abnormalities and activation of this protein in human sepsis syndrome have been reported for more than a decade, although its role in the pathogenesis and as a biomarker of ARDS has recently attracted renewed attention. Sustained elevations of plasma LBP at 48 hours postadmission to an ICU were associated with ARDS (not ALI) but no ROC curves were generated to specify a particular cutoff in LBP levels to predict ARDS.[87] In addition, admission LBP had no discriminatory value between survivors or nonsurvivors.

COMBINING BIOMARKERS FOR DIAGNOSIS OF ALI

Given the failure of a single biomarker to discriminate ALI with high accuracy, the question arises whether a composite of biomarkers that represent the most commonly identified and clinically validated biologic ontologies (inflammation, endothelial activation, lung epithelial injury, and coagulation/altered fibrinolysis) might have better performance than any individual biomarker for diagnosis for ALI. As discussed previously, Fremont and colleagues[76] posed this question with regards to the diagnosis of ALI secondary to trauma. Using a backward elimination model, 21 biomarkers were reduced to the top-performing 7: RAGE, PCP III, brain natriuretic peptide, Ang-2, TNF-α, IL-10, and IL-8. A model that utilized these 7 biomarkers generated an AUC of 0.86 for differentiating ALI/ARDS from a group of critically ill trauma patients without ALI who had normal chest radiographs or hydrostatic pulmonary edema. The top 3 performing markers (RAGE, PCP III, and IL-8) had an AUC of 0.83 and excellent discriminatory power (see **Fig. 1**).

PROTEIN BIOMARKERS FOR PREDICTING OUTCOME IN ALI

Much of the strongest evidence in the field of ALI biomarkers comes from outcome prediction. Several biomarkers belonging to the biologic ontologies (discussed previously) have been validated in large multicenter clinical trials principally from ARDSNet. The outcomes most commonly predicted are hospital, 30-day, 60-day, or 180-day mortality; ventilator-free and organ-failure–free days; and assessment of response to low-tidal volume ventilation. The majority of this work has been performed in the past 10 years and is the strongest measure of progress in the field.

Markers of endothelial injury (vWF), epithelial injury (SP-D), leukocyte-endothelial interaction (ICAM-1), inflammation (IL-6, IL-8, and TNF-R1) and alterations in coagulation/fibrinolysis (protein C and PAI-1) have the most robust associations with clinical outcomes such as mortality.

Elevations in plasma levels of vWF were independently associated with hospital mortality to day 180 in ALI in 559 patients even after controlling for illness severity, sepsis, and ventilator strategy.[88] vWF levels were not responsive to a lower tidal volume strategy, however. Similarly, higher plasma SP-D levels in 565 patients were also independently associated with 180-day mortality and reduced ventilator-free and organ-failure free days.[3] ICAM-1 in the larger multicenter arm of the study by Calfee and colleagues[80] involving 778 patients again showed an independent association with the same outcomes listed previously. The same independent association of lower levels with survival and more ventilator-free and organ failure–free days were replicated in 593 patients with ALI for IL-6, IL-8, and sTNF-R1.[89] Finally in 779 patients, Ware and colleagues[9] showed that lower enrollment levels of protein C and higher levels of PAI-1 were independently and synergistically associated with mortality and organ failure–free days (**Fig. 3**).

Decoy Receptor 3

Decoy receptor 3 (DcR 3) is a soluble, pleiotropic, immunomodulator member of the TNF superfamily that binds Fas ligand and LIGHT (a lymphotoxin receptor)[90] with an as-yet unknown role in ALI. Chen and colleagues[91] evaluated a panel of biomarkers (TNF-α, IL-6, and soluble triggering receptor expressed on myeloid cells 1 [sTREM]), including DcR 3, in 88 patients with ARDS and obtained ROC curves for mortality prediction for each biomarker. DcR 3 had the best performance and the highest odds ratio for mortality in this patient cohort. Its performance need to be assessed under different clinical conditions and against other markers but its use warrants further study.

C-reactive protein, procalcitonin, and bilirubin

C-reactive protein (CRP) is a biomarker in common clinical use to delineate the activity of a host of inflammatory conditions, such as sepsis, cardiovascular disease, and rheumatologic disorders. ARDS is broadly an inflammatory condition of the lung. Bajwa and colleagues[92] studied the impact of CRP levels on mortality in ARDS patients. They found an association between higher CRP levels and better outcomes, including 60-day mortality, organ failure, and duration of mechanical ventilation. The biologic rationale for this finding is unclear although it might be due to reduced neutrophil chemotaxis induced by CRP at higher levels, thus potentially reducing the inflammatory burden. The same group measure serum bilirubin levels in a larger cohort of 1006 patients and demonstrated a significant association with ARDS incidence and mortality with levels greater than 2.0 mg/dL.[93]

In contrast to the data on CRP, a smaller study by Tseng and colleagues[94] examined the related inflammatory molecule, procalcitonin, and identified it as a prognostic marker of mortality in pneumonia-induced ARDS. Whether this association still holds for other causes of ARDS or in a direct comparison with CRP is unknown.

Combining biomarkers for prognosis and pathogenesis

Drawing on the large numbers of biomarkers measured at enrollment in the ARDSNet low tidal volume study, Ware and colleagues[12] tested the ability of a panel of 8 biomarkers previously associated with mortality (vWF, SP-D, TNF-R1, IL-6, IL-8,

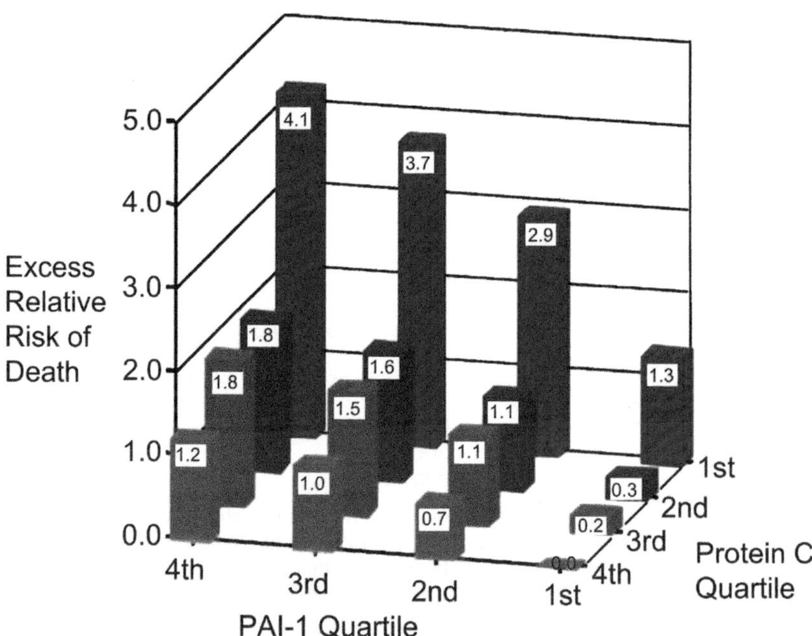

Fig. 3. Multidimensional representation charting plasma protein C and PAI-1 levels by quartile against excessive relative risk of death calculated as the difference between the highest PAI-1 and lowest protein C quartiles in 779 patients with ALI. (*Reproduced from* Ware LB, Matthay MA, Parsons PE, et al. Pathogenetic and prognostic significance of altered coagulation and fibrinolysis in acute lung injury/acute respiratory distress syndrome. Crit Care Med 2007;35(8):1826; with permission.)

ICAM-1, protein C, and PAI-1) and 6 clinical predictors (age, cause of lung injury, Acute Physiology and Chronic Health Evaluation [APACHE] III score, plateau pressure, organ failures, and alveolar-arterial difference) to discriminate 60-day mortality in patients with ALI/ARDS enrolled in the high positive end-expiratory pressure versus low positive end-expiratory pressure trial.[95] Using the clinical predictors only, a logistic regression model had an AUC of 0.815. A model combining the 8 biomarkers with the 6 clinical predictors had improved discrimination with an AUC of 0.850, suggesting a modest benefit in terms of adding biomarkers. A reduced model with APACHE III score, age, SP-D, and IL-8 had an AUC of 0.834 (**Fig. 4**). In this study, the best performing biomarkers were markers of alveolar epithelial injury (SP-D) and inflammation/neutrophil chemotaxis (IL-8), highlighting the importance of these mechanisms in the pathogenesis of ALI.

A similar analysis was undertaken with preselected biomarkers of inflammation and coagulation to investigate if these markers were still predictive of clinical outcomes after the widespread institution of low tidal volume ventilation.[96] In 50 patients with early ALI, the 3 top markers out of a broad panel were IL-8, ICAM-1, and protein C, of which the 2 former were independently associated with increased mortality in ALI. SP-D was not measured in this cohort. IL-8 featured prominently in both data sets that have a combination of biomarkers.[12,76]

Risk Reclassification with Multiple Biomarkers

Risk reclassification is a relatively new statistical approach that was developed to overcome deficiencies with ROC-based methods, which typically require large odds

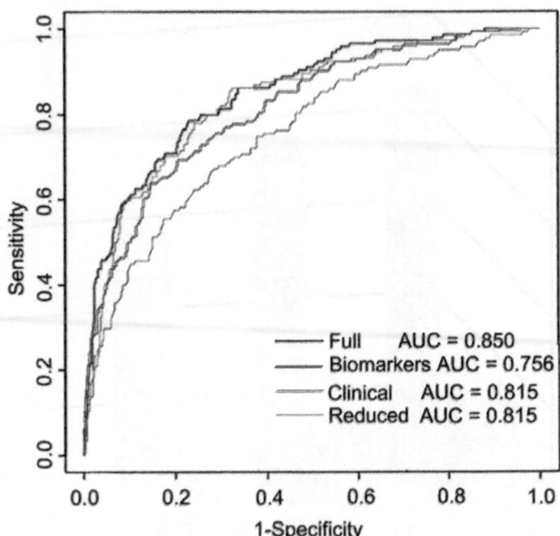

Fig. 4. ROC curve for multiple mortality prediction models in patients with ALI. Full model includes 6 clinical predictors (age, cause of injury, APACHE III, plateau pressure, organ failures, alveolar-arterial difference) and 8 biomarkers (IL-8, IL-6, TNF-R1, SP-D, protein C, PAI-1, and ICAM-1) and has an AUC 0.850. The reduced model includes APACHE III score, age, SP-D, and IL-8 with an AUC 0.834. (*From* Ware LB, Koyama T, Billheimer DD, et al. Prognostic and pathogenetic value of combining clinical and biochemical indices in patients with acute lung injury. Chest 2010;137(2):292; with permission.)

ratios to demonstrate improvements in the AUC with addition of a novel biomarker to established predictors. Risk reclassification compares the predictive accuracy of 2 models—a baseline model and a secondary model putatively improved by additional variables, such as biomarker data. This comparison generates a net reclassification improvement index based on the proportion of patients newly reclassified to a risk category more closely allied with the outcome examined.[97] Working with biomarkers measured in the first 2 ARDSNet clinical trials, Calfee and colleagues[98] showed that a panel of 5 biomarkers (ICAM, vWF, IL-8, SP-D, and sTNF-R1) significantly improved risk prediction for mortality when compared with a clinical prediction model using APACHE III scores only. This method also was superior in detecting differences in outcome prediction that were not detected with the ROC-based approach.

BEYOND PROTEIN BIOMARKERS: NOVEL PREDICTORS IN ALI

Stem Cells

Adult-derived stem cells have been studied as biomarkers in ALI. Circulating endothelial progenitor cells have attracted attention recently as prognostic as well as potential therapeutic targets in ALI.[99] A handful of studies have shown a small but consistent effect linking higher circulating levels of endothelial progenitor cells with survival from ALI,[100,101] suggesting that mobilization of endothelial progenitor cells in periods of acute stress may be beneficial.

Exhaled Breath Condensate

The exhaled breath condensate (EBC) is a novel, noninvasive method for analyzing byproducts of metabolism as the lung excretes them. The underlying biologic principal is that injury to the lung leads to differential release of metabolites, which can be recovered in the EBC. Both physical characteristics of the EBC, such as pH and metabolites, including products of nitric oxide metabolism (nitrosative stress), isoprostanes, hydrogen peroxide, and cytokines, have been studied. It is not unclear whether these measurements reflect systemic or lung-specific production of metabolites or the anatomic region of the respiratory tract from which they arise. Acidification of the EBC and increases in nitric oxide metabolites has been associated with overdistention from mechanical ventilation.[102] A lower EBC pH was also inversely related to the Lung Injury Severity Score.[103] Overall, there is still a lack of data but the use of EBC is appealing because unlike BAL, it samples the lung compartment noninvasively. Coupling measurements of EBC to emerging metabolomic techniques is an avenue of future research.

Genetic Approaches

The role of genetic polymorphisms as biomarkers of risk for ALI or poor prognosis is beginning to be explored. The study of genetic markers in ALI encounters many of the same methodologic issues as the candidate protein biomarker approach, including phenotype definition, power estimation, quality control, population stratification, and relevant control identification. These methodologic issues may take on higher significance given the relatively modest predicted contribution of single gene polymorphisms to ALI.[25]

Two approaches are used in genetic studies of ALI: the candidate gene approach and the powerful but labor-intensive genome-wide approach to identifying susceptibility loci or genes. The candidate approach is hypothesis-driven and involves choosing candidate genes that may be of likely relevance to the disease process, based on knowledge gained from experimental and clinical studies and testing for an association with ALI. As recently reviewed,[25] only 31 genetic associations, 21 of which have been replicated, have been shown to have associations with the ALI phenotype. Many of the genes corroborate what is known about the pathophysiology of ALI from individual biomarkers. For example, polymorphisms in cytokines, both proinflammatory (TNFA, IL-6, and IL-8)[104,105] and anti-inflammatory (IL-10)[106]; epithelial markers (SP-B)[107]; cell signaling (mannose-binding lectin[108]); and the deep internal machinery of the cell (NF of κ light polypeptide gene enhancer in B-cells 1)[109] have been demonstrated. The most widely replicated polymorphisms are in the genes for IL-6, SP-B, and angiotensin 1 converting enzyme.[25] Pathogenic concepts, such as dysregulated iron metabolism, have been revived by genetic association studies as evidenced in the recently reported ferritin light chain polymorphism.[110]

Conversely, genome-wide association studies are not a priori hypothesis-driven and thus offer a potentially less-biased avenue to genetic marker discovery. This approach requires substantial increases in sample size and data analysis, but because of the relative reduction in genotyping costs and development of more standardized approaches to genome-wide association studies data analysis, this approach is becoming increasingly popular for discovery and replication studies of complex diseases. The output of genome-wide association studies is candidate genes that can be supported by other genome-wide approaches, such as expression array and proteomic profiling.

Gene Expression Studies

Howrylak and colleagues[111] explored a gene expression signature for ALI due to sepsis as opposed to sepsis alone that would identify a set of genes uniquely activated in ALI regardless of genetic predisposition. Using an innovative group of classification algorithms, they arrived at an 8-gene expression profile in whole blood that was characteristic of ALI. This model had a within-study accuracy of 100% for diagnosis of ALI and when validated still had 89% accuracy albeit with n = 9. A similar approach was used to study differential gene expression between the early and late phases of ARDS. Peptidase inhibitor 3 (PI3) or pre-elafin (a neutrophil elastase inhibitor) gene expression became progressively silenced from acute to recovery stages of ARDS.[112] A follow-up validation study examined the clinical significance of this finding in relation to the ratio of human neutrophil elastase (HNE) to PI3 in the plasma of ICU patients at risk for ARDS. An increase in HNE to PI3 ratio from pre-ARDS to early ARDS in patients developing the syndrome was observed. In contrast, the ratio fell in an at-risk patient cohort who remained free of ARDS. Thus, a change in HNE:PI3 balance might be a useful indicator of imminent ARDS.[113]

In summary, gene expression analysis is a promising methodology for identification of novel biomarkers of ALI. The gene expression profile generated depends, however, to a large extent on the cellular mix present in the sample, a factor of particular concern in whole blood gene expression studies.

Proteomics and Metabolomics

Proteomics is a systems-based methodology for mining the complex changes in protein expression and post-translational modifications present in biologic samples that can occur with disease processes. A variety of approaches have been used, including 2-D electrophoresis methods as well as the more powerful approach of liquid chromatography–tandem mass spectrometry. Insulinlike growth factor–binding protein 3, a marker of apoptosis, and S100 proteins A8 and A9 (markers of inflammation) have been identified in this way.[114,115] The next frontier is to move forward from descriptive lists of differentially expressed proteins to mechanistic insights, making use of a plethora of cutting-edge analytic tools, such as principal component analysis, gene-ontology, and network analysis to identify nodal points of protein-protein interaction.[116,117]

The nascent field of metabolomics may also be an avenue for biomarker discovery. Downstream metabolic profiles are analyzed to characterize a physiologic or disease-specific state. Critically, metabolomics allows real-time integration of upstream genomic and proteomic data.[118] This approach was explored in a small sample of major trauma patients admitted to an emergency department using nuclear MRI–based metabolomics on whole blood to establish a differential metabolic fingerprint between survivors and nonsurvivors.[119] Similarly, Stringer and colleagues[120] performed a feasibility study to identify metabolites associated with sepsis-induced ALI. They found quantitative differences in 4 metabolites: total glutathione, adenosine, phosphatidylserine, and sphingomyelin between healthy controls and a small cohort with sepsis-induced ALI. It is premature to assess the potential impact of this methodology but newer more quantitative methodologies should advance the field.

SUMMARY

Is progress being made? This review has identified 4 areas where significant progress has been made over the last 10 years. The first area is the large-scale validation of several candidate biomarkers from a range of biologic pathways (IL-8, IL-6, vWF, protein C, PAI-1, and SP-D) for prognostication and mortality prediction. The second area is several novel predictors still requiring validation, mediating endothelial permeability (Ang-2), epithelial cell injury (CC-16), and inflammation (DcR 3), that seem to have strong translational potential or be of particular scientific interest, such as endothelial progenitor cells. Only 2% of the proteome has been fully characterized, which helps to contextualize the current state of ALI biomarker research. The third area is the advent of genomics and proteomics allied to computationally intensive methods in the field of bioinformatics. These high-dimensional methodologies hold great promise for integrating vast arrays of information, to make predictions about those at risk or those with early disease from genomic or proteomic signatures and to identify novel biomarkers. The final area has been the ability to combine and test all of the above biomarkers into prognostic indices capable of outperforming individual biomarkers alone.

Although much progress has been made, further progress is dependent on the availability of large well-phenotyped databases of clinical data and biologic samples from patients at risk for and with established ALI. Only with large samples sizes and excellent clinical phenotyping will full operationalization of candidate and novel biomarkers be possible, transforming candidate into clinic-worthy biomarkers, so that patients may ultimately benefit.

REFERENCES

1. Hudson LD, Martin TR. Predicting ARDS: problems and prospects. Lancet 1997;349(9068):1783.
2. The Acute Respiratory Distress Syndrome Network. Ventilation with lower tidal volumes as compared with traditional tidal volumes for acute lung injury and the acute respiratory distress syndrome. N Engl J Med 2000;342(18):1301–8.
3. Eisner MD, Parsons P, Matthay MA, et al. Plasma surfactant protein levels and clinical outcomes in patients with acute lung injury. Thorax 2003;58(11):983–8.
4. Biomarkers and surrogate endpoints: preferred definitions and conceptual framework. Clin Pharmacol Ther 2001;69(3):89–95.
5. WHO International Programme on Chemical Safety. Biomarkers in risk assessment: validity and validation. 2001. Available at: http://www.inchem.org/documents/ehc/ech/ech222.htm. Accessed October 20, 2010.
6. WHO International Programme on Chemical Safety. Biomarkers in risk assessment: validity and validation. 1993. Available at: http://www.inchem.org/documents/ehc/ech/ech155.htm. Accessed October 20, 2010.
7. Strimbu K, Tavel JA. What are biomarkers? Curr Opin HIV AIDS 2010;5(6):463–6.
8. Spragg RG, Bernard GR, Checkley W, et al. Beyond mortality: future clinical research in acute lung injury. Am J Respir Crit Care Med 2010;181(10):1121–7.
9. Ware LB, Matthay MA, Parsons PE, et al. Pathogenetic and prognostic significance of altered coagulation and fibrinolysis in acute lung injury/acute respiratory distress syndrome. Crit Care Med 2007;35(8):1821–8.
10. Marshall JC, Reinhart K. Biomarkers of sepsis. Crit Care Med 2009;37(7):2290–8.
11. Willson DF, Thomas NJ, Markovitz BP, et al. Effect of exogenous surfactant (calfactant) in pediatric acute lung injury: a randomized controlled trial. JAMA 2005;293(4):470–6.
12. Ware LB, Koyama T, Billheimer DD, et al. Prognostic and pathogenetic value of combining clinical and biochemical indices in patients with acute lung injury. Chest 2010;137(2):288–96.
13. Tzouvelekis A, Pneumatikos I, Bouros D. Serum biomarkers in acute respiratory distress syndrome an ailing prognosticator. Respir Res 2005;6:62.
14. Olman MA, White KE, Ware LB, et al. Pulmonary edema fluid from patients with early lung injury stimulates fibroblast proliferation through IL-1 beta-induced IL-6 expression. J Immunol 2004;172(4):2668–77.

15. Soreide K. Receiver-operating characteristic curve analysis in diagnostic, prognostic and predictive biomarker research. J Clin Pathol 2009;62(1):1–5.
16. Zhu W, Zeng N, Wang N. Sensitivity, Specificity, Accuracy, Associated Confidence Interval and ROC Analysis with Practical SAS Implementations. 2010. Available at: http://www.nesug.org/Proceedings/nesug10/hl/hl07.pdf. Accessed November 14, 2010.
17. Shehabi Y, Seppelt I. Pro/Con debate: is procalcitonin useful for guiding antibiotic decision making in critically ill patients? Crit Care 2008;12(3):211.
18. Kaufman RA, Oakley-Brown H, Watkins R, et al. Strategic planning for success: aligning people, performance, and payoffs. 2003.
19. Ware LB, Matthay MA. The acute respiratory distress syndrome. N Engl J Med 2000;342(18):1334–49.
20. Levitt JE, Gould MK, Ware LB, et al. The pathogenetic and prognostic value of biologic markers in acute lung injury. J Intensive Care Med 2009;24(3):151–67.
21. Imai Y, Kuba K, Rao S, et al. Angiotensin-converting enzyme 2 protects from severe acute lung failure. Nature 2005;436(7047):112–6.
22. Tejera P, Wang Z, Zhai R, et al. Genetic polymorphisms of peptidase inhibitor 3 (elafin) are associated with acute respiratory distress syndrome. Am J Respir Cell Mol Biol 2009;41(6):696–704.
23. Parsons PE, Matthay MA, Ware LB, et al. Elevated plasma levels of soluble TNF receptors are associated with morbidity and mortality in patients with acute lung injury. Am J Physiol Lung Cell Mol Physiol 2005;288(3):L426–31.
24. Okajima K, Harada N, Sakurai G, et al. Rapid assay for plasma soluble E-selectin predicts the development of acute respiratory distress syndrome in patients with systemic inflammatory response syndrome. Transl Res 2006;148(6):295–300.
25. Gao L, Barnes KC. Recent advances in genetic predisposition to clinical acute lung injury. Am J Physiol Lung Cell Mol Physiol 2009;296(5):L713–25.
26. Matthay MA, Zimmerman GA. Acute lung injury and the acute respiratory distress syndrome: four decades of inquiry into pathogenesis and rational management. Am J Respir Cell Mol Biol 2005;33(4):319–27.
27. Bastarache JA, Ware LB, Bernard GR. The role of the coagulation cascade in the continuum of sepsis and acute lung injury and acute respiratory distress syndrome. Semin Respir Crit Care Med 2006;27(4):365–76.
28. Ware LB, Fremont RD, Bastarache JA, et al. Determining the aetiology of pulmonary oedema by the oedema fluid-to-plasma protein ratio. Eur Respir J 2010;35(2):331–7.
29. Kitano H. Systems biology: a brief overview. Science 2002;295(5560):1662–4.
30. Meduri GU, Headley S, Kohler G, et al. Persistent elevation of inflammatory cytokines predicts a poor outcome in ARDS. Plasma IL-1 beta and IL-6 levels are consistent and efficient predictors of outcome over time. Chest 1995;107(4):1062–73.
31. Park WY, Goodman RB, Steinberg KP, et al. Cytokine balance in the lungs of patients with acute respiratory distress syndrome. Am J Respir Crit Care Med 2001;164(10 Pt 1):1896–903.
32. Parsons PE, Moss M, Vannice JL, et al. Circulating IL-1ra and IL-10 levels are increased but do not predict the development of acute respiratory distress syndrome in at-risk patients. Am J Respir Crit Care Med 1997;155(4):1469–73.
33. Bouros D, Alexandrakis MG, Antoniou KM, et al. The clinical significance of serum and bronchoalveolar lavage inflammatory cytokines in patients at risk for Acute Respiratory Distress Syndrome. BMC Pulm Med 2004;4:6.
34. Pittet JF, Mackersie RC, Martin TR, et al. Biological markers of acute lung injury: prognostic and pathogenetic significance. Am J Respir Crit Care Med 1997; 155(4):1187–205.

35. Suter PM, Suter S, Girardin E, et al. High bronchoalveolar levels of tumor necrosis factor and its inhibitors, interleukin-1, interferon, and elastase, in patients with adult respiratory distress syndrome after trauma, shock, or sepsis. Am Rev Respir Dis 1992;145(5):1016–22.
36. Takala A, Jousela I, Takkunen O, et al. A prospective study of inflammation markers in patients at risk of indirect acute lung injury. Shock 2002;17(4): 252–7.
37. Donnelly SC, Strieter RM, Kunkel SL, et al. Interleukin-8 and development of adult respiratory distress syndrome in at-risk patient groups. Lancet 1993; 341(8846):643–7.
38. Cohen MJ, Brohi K, Calfee CS, et al. Early release of high mobility group box nuclear protein 1 after severe trauma in humans: role of injury severity and tissue hypoperfusion. Crit Care 2009;13(6):R174.
39. Ley K, Laudanna C, Cybulsky MI, et al. Getting to the site of inflammation: the leukocyte adhesion cascade updated. Nat Rev Immunol 2007;7(9): 678–89.
40. van Meurs M, Kumpers P, Ligtenberg JJ, et al. Bench-to-bedside review: angiopoietin signalling in critical illness - a future target? Crit Care 2009;13(2):207.
41. Fiedler U, Augustin HG. Angiopoietins: a link between angiogenesis and inflammation. Trends Immunol 2006;27(12):552–8.
42. Jones PF. Not just angiogenesis—wider roles for the angiopoietins. J Pathol 2003;201(4):515–27.
43. Gallagher DC, Parikh SM, Balonov K, et al. Circulating angiopoietin 2 correlates with mortality in a surgical population with acute lung injury/adult respiratory distress syndrome. Shock 2008;29(6):656–61.
44. Christie JD, Wurfel MM, Keefe GE, et al. Genome wide association (gwa) identifies functional susceptibility loci for trauma-induced acute lung injury. Am J Respir Crit Care Med 2010;181:A1205.
45. Meyer NJ, Li M, Shah CV, et al. Large scale genotyping in an African American trauma population identifies angiopoeitin-2 variants associated with ALI. Am J Respir Crit Care Med 2010;179:A3879.
46. Meyer NJ, Li M, Feng R, et al. ANGPT2 genetic variant is associated with trauma-associated acute lung injury and altered plasma angiopoietin-2 isoform ratio. Am J Respir Crit Care Med 2011. [Epub ahead of print].
47. Medford AR, Millar AB. Vascular endothelial growth factor (VEGF) in acute lung injury (ALI) and acute respiratory distress syndrome (ARDS): paradox or paradigm? Thorax 2006;61(7):621–6.
48. Oh H, Takagi H, Suzuma K, et al. Hypoxia and vascular endothelial growth factor selectively up-regulate angiopoietin-2 in bovine microvascular endothelial cells. J Biol Chem 1999;274(22):15732–9.
49. Findley CM, Cudmore MJ, Ahmed A, et al. VEGF induces Tie2 shedding via a phosphoinositide 3-kinase/Akt dependent pathway to modulate Tie2 signaling. Arterioscler Thromb Vasc Biol 2007;27(12):2619–26.
50. Ware LB, Kaner RJ, Crystal RG, et al. VEGF levels in the alveolar compartment do not distinguish between ARDS and hydrostatic pulmonary oedema. Eur Respir J 2005;26(1):101–5.
51. van der Heijden M, van Nieuw Amerongen GP, Koolwijk P, et al. Angiopoietin-2, permeability oedema, occurrence and severity of ALI/ARDS in septic and nonseptic critically ill patients. Thorax 2008;63(10):903–9.
52. Franchini M, Lippi G. Von Willebrand factor and thrombosis. Ann Hematol 2006; 85(7):415–23.

53. Rubin DB, Wiener-Kronish JP, Murray JF, et al. Elevated von Willebrand factor antigen is an early plasma predictor of acute lung injury in nonpulmonary sepsis syndrome. J Clin Invest 1990;86(2):474–80.
54. Bajaj MS, Tricomi SM. Plasma levels of the three endothelial-specific proteins von Willebrand factor, tissue factor pathway inhibitor, and thrombomodulin do not predict the development of acute respiratory distress syndrome. Intensive Care Med 1999;25(11):1259–66.
55. Moss M, Ackerson L, Gillespie MK, et al. von Willebrand factor antigen levels are not predictive for the adult respiratory distress syndrome. Am J Respir Crit Care Med 1995;151(1):15–20.
56. Langer HF, Chavakis T. Leukocyte-endothelial interactions in inflammation. J Cell Mol Med 2009;13(7):1211–20.
57. Newman W, Beall LD, Carson CW, et al. Soluble E-selectin is found in supernatants of activated endothelial cells and is elevated in the serum of patients with septic shock. J Immunol 1993;150(2):644–54.
58. Donnelly SC, Haslett C, Dransfield I, et al. Role of selectins in development of adult respiratory distress syndrome. Lancet 1994;344(8917):215–9.
59. Matthay MA, Zemans RL. The acute respiratory distress syndrome: pathogenesis and treatment. Annu Rev Pathol 2011;6:147–63.
60. Calfee CS, Ware LB, Eisner MD, et al. Plasma receptor for advanced glycation end products and clinical outcomes in acute lung injury. Thorax 2008;63(12):1083–9.
61. Nakashima T, Yokoyama A, Inata J, et al. Mucins carrying selectin ligands as predictive biomarkers of disseminated intravascular coagulation complication in ARDS. Chest 2011;139(2):296–304.
62. Pastva AM, Wright JR, Williams KL. Immunomodulatory roles of surfactant proteins A and D: implications in lung disease. Proc Am Thorac Soc 2007;4(3):252–7.
63. Chroneos ZC, Sever-Chroneos Z, Shepherd VL. Pulmonary surfactant: an immunological perspective. Cell Physiol Biochem 2010;25(1):13–26.
64. Greene KE, Wright JR, Steinberg KP, et al. Serial changes in surfactant-associated proteins in lung and serum before and after onset of ARDS. Am J Respir Crit Care Med 1999;160(6):1843–50.
65. Greene KE, Ye S, Mason RJ, et al. Serum surfactant protein-A levels predict development of ARDS in at-risk patients. Chest 1999;116(Suppl 1):90S–1S.
66. Bersten AD, Hunt T, Nicholas TE, et al. Elevated plasma surfactant protein-B predicts development of acute respiratory distress syndrome in patients with acute respiratory failure. Am J Respir Crit Care Med 2001;164(4):648–52.
67. Broeckaert F, Bernard A. Clara cell secretory protein (CC16): characteristics and perspectives as lung peripheral biomarker. Clin Exp Allergy 2000;30(4):469–75.
68. Determann RM, Millo JL, Waddy S, et al. Plasma CC16 levels are associated with development of ALI/ARDS in patients with ventilator-associated pneumonia: a retrospective observational study. BMC Pulm Med 2009;9:49.
69. Kropski JA, Fremont RD, Calfee CS, et al. Clara cell protein (CC16), a marker of lung epithelial injury, is decreased in plasma and pulmonary edema fluid from patients with acute lung injury. Chest 2009;135(6):1440–7.
70. Thygesen K, Alpert JS, White HD, et al. Universal definition of myocardial infarction. Circulation 2007;116(22):2634–53.
71. Bernard GR, Artigas A, Brigham KL, et al. The American-European Consensus Conference on ARDS. Definitions, mechanisms, relevant outcomes, and clinical trial coordination. Am J Respir Crit Care Med 1994;149(3 Pt 1):818–24.

72. Phua J, Stewart TE, Ferguson ND. Acute respiratory distress syndrome 40 years later: time to revisit its definition. Crit Care Med 2008;36(10):2912–21.
73. Aman J, van der Heijden M, van Lingen A, et al. Plasma protein levels are markers of pulmonary vascular permeability and degree of lung injury in critically ill patients with or at risk for acute lung injury/acute respiratory distress syndrome. Crit Care Med 2011;39(1):89–97.
74. Creagh-Brown BC, Quinlan GJ, Evans TW, et al. The RAGE axis in systemic inflammation, acute lung injury and myocardial dysfunction: an important therapeutic target? Intensive Care Med 2010;36(10):1644–56.
75. Uchida T, Shirasawa M, Ware LB, et al. Receptor for advanced glycation end-products is a marker of type I cell injury in acute lung injury. Am J Respir Crit Care Med 2006;173(9):1008–15.
76. Fremont RD, Koyama T, Calfee CS, et al. Acute lung injury in patients with traumatic injuries: utility of a panel of biomarkers for diagnosis and pathogenesis. J Trauma 2010;68(5):1121–7.
77. Tzu J, Marinkovich MP. Bridging structure with function: structural, regulatory, and developmental role of laminins. Int J Biochem Cell Biol 2008;40(2):199–214.
78. Katayama M, Ishizaka A, Sakamoto M, et al. Laminin gamma2 fragments are increased in the circulation of patients with early phase acute lung injury. Intensive Care Med 2010;36(3):479–86.
79. Muller WA. Mechanisms of transendothelial migration of leukocytes. Circ Res 2009;105(3):223–30.
80. Calfee CS, Eisner MD, Parsons PE, et al. Soluble intercellular adhesion molecule-1 and clinical outcomes in patients with acute lung injury. Intensive Care Med 2009;35(2):248–57.
81. Conner ER, Ware LB, Modin G, et al. Elevated pulmonary edema fluid concentrations of soluble intercellular adhesion molecule-1 in patients with acute lung injury: biological and clinical significance. Chest 1999;116(Suppl 1):83S–4S.
82. Prabhakaran P, Ware LB, White KE, et al. Elevated levels of plasminogen activator inhibitor-1 in pulmonary edema fluid are associated with mortality in acute lung injury. Am J Physiol Lung Cell Mol Physiol 2003;285(1):L20–8.
83. Pugin J, Verghese G, Widmer MC, et al. The alveolar space is the site of intense inflammatory and profibrotic reactions in the early phase of acute respiratory distress syndrome. Crit Care Med 1999;27(2):304–12.
84. Chesnutt AN, Matthay MA, Tibayan FA, et al. Early detection of type III procollagen peptide in acute lung injury. Pathogenetic and prognostic significance. Am J Respir Crit Care Med 1997;156(3 Pt 1):840–5.
85. Meduri GU, Tolley EA, Chinn A, et al. Procollagen types I and III aminoterminal propeptide levels during acute respiratory distress syndrome and in response to methylprednisolone treatment. Am J Respir Crit Care Med 1998;158(5 Pt 1): 1432–41.
86. Dentener MA, Vreugdenhil AC, Hoet PH, et al. Production of the acute-phase protein lipopolysaccharide-binding protein by respiratory type II epithelial cells: implications for local defense to bacterial endotoxins. Am J Respir Cell Mol Biol 2000;23(2):146–53.
87. Villar J, Perez-Mendez L, Espinosa E, et al. Serum lipopolysaccharide binding protein levels predict severity of lung injury and mortality in patients with severe sepsis. PLoS One 2009;4(8):e6818.
88. Ware LB, Eisner MD, Thompson BT, et al. Significance of von Willebrand factor in septic and nonseptic patients with acute lung injury. Am J Respir Crit Care Med 2004;170(7):766–72.

89. Parsons PE, Eisner MD, Thompson BT, et al. Lower tidal volume ventilation and plasma cytokine markers of inflammation in patients with acute lung injury. Crit Care Med 2005;33(1):1–6 [discussion: 230–2].
90. Ware CF. Targeting the LIGHT-HVEM pathway. Adv Exp Med Biol 2009;647: 146–55.
91. Chen CY, Yang KY, Chen MY, et al. Decoy receptor 3 levels in peripheral blood predict outcomes of acute respiratory distress syndrome. Am J Respir Crit Care Med 2009;180(8):751–60.
92. Bajwa EK, Khan UA, Januzzi JL, et al. Plasma C-reactive protein levels are associated with improved outcome in ARDS. Chest 2009;136(2):471–80.
93. Zhai R, Sheu CC, Su L, et al. Serum bilirubin levels on ICU admission are associated with ARDS development and mortality in sepsis. Thorax 2009;64(9):784–90.
94. Tseng JS, Chan MC, Hsu JY, et al. Procalcitonin is a valuable prognostic marker in ARDS caused by community-acquired pneumonia. Respirology 2008;13(4): 505–9.
95. Brower RG, Lanken PN, MacIntyre N, et al. Higher versus lower positive end-expiratory pressures in patients with the acute respiratory distress syndrome. N Engl J Med 2004;351(4):327–36.
96. McClintock D, Zhuo H, Wickersham N, et al. Biomarkers of inflammation, coagulation and fibrinolysis predict mortality in acute lung injury. Crit Care 2008; 12(2):R41.
97. Pencina MJ, D'Agostino RB Sr, D'Agostino RB Jr, et al. Evaluating the added predictive ability of a new marker: from area under the ROC curve to reclassification and beyond. Stat Med 2008;27(2):157–72 [discussion: 207–12].
98. Calfee CS, Ware L, Glidden DV, et al. Use of risk reclassification with multiple biomarkers improves mortality prediction in acute lung injury. Critical Care Medicine 2011. [Epub ahead of print].
99. Matthay MA, Thompson BT, Read EJ, et al. Therapeutic potential of mesenchymal stem cells for severe acute lung injury. Chest 2010;138(4):965–72.
100. Burnham EL, Mealer M, Gaydos J, et al. Acute lung injury but not sepsis is associated with increased colony formation by peripheral blood mononuclear cells. Am J Respir Cell Mol Biol 2010;43(3):326–33.
101. Burnham EL, Taylor WR, Quyyumi AA, et al. Increased circulating endothelial progenitor cells are associated with survival in acute lung injury. Am J Respir Crit Care Med 2005;172(7):854–60.
102. Owens RL, Stigler WS, Hess DR. Do newer monitors of exhaled gases, mechanics, and esophageal pressure add value? Clin Chest Med 2008;29(2): 297–312, vi–vii.
103. Gessner C, Hammerschmidt S, Kuhn H, et al. Exhaled breath condensate acidification in acute lung injury. Respir Med 2003;97(11):1188–94.
104. Gong MN, Zhou W, Williams PL, et al. -308GA and TNFB polymorphisms in acute respiratory distress syndrome. Eur Respir J 2005;26(3):382–9.
105. Sutherland AM, Walley KR, Manocha S, et al. The association of interleukin 6 haplotype clades with mortality in critically ill adults. Arch Intern Med 2005; 165(1):75–82.
106. Gong MN, Thompson BT, Williams PL, et al. Interleukin-10 polymorphism in position -1082 and acute respiratory distress syndrome. Eur Respir J 2006;27(4): 674–81.
107. Gong MN, Wei Z, Xu LL, et al. Polymorphism in the surfactant protein-B gene, gender, and the risk of direct pulmonary injury and ARDS. Chest 2004;125(1): 203–11.

108. Gong MN, Zhou W, Williams PL, et al. Polymorphisms in the mannose binding lectin-2 gene and acute respiratory distress syndrome. Crit Care Med 2007; 35(1):48–56.
109. Zhai R, Zhou W, Gong MN, et al. Inhibitor kappaB-alpha haplotype GTC is associated with susceptibility to acute respiratory distress syndrome in Caucasians. Crit Care Med 2007;35(3):893–8.
110. Lagan AL, Quinlan GJ, Mumby S, et al. Variation in iron homeostasis genes between patients with ARDS and healthy control subjects. Chest 2008;133(6): 1302–11.
111. Howrylak JA, Dolinay T, Lucht L, et al. Discovery of the gene signature for acute lung injury in patients with sepsis. Physiol Genomics 2009;37(2):133–9.
112. Wang Z, Beach D, Su L, et al. A genome-wide expression analysis in blood identifies pre-elafin as a biomarker in ARDS. Am J Respir Cell Mol Biol 2008;38(6): 724–32.
113. Wang Z, Chen F, Zhai R, et al. Plasma neutrophil elastase and elafin imbalance is associated with acute respiratory distress syndrome (ARDS) development. PLoS One 2009;4(2):e4380.
114. Schnapp LM, Donohoe S, Chen J, et al. Mining the acute respiratory distress syndrome proteome: identification of the insulin-like growth factor (IGF)/IGF-binding protein-3 pathway in acute lung injury. Am J Pathol 2006;169(1):86–95.
115. de Torre C, Ying SX, Munson PJ, et al. Proteomic analysis of inflammatory biomarkers in bronchoalveolar lavage. Proteomics 2006;6(13):3949–57.
116. Ware LB, Matthay MA. Beyond fishing: the role of discovery proteomics in mechanistic lung research. Am J Physiol Lung Cell Mol Physiol 2009;296(1):L12–3.
117. Gerszten RE, Accurso F, Bernard GR, et al. Challenges in translating plasma proteomics from bench to bedside: update from the NHLBI Clinical Proteomics Programs. Am J Physiol Lung Cell Mol Physiol 2008;295(1):L16–22.
118. Lacy P. Metabolomics of sepsis-induced acute lung injury: a new approach for biomarkers. Am J Physiol Lung Cell Mol Physiol 2011;300(1):L1–3.
119. Cohen MJ, Serkova NJ, Wiener-Kronish J, et al. 1H-NMR-based metabolic signatures of clinical outcomes in trauma patients–beyond lactate and base deficit. J Trauma 2010;69(1):31–40.
120. Stringer KA, Serkova NJ, Karnovsky A, et al. Metabolic consequences of sepsis-induced acute lung injury revealed by plasma (1)H-nuclear magnetic resonance quantitative metabolomics and computational analysis. Am J Physiol Lung Cell Mol Physiol 2011;300(1):L4–11.

Recovery and Long-Term Outcome in Acute Respiratory Distress Syndrome

Margaret S. Herridge, MD, MPH

KEYWORDS

- Acute respiratory distress syndrome • Outcome
- ICU-acquired weakness • Health care use • Cost
- Pulmonary function • Psychological • Psychiatric

Interest in longer-term outcomes after acute respiratory distress syndrome (ARDS) and the understanding of patterns of recovery have increased enormously over the past 10 years. Historically, the outcome of greatest interest after ARDS was pulmonary function and, ironically, the respiratory system may be one of the more resilient organ systems after an episode of severe lung injury. The evaluation of generic and disease-specific health-related quality of life (HRQOL) measures after ARDS has evolved to include a detailed evaluation of functional outcome, exercise capacity, neuropsychological morbidity, and in-person follow-up to catalog and describe the varied consequences of an episode of ARDS and its longer-term repercussions for patients and family.

Most patients who survive an episode of ARDS will sustain some degree of permanent disability[1,2] and reduction in HRQOL as a consequence of intensive care unit (ICU)-acquired weakness, in addition to a spectrum of other physical disabilities.[1–10] Patients may also develop significant new neurologic morbidity, including neurocognitive impairments, and psychiatric disorders.[11–15] This legacy of muscle, nerve, and brain dysfunction comes at significant additional cost, with some reports stating that health care use after critical illness is similar to that of patients with chronic disease,[2,10,16,17] which may represent an important public health concern.

This article highlights important advances in outcomes after ARDS and describes pulmonary outcomes, the most recent data on functional and neuropsychological

---

This work was supported by grants from the Canadian Institutes of Health Research, Physicians' Services Incorporated Foundation, Ontario Thoracic Society, and Canadian Intensive Care Foundation.

The author has nothing to disclose.

Division of Respiratory and Interdepartmental Division of Critical Care Medicine, Toronto General Hospital, University of Toronto, 11C-1180 585 University Avenue, Toronto, Ontario M5G 2C4, Canada

E-mail address: margaret.herridge@uhn.on.ca

Crit Care Clin 27 (2011) 685–704
doi:10.1016/j.ccc.2011.04.003
criticalcare.theclinics.com

disability in patients, health care cost, family caregivers, and early models of rehabilitation and intervention.

LONG-TERM OUTCOME MEASURES AFTER ARDS

Survivors of acute lung injury or ARDS (ALI/ARDS) represent an important subset of complex critically ill and long-stay ICU patients.[18] Most patients with ARDS spend weeks in the ICU and therefore constitute a subgroup of the chronically critically ill patient population, helping to highlight the enormous heterogeneity in outcomes within the chronically critically ill population. ALI/ARDS is estimated to affect 190,600 people per year in the United States and to be associated with 74,500 deaths and 3.6 million hospital days.[19] More than 100,000 patients will survive ALI/ARDS each year,[19] and this condition is now recognized as an important public health concern.

Pulmonary Function

After the initial description of ARDS by Ashbaugh and colleagues[20] in 1967, a flurry of articles described pulmonary outcome in ARDS survivors over the first several months after ICU discharge. Overwhelmingly, these were case series or involved small cohorts, and reported good pulmonary recovery with a mild restrictive or obstructive pattern, or normal volumes and spirometry and a mild to moderate reduction in diffusion capacity.[21–23] Given the subtlety of most reported derangements in pulmonary function after ARDS, the extent to which this influences functional and HRQOL outcomes, even though statistical associations were noted, may be difficult to determine. Furthermore, in most studies, the extent to which patients had preexisting pulmonary disease was unclear, and how underlying lung dysfunction might interact with severe lung injury, both during the acute critical illness and over the subsequent months to years while the lung is remodeling, remains uncertain.

McHugh and colleagues[6] evaluated pulmonary function in 37 ARDS survivors at 3, 6, and 12 months after extubation and noted that pulmonary function improved substantially by 6 months, but little thereafter, and that greater severity of lung injury was associated with impaired return to normal lung volumes. They also noted that the Sickness Impact Profile (SIP) score paralleled the pulmonary function, but that most patients did not attribute their current health problems to breathing difficulties.

Schelling and colleagues[15] noted a relationship between the number of pulmonary function impairments and a reduction in HRQOL scores, and also found that these patients were less likely to return to work. Of all the pulmonary measures, the diffusing capacity of the lung for carbon monoxide (DLCO) was the only pulmonary function parameter that correlated with HRQOL. Heyland and colleagues[24] noted a correlation between the physical function domain of the Medical Outcomes Study 36-item short-form health survey (SF-36) and FEV_1, but this had reached the lower bound of normal by 6-month follow-up. Similar to the observation by McHugh and colleagues,[6] their data suggested that pulmonary function was associated with the severity of lung injury in the ICU, although no data currently correlate ventilatory strategy with longer-term pulmonary outcome.[25]

Neff and collaborators[26] described a mix of restrictive and obstructive findings and a reduction in diffusing capacity in their report on 16 survivors of severe lung injury after trauma, and Orme and colleagues[8] reported relatively preserved lung volumes and spirometry in their follow-up of 66 patients, and noted a persistent reduction in diffusing capacity. A more recent study by Masclans and colleagues[27] again confirmed that some patients had mild restrictive disease 6 months after ARDS.

Pulmonary function data from the Toronto ARDS cohort study showed that most patients had recovery to normal or near normal spirometry within 6 to 12 months after ICU discharge, and that pulmonary function remained stable through to 5-year follow-up. Because approximately 40% of this cohort was seen in the home, data for lung volumes and DLCO were incomplete. Furthermore, this cohort was relatively young and had minimal reported preexisting pulmonary morbidity, although approximately half reported ever smoking.[1,10]

Nobauer-Huhmann and colleagues[28] were the first to perform imaging on patients with ARDS at 6 to 10 months after illness. In their sample of 15 patients, they noted that most had localized changes in the nondependent lung zones, and the investigators were able to document some association between severity of lung injury and duration of mechanical ventilation.[29] Subsequently, Desai and colleagues[30] reported CT findings in patients with ARDS 3 years after their illness and noted that reticular changes were most common but that areas of decreased attenuation and ground glass opacities were also observed, primarily in the anterior lung zones. Duration of mechanical ventilation was also associated with radiographic findings in this group, suggesting that this may reflect ventilator-induced lung injury.

Two ARDS cohorts have captured radiographic follow-up data after ARDS up to 5 years.[10,31] The Toronto ARDS cohort study[10] evaluated 25 patients through CT of the thorax at 5-year follow-up, with most scans showing radiologic abnormalities, the most common being nondependent minor pulmonary fibrosis consistent with ventilator-induced lung injury. Approximately one-third of these patients also had evidence of bronchiectasis or new pulmonary fibrosis associated with symptoms of dyspnea, sputum production, or minor obstructive or restrictive changes on pulmonary function. Linden and colleagues[31] also documented a predominantly reticular pattern on CT imaging in 21 patients. This finding was consistent with fibrosis, but because these patients all received extracorporeal membrane oxygenation (ECMO), no ventral distribution was observed, and most had spirometry within the lower bound of normal. Greater duration of ECMO was associated with a reduction in the total lung capacity.

Pulmonary function outcomes may be heterogeneous after an episode of ARDS, but most young patients without documented preexisting lung disease regain normal or near-normal function with a persistent mild reduction in diffusion capacity. These patients seem to maintain stable pulmonary function up to 5 years after the initial episode of severe lung injury.[10] The current spectrum of results suggests possible variability by smoking history, preexisting obstructive or restrictive pulmonary disease, physiologic restriction related to ICU-acquired weakness affecting respiratory muscles, presence of other pulmonary processes that fulfill the ARDS definition but have a different natural history (eg, cryptogenic organizing pneumonia), and loss to follow-up that continues to challenge validity and interpretation of follow-up data. Most outcome studies found that ARDS survivors are often unable to resume their prior physical function, but the degree of pulmonary dysfunction documented across studies does not solely explain this degree of functional limitation.

Functional Disability

Over the past several years, research has highlighted the concept of a continuum of weakness that begins within hours of mechanical ventilation,[32] is evident through bedside evaluation within 1 week of ICU admission using the Medical Research Council scoring system,[33] and may persist with incomplete recovery for years after ICU discharge (**Fig. 1**). A recent 5-year ARDS outcomes study illustrates that relatively young (median age, 45 years) previously working patients with few comorbidities may not regain their pre–critical illness functional status nor HRQOL by 5 years after ICU

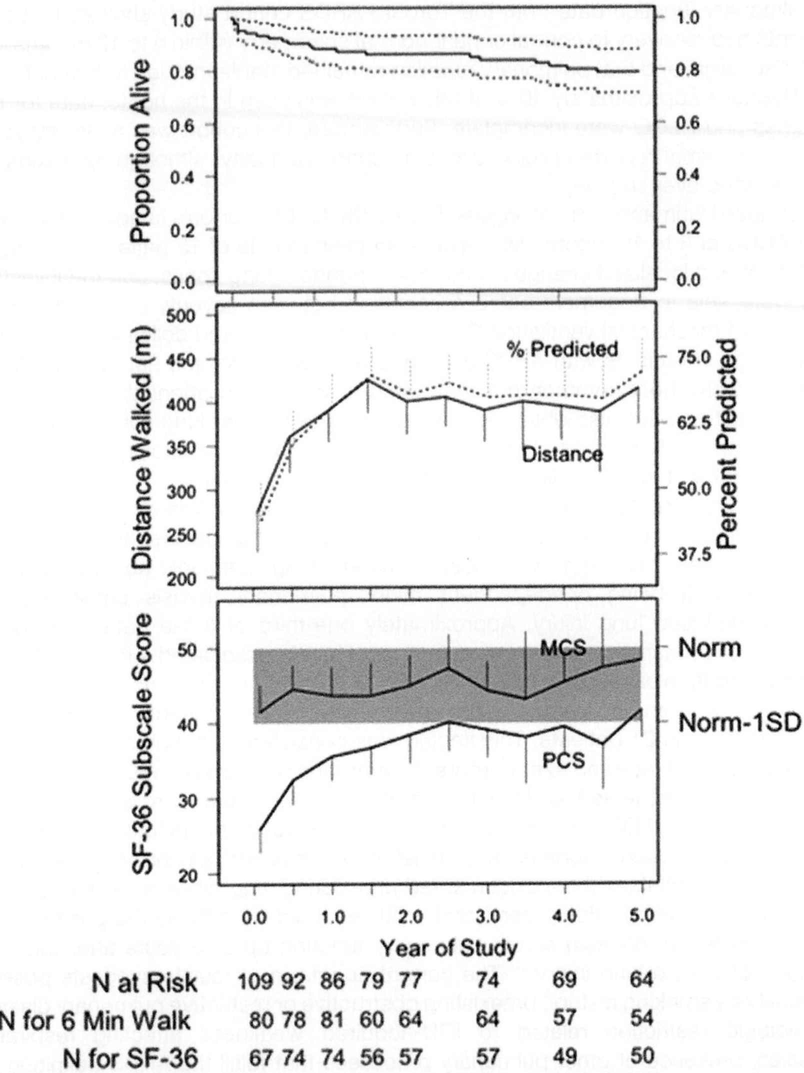

Fig. 1. Survival, 6-minute walk distance and quality of life to 5 years after ICU discharge. Exact survival times were used for these analyses, whereas deaths indicated in the consort diagram were included between scheduled follow-up visits. Top panel: Kaplan-Meier curve to 5 years. Dashed lines represent the 95% CI. Middle panel: Distance walked in 6 minutes (meters and percent predicted); distance in meters is a solid line and percent predicted is a dashed line. Bottom panel: SF-36 subscale scores for physical component score and mental component score. (*From* Herridge MS, Tansey CM, Matté A, et al. Functional disability 5 years after acute respiratory distress syndrome. N Engl J Med 2011;364(14):1299; with permission.)

discharge. The concept of ICU-acquired weakness has gained momentum over the past several years, but investigators have recently observed that it may cause irreversible functional disability. Furthermore, this persistent dysfunction may also be influenced by a spectrum of other physical and neuropsychological disabilities that continue to plague patients over the longer term.

Neuromuscular Dysfunction

Muscle weakness and impaired function constitute an important morbidity of severe critical illness and have been described in most detail in ARDS survivors, but similar reports of functional disability in survivors of sepsis and chronic critical illness have been increasing, and clearly these conditions overlap. Reported disability and reduction in activities of daily living have been inferred to be a consequence of ICU-acquired muscle wasting and weakness syndrome.[16,34]

Accurate characterization and potential intervention in neuromuscular disability after critical illness has many challenges. First, significant heterogeneity exists across different critically ill patient populations in terms of susceptibility and risk factors for neuromuscular dysfunction, and no validated measures currently help stratify patients according to risk and subsequent degree of acquired physical disability. Adding to the confusion, several different terminologies are used in the literature, including critical illness polyneuropathy, critical illness polyneuropathy and myopathy, ICU-acquired paresis, critical illness myopathy and/or neuropathy, ICU-acquired weakness, and critical illness neuropathy and myopathy (CINMA). Furthermore, muscle and nerve lesions often coexist, complicating the ability to understand discrete risk factors or natural history. Obstacles also exist in terms of testing methods, criteria for diagnosis, surveillance, and selection bias in evaluation and reporting. Sensory and motor evaluations are limited in heavily sedated patients, and clinical bedside testing and determination of the prevalence of these lesions may be unreliable. Despite these limitations, some excellent models for classifying these lesions were recently proposed.[35]

A recent review of risk factors and prevention of ICU-acquired weakness[28] highlights nonmodifiable factors, including multiple organ failure and severity of illness, and modifiable factors, such as muscle immobilization, hyperglycemia, and corticosteroid and neuromuscular blocker use. This long-term morbidity may be modified through changes in current ICU practice patterns but this awaits further study. The next section describes the muscle and nerve injuries relevant to survivors of ARDS that constitute the wasting and weakness syndrome observed after critical illness.

Critical Illness Polyneuropathy

Background and incidence

In 1984, Bolton and his Canadian colleagues published a landmark article describing challenges in liberating 5 critically ill patients from mechanical ventilation.[36] These patients had a primary axonopathy on electrophysiologic testing which presented as a mixed sensorimotor neuropathy. It is now clear that CIP is very common in patients with the systemic inflammatory response syndrome (SIRS) and sepsis which frequently co-exist with ARDS. There are reports of an occurrence of CIP in 70% to 100% of longer stay ICU patients. It remains challenging to capture the true incidence of CIP because of poor consensus on surveillance, unclear criteria for definition and diagnosis, as well as timing and nature of testing. Where patients were evaluated solely on the basis of weakness, studies have reported an incidence of 25% to 36%.[32,37] A rigorous systematic review on over 1400 critically ill patients, reported an incidence of CINMA of close to 50% (95% confidence interval 43–49%).[38] These authors defined patients as having CINMA if they were evaluated using diagnostic tests (nerve conduction velocities, needle electromyography, direct muscle stimulation, histopathology of muscle or nerve tissue) or a combination of these test findings and clinical findings of muscle weakness, decreased or absent deep tendon reflexes, and or failure to liberate from mechanical ventilation. It is often very challenging to identify weakness in unresponsive or minimally interactive critically ill patients. However, electromyography (EMG) testing will demonstrate abnormalities showing an initial primary axonal degeneration of the motor neurons, followed by the sensory neural fibers and this coincides with acute and chronic changes of denervation noted on muscle biopsies in affected patients.[39] The impetus to screen for this lesion implies that it is important to detect this early to facilitate intervention. However, the ability to intervene in this process, the nature of an intervention and the natural history of this lesion is not currently known.

Critical Illness Myopathy

Background and incidence

The term critical illness myopathy (CIM) currently includes critical illness myopathy, acute quadriplegic myopathy, thick filament myopathy and necrotizing myopathy. This rather heterogeneous grouping has a reported incidence varying from 48% and 96% in prospective studies, some of which have included muscle biopsy.[40] The pathology of CIM is that of a diffuse, non-necrotizing myopathy associated with fatty degeneration of muscle fibers, fiber atrophy and fibrosis.[41] This has been described in patients with sepsis/ARDS but also in those receiving treatment with neuromuscular blockers and/or corticosteroids. The diagnosis of CIM distinct from CIP can be difficult since the phenotype of paresis with difficulty in weaning may virtually overlap and this is further compounded by the fact that these lsions often co-exist. Muscle biopsy may allow differentiation between these. A small case series of biopsies from survivors of severe ARDS showed chronic myopathic changes up to 2 years after the episode of critical illness thereby raising the possibility of residual muscle injury as the sole correlate for chronic functional disability observed in these patients.[42]

The thick filament myopathy is characterized by loss of myosin filaments in the context of significant corticosteroid or neuromuscular blocker exposure and immobility.[43] There has been speculation that this may represent a precursor to acute necrotizing myopathy since this form of CIM may show progression to myonecrosis. Acute necrotizing myopathy is distinguished by extensive myonecrosis with vacuolization and phagocytosis of muscle fibers and has also been associated with corticosteroid and neuromuscular blocker exposure. It is important to emphasize that steroids and paralytics may not necessarily be causally linked to this process since they will frequently be employed in sicker patients with multiple failed organ systems.[44]

Additional Physical Morbidities

Several other physical sequelae may also influence functional outcomes, physical HRQOL, need for subsequent hospitalization, and accrued costs over time. These conditions have been studied in the most detail in survivors of ARDS and cataloged in recent ARDS publications.[1,10] These sequelae include tracheal stenosis with subsequent need for tracheal resection complicated by malacia and T-tube placement, heterotopic ossification, contractures, frozen shoulders, hoarseness and voice changes, tooth loss, sensorineural hearing loss, and tinnitus, and these contributed to emotional outcomes, social isolation, and sexual dysfunction.

Entrapment neuropathy

The Toronto ARDS cohort study observed a 6% prevalence of peroneal and ulnar nerve palsies at 1-year follow-up.[1] Although this represents only a small proportion of patients, these nerve palsies complicated rehabilitation therapy and precluded return to original work in some cases. By 5 years, these had resolved, as had foot drop in all patients.

Heterotopic ossification

Heterotopic ossification is the deposition of para-articular ectopic bone and has been previously associated with polytrauma, burns, pancreatitis, and ARDS.[45] Heterotopic ossification is associated with paralysis and prolonged immobilization. A 5% prevalence of heterotopic ossification was reported at 1 year in ARDS survivors, with all patients having large joint immobilization and subsequent functional limitation.[1] Heterotopic ossification is remediable with appropriate surgical intervention, and screening for this condition may help improve long-term functional outcomes. However, patients may be reluctant to undergo any surgical procedure after a severe critical illness because of fear of complications, and this may represent an important barrier to rehabilitation and return to prior functional status.

Cosmesis

The physical devastation after ARDS and critical illness cannot be overstated, and the way in which patients are transformed and struggle with dramatically changed appearance has significant long-term implications. Many patients experience often-devastating emotional effects related to their altered appearance. Recent 5-year data show that patients describe ongoing concerns about cosmesis, including scars from laparotomy, chest tube, central line, arterial line and tracheostomy insertion, burns, striae from volume overload, and facial scars from prolonged noninvasive mask ventilation. Many of these patients underwent tracheostomy revision. Patients reported that cosmetic concerns contributed to social isolation and sexual dysfunction.

ARDS and Brain Injury

Neurocognitive impairments

In their groundbreaking paper from 1999, Hopkins and colleagues[11] evaluated 55 survivors of ARDS at 1 year after ICU discharge. At hospital discharge, all patients experienced cognitive impairments, including problems with memory, attention, or concentration, and a global loss of cognitive function. By 1-year follow-up, most patients showed improvement in overall cognitive function, but 30% still showed deficits on the Wechsler Adult Intelligence Scale–Revised; 78% had impairment of at least one cognitive function, including memory, attention, or concentration; and 48% experienced a decreased speed of mental processing.[11] In the 2-year follow-up of this cohort, these same investigators reported no additional improvement in neurocognitive sequelae beyond 1 year (**Fig. 2**).[12] Since these landmark papers, the literature continues to document an important prevalence of neurocognitive dysfunction in ARDS survivors and other groups of critically ill patients, and the important impact this has on HRQOL. Hopkins and colleagues[11] were the first to report the significant effect this had on reported HRQOL outcomes, and Rothenhausler and colleagues[14] also noted that ARDS survivors with neurocognitive sequelae had worse quality of life than individuals without neuropsychological dysfunction.

Currently, close to 1000 patients in 15 different cohorts have undergone neurocognitive evaluation after critical illness.[9,11,14,46–51] Similar to the landmark findings from the Hopkins studies, other reports have documented cognitive impairments in 100% of patients at hospital discharge and in large numbers of patients up to 6 years.[9–12,14,49,50,52–55] In most cases, impairments seem to improve most rapidly in the first 6 to 12 months after hospital discharge. Additional outcomes data in patients without ARDS help highlight the observation that different neurocognitive domains may be impaired in different ICU survivors, depending on the nature of the injury acquired during the episode of critical illness and its treatment, the presence of

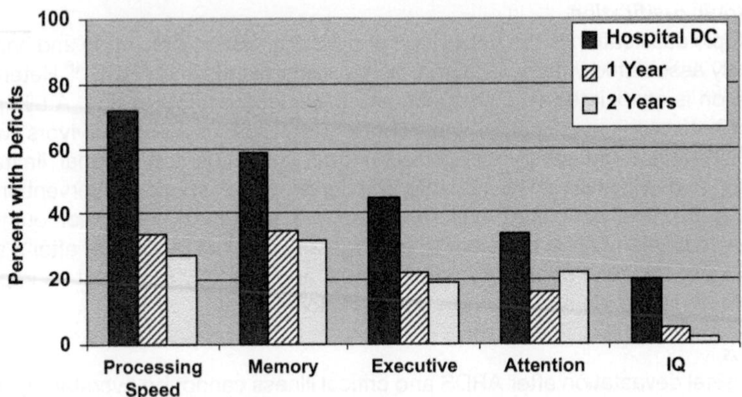

Fig. 2. Cognitive outcomes after ARDS (*Data from* Hopkins RO, Weaver LK, Pope D, et al. Neuropsychological sequelae and impaired health status in survivors of severe acute respiratory distress syndrome. Am J Respir Crit Care Med 1999;160:50–6; and Hopkins RO, Weaver LK, Collingridge D, et al. Two-year cognitive, emotional, and quality-of-life outcomes in acute respiratory distress syndrome. Am J Respir Crit Care Med 2005;171:340–7.)

underlying neurocognitive abnormalities, and other patient-specific vulnerabilities, including older age.

The effect of acute care hospitalization and critical illness on the brain remains poorly understood. It is unclear whether critical illness itself or its associated treatment causes the decline in cognitive function or simply further compromises preexisting brain dysfunction. In a recent report by Ehlenbach and colleagues,[56] older adults without neurocognitive impairments or dementia underwent neurocognitive assessment before and after an acute care or ICU hospitalization. Those who had acute care or critical illness hospitalization experienced a greater decline in neurocognitive function and new incident dementia compared with individuals who were not hospitalized. These data suggest that the acute or critical illness may cause a significant decrement in neurocognitive function. Iwashyna and colleagues[37] evaluated cognitive impairment in a group of patients with sepsis derived from the Health and Retirement Study and confirmed the observations outlined earlier. This longitudinal cohort showed that patients with severe sepsis developed new, important, and persistent neurocognitive dysfunction. The data from these studies suggest that an episode of acute or critical illness may be causally linked to a new compromise in neurocognition in older patients.[34,56]

There remains little general awareness about neurocognitive dysfunction after critical illness, and no formal educational programs to assist patients, caregivers, or physicians caring for these patients. As physical rehabilitation programs become part of the ICU continuum of care, the importance of referral for neurocognitive rehabilitation may also need to be considered.

Psychiatric Morbidity

Psychiatric conditions after critical illness and ICU treatment are common. The range of depression reported in survivors of ARDS is 17% to 58%, and reports have suggested that patients with ARDS may experience a greater degree of depression compared with populations of general critically ill patients.[3,4,46,57] Prospective evaluation of risk factors associated with depression in patients with ARDS showed relationships with longer duration of mechanical ventilation, ICU length of stay, and sedation. A recent study assessing risk factors for depression and anxiety in ARDS survivors found that at 1 year, alcohol dependence, female gender, and younger age were predictors of depression,[58] and that ratio of arterial oxygen tension to inspired oxygen fraction and duration of mechanical ventilation were predictors of anxiety. Predictors of depression at 2 years were depression and neurocognitive sequelae at 1 year, whereas the predictor of anxiety at 2 years was anxiety at 1 year.[58] A recent study found that hypoglycemia may be an important risk factor for depression in ARDS survivors, and this warrants further study.[59] The rates of depression in critically ill patients are similar to the 22% to 33% observed in chronically ill medical inpatients[60] and 25% to 28% in patients with cardiac and pulmonary disorders.[61]

In a recent systematic summary, Davydow and colleagues[62] reported that 28% of ICU survivors had clinically significant depression, but sex, age, or severity of illness at ICU admission were not consistent risk factors for this. Early post-ICU depressive symptoms were a strong risk factor for subsequent depressive symptoms, and post-ICU depressive symptoms were associated with substantially lower HRQOL. In addition, episodes of depression may occur years after the critical illness. In the Toronto ARDS cohort study,[33] more than 50% of patients had a physician-diagnosed episode of depression or anxiety between 2 and 5 years after ICU discharge.

The depression and anxiety observed after ICU treatment are likely multifactorial. Additional study is needed to better understand patient vulnerability, illness, and ICU treatment-specific determinants of mood and psychiatric disorders, and appropriate tools for diagnosis, treatment, and ongoing management.

Posttraumatic stress disorder is defined as a set of characteristic symptoms occurring after a traumatic event(s) where triggers include intense helplessness, fear or personal threat a serious personal threat.[63] Diagnostic criteria include a history of traumatic event(s) associated with symptoms from each of three symptom clusters: hyperarousal symptoms, intrusive recollections and avoidant/numbing symptoms. A number of studies have examined the asssociation between severe critical illness, its treatment and PTSD development. Schelling and colleagues pioneered this work and were the first to highlight the importance of PTSD to the critical care community.[64] In a cohort of 80 ARDS survivors 4 years following discharge from the ICU, these investigators documented that almost one third of the ARDS survivors reported compromised memory, disturbing dreams, anxiety, and sleeping difficulties after ICU discharge, and 28% prevalence of PTSD. In this study, PTSD was associated with the number of adverse ICU-related memories recalled by patients.

In a different study sample, Kapfhammer and colleagues showed that 44% of critically ill patients fulfilled criteria for PTSD at hospital discharge and in 24% of patients, these persisted up to 8 years or longer.[13] Davydow and colleagues reported that the median point prevalence of questionnaire-ascertained "clinically significant" PTSD symptoms was 22%, and the median point prevalence of clinician-diagnosed PTSD was 19% in populations of general critically ill patients.[57] Predictors of post-ICU PTSD included history of psychopathology, greater ICU benzodiazepine exposure and post-ICU memories of in-ICU disturbing and/or psychotic experiences.

These authors also noted that female sex and younger age were less consistent predictors, and severity of critical illness was not a predictor. Post-ICU PTSD was associated with substantially lower HRQL. The occurrence of PTSD in patients with ARDS may be higher, with Psychiatrist-diagnosed PTSD prevalence ranging from 445 at hospital discharge to 24% at 8 year follow-up.[57,65] Memory for nightmares or delusions while in ICU as well as a complete absence of any ICU memories have also been noted as risks for PTSD.[13] PTSD is currently considered another significant sequela of critical illness/ARDS with an important contribution to job loss and long-term disability.[13,57,66]

Psychiatric disorders after critical illness may be a consequence of brain injury sustained from critical illness or its treatments, a psychological reaction to the emotional and physiologic stress of critical illness, or caused by other unknown factors. Additional candidate contributors may include medications, physiologic changes, pain, altered sensory inputs, sleep derangement, and an unfamiliar environment.[67–69] A recent review article found an association between recall of delusional memories after ICU discharge and PTSD-related symptoms, depression, and anxiety.[70] Although some suggestion has been made that factual memories could protect surviving patients from developing symptoms of PTSD, a recent study suggests otherwise. Myhren and colleagues[71] evaluated 194 patients and found that 27% had symptoms of PTSD, and that the predictors in this study sample were higher education level, optimism, factual recall, and memory of pain.

How longstanding and debilitating psychiatric disorders may be after critical illness and the important deleterious impact they have on HRQOL, functional, and family caregiver outcomes are just starting to be appreciated. In response to these reports of significant mental health challenges, literature is now emerging evaluating potential interventions to prevent or reduce these psychiatric sequelae. A recent review article suggests that corticosteroid administration may protect patients against post-ICU PTSD.[72] A novel and important study that used ICU diaries, which contained information and photographs from the ICU stay, suggested that these may reduce the incidence of PTSD.[73] Of the patients who received the diary, only 5% had clinically significant PTSD symptoms compared with 13% of controls. This intervention seemed to be most effective for those with important early PTSD symptoms.[73]

HRQOL

HRQOL is defined as a set of causally linked dimensions of health, including biologic/physiologic, mental, physical, social, and neurocognitive functions, and health perception.[4] Measures of HRQOL assess how disease and its treatment are related to physical, social, emotional, and neurocognitive functioning and have emerged as an important patient-centered metric of recovery from critical illness. Emerging evidence suggests that the degree of disability acquired during critical illness and the resultant decrement in HRQOL may be variable across patient populations and relate to differences in premorbid functional status, burden of comorbid illness, and nature and duration of critical illness and its treatment. This heterogeneity is important to consider when attempting to risk stratify patients for within-ICU and post-ICU rehabilitation interventions.

Considerable homogeneity in HRQOL outcomes exists across different cohorts of patients with ARDS,[5] and the following is a brief, historical overview of the emergence of the literature on ARDS HRQOL outcomes, including recent data on 5-year outcomes.

In 1994, McHugh and colleagues[6] prospectively evaluated pulmonary function and quality of life to assess recovery over time and evaluate the relationship between pulmonary function and functional disability. These investigators found that the SIP scores (Sickness Impact Profile-generic quality-of-life measure of the patient's self-perceived physical and psychological condition) were low at extubation, rose significantly in the first 3 months, with only slight improvement to 1 year. When quality of life was assessed using a lung-related SIP score, only a modest proportion of the patients' overall dysfunction was attributed to residual pulmonary problems. Weinert and colleagues[4] administered the SF-36, which yields scores in eight domains, including physical and social functioning, role limitations because of emotional or physical problems, mental health, vitality, bodily pain, and general health perceptions.[74] Although they observed that all domains of the SF-36 were substantially reduced, the largest decrements occurred in role-physical and physical functioning. Some of the decrement in quality of life was attributed to pulmonary dysfunction, but most patients attributed reduced quality of life to generalized disability. Schelling and colleagues[64] made similar observations about impaired physical functioning and inferred that disability was caused by pulmonary dysfunction; however, they did not assess this directly in their study. Davidson and colleagues[7] assessed differences in HRQOL in ARDS survivors and comparably ill controls using the SF-36 and a pulmonary disease–specific measure (St. Georges Respiratory Questionnaire [SGRQ]) to determine the degree to which perceived physical disability in ARDS survivors was related to pulmonary dysfunction. Similar to previous reports, all domains of the SF-36 were reduced and the largest decrement was in the role-physical domain. ARDS survivors had significantly worse scores on the SGRQ compared with critically ill controls, which was postulated to suggest an ARDS-specific degree of physical disability. However, SGRQ was validated in patients with structural lung disease, and the three domains of the questionnaire—symptoms, activity and impacts—may also be influenced by nonpulmonary factors, including ICU-acquired weakness and other physical disabilities documented in patients with ARDS. Therefore, the appropriateness and applicability of this measure in ARDS patients remains uncertain.

In a prospective cohort study of ARDS survivors, Angus and colleagues[3] used the Quality of Well-Being (QWB) scale to measure quality-adjusted survival in the first year after hospital discharge. The mean QWB scores for the patients at 6 and 12 months were significantly lower than a control population of patients with cystic fibrosis. When QWB was disaggregated into its component subscores, the symptom component scores accounted for 70% of the decrement in perfect health at 6 and 12 months. Although respiratory symptoms were reported in almost half of the patients, the most common complaints were musculoskeletal and constitutional.

Orme and colleagues[8] evaluated HRQOL and pulmonary function outcomes in a prospective cohort study of 78 ARDS survivors treated with higher tidal volume versus lower tidal volume ventilation strategies. Both groups (higher and lower tidal volumes) reported decreased HRQOL in physical functioning, physical ability to maintain their roles (role-physical), bodily pain, general health, and vitality (energy) on the SF-36. The pulmonary function abnormalities correlated with decreased HRQOL in domains reflecting physical function and were not related to ventilation strategy. An earlier paper by Cooper and investigators[25] also failed to show any relationship between ventilation strategy and longer-term pulmonary, functional, or HRQOL outcomes.

A fairly recent meta-analysis of HRQOL studies in patients with ARDS found lower quality-of-life scores for ARDS survivors, consistent with previous reports.[5] Of additional interest, the recovery of HRQOL in ARDS survivors may vary significantly across domains and over time, consistent with data from Hopkins and colleagues.[12] Despite early improvement in the mental health domains, physical quality of life in ARDS survivors remains significantly lower compared with healthy populations years after ICU discharge.[5]

Data on ARDS survivors are consistent with findings of studies involving more general populations of critically ill patients. A meta-analysis of quality-of-life studies in these patients consistently found lower quality-of-life scores compared to matched, normative controls at all time points (from hospital discharge to 66 months later) after ICU discharge.[75] Furthermore, the investigators found larger decrements in the four physical domains (physical functioning, role-physical, bodily pain, and general health perceptions) than in the mental domains (vitality, social functioning, role-emotional, and mental health). The greatest gains occur in physical functioning, social functioning, and role-physical in the first 6 months, with only modest additional improvements thereafter.[75] Recent ARDS outcomes data confirm these observations in a single cohort followed up for 5-years, with minimal loss to follow-up. This study shows little change in mental health domains over years, but an improvement in the physical component score of the SF-36 to approximately 2 years after ICU discharge, with a plateau below normal predicted values to 5 years. The most persistently affected domains at 5 years were those of general health and vitality (see **Fig. 1**).[10]

Iwashyna and colleagues[34] recently noted similar outcomes, They found a persistent reduction in functional status after sepsis and critical illness. In their older patient study sample (median age, 77 years), they observed a high rate of new functional limitations in those who had no limits before their episode of sepsis (mean, 1.57 new limitations; 95% CI, 0.99–2.15). In those with reductions in activities of daily living before sepsis, the investigators noted an important further decrement in function. They observed that neurocognitive and physical decline persisted for at least 8 years after the episode of sepsis and that the episode of critical illness represented an important decline in the patients' ability to live independently.[34]

The theme of acquired and persistent morbidity after an episode of critical illness is echoed further in a recent report on outcomes in chronically critically ill patients. Unroe and colleagues[16] evaluated the trajectories of care and resource use for 126 patients with a median age of 55 years. These patients had an average of two comorbid conditions, and most were not employed at the time of ICU admission or were retired or disabled and receiving prolonged mechanical ventilation. At 1 year, only 11 patients (9% of the cohort) were alive and without functional dependency. Patients with poor outcomes were older, had more comorbid conditions, and were more frequently discharged to a post–acute care facility. The mean cost per patient was $306,135 (standard deviation [SD], $285,467), and the total cohort cost was $38.1 million, for an estimated $3.5 million per independently functioning survivor at 1 year.

These data indicate that HRQOL in ARDS survivors is adversely influenced by physical and neuropsychological morbidities and that an episode of severe lung injury changes the trajectory of functional outcome and may necessitate a change in employment and disposition in the case of poor premorbid function or organ reserve. The HRQOL data have helped raise awareness among the critical care community regarding long-term morbidity, and more recent in-person natural history cohort data have helped to "fill in the blanks" in terms of the specific determinants of these important decrements in function that persist for years after critical illness and that may represent permanent disability in many cases. Data from other ARDS cohorts with different study samples will help elucidate how robust these HRQOL and other outcomes are.[76]

Health Care Use and Cost

Limited data are available on the health care costs in patients with ARDS, with most data derived from the index hospitalization, and much less information on rehospitalization and accrued outpatient costs years after the critical illness. Angus and colleagues[17] evaluated health care costs and long-term outcome after ARDS as part of their phase III study on nitric oxide. In their relatively young cohort (mean age, 50 years) with very few comorbidities at ICU admission and excellent premorbid functional status, the investigators observed hospital costs of approximately $50,000 exclusive of physician costs, and almost half of patients were discharged to another health care facility or to home with professional help. Of these patients, 24% were readmitted within 6 months and QWB scores were low, with most patients sustaining important decrements in function compared with baseline.

Costs were also reported by Cheung and colleagues[2] in their 2-year ARDS outcomes study. Similar to the study by Angus and colleagues,[3] this cohort was also relatively young and had few baseline comorbidities and, on average, spent several weeks in the ICU. Two-year mean costs, including those from the ICU stay, ward, and post-hospital discharge to 2 years were $97,810, $31,640, and $28,350, respectively. In the ICU, patients with more organ dysfunction acquired during their ICU stay, slower resolution of lung injury, burns, and an informal caregiver present had higher costs. Postdischarge costs were influenced most by the need for subsequent hospitalizations and inpatient rehabilitation. These hospitalizations were related to the risk factor for ARDS. These costs were similar to those previously reported by Valta and colleagues[77] in a 1999 study on 59 Finnish patients with ARDS ($127,900 in Canadian 2002 dollars) and Hamel and colleagues[78] in 2000 for 963 patients with ARDS or acute respiratory failure in the SUPPORT study ($94,500–$112,100 in Canadian 2002 dollars).

In the 5-year follow-up of the Toronto ARDS cohort study, outpatient costs continued to decrease to approximately $6000 to year 3 after ICU discharge but did not decrease beyond this in years 4 and 5. Medication costs and rehospitalization costs seemed to contribute most to these costs and were approximately three- to fourfold more than what one would expect for an age- and sex-matched patient population. This health care use was more consistent with the lower bound of that reported for chronic disease.[10] Patients with a greater burden of comorbid illness had a greater rate of increase in cumulative cost over time (**Fig. 3**).

Caregiver and Family Burden in Critical Illness

The caregiver in critical illness experiences a twofold insult. Initially, they perform a bedside vigil for their loved one during the ICU stay and then are asked to assume complete responsibility for their family member who is often discharged home with complex medical needs, perhaps unresolved delirium, and compromised mobility. That many of these folks are unable to cope, and feel isolated and overwhelmed is hardly surprising.

Researchers have begun to focus on the importance of caregiver outcomes and interactions with caregivers of ICU survivors to understand the effect of critical illness on the family unit. Recent work indicates that close to 60% of ICU survivors who received long-term mechanical ventilation still required the assistance of a family caregiver 1 year after the critical illness.[79] Existing evidence suggests that providing this care may have a deleterious impact on caregivers, and may compromise HRQOL compared with age- and sex-matched persons.[80] Furthermore, significant mental health issues have been reported among caregivers, including PTSD,[81] emotional distress,[80,82–84] caregiver burden,[85] depression,[86] and anxiety.[87]

In a recent review, Johnson and colleagues[88] concluded that caregivers experience burden from the patient's physical and psychological dysfunction and the challenges of managing complex care in the home. Lifestyle disruption and provision of high levels of care[80] also contribute to poor caregiver outcome.[80,84] Much of the current research has been limited by the cross-sectional design and follow-up of 1 year after hospital discharge.[2] Caregiver needs will likely change over time as patients move through different transitions in their recovery and attempt reintegration into their prior lifestyle or return to work; very little is currently known about these longer-term transitions and the support or educational needs of the caregiver.

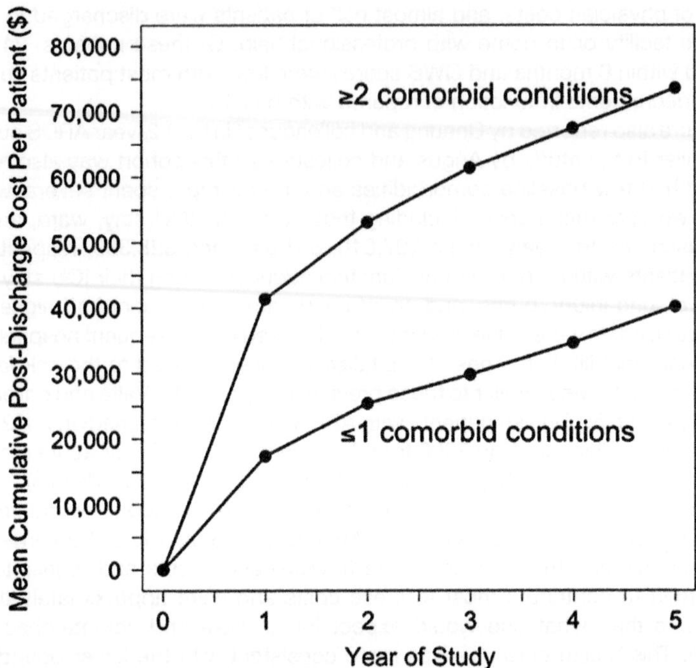

Fig. 3. Cumulative costs to 5 years after ICU discharge stratified by number of comorbid conditions at ICU admission. Lower line is ≤1 comorbid condition and upper line is ≥2 comorbid conditions. (*From* Herridge MS, Tansey CM, Matté A, et al. Functional disability 5 years after acute respiratory distress syndrome. N Engl J Med 2011;364(14):1302; with permission.)

Treatment: ICU and Post-ICU Rehabilitation

Perhaps one of the most fundamental limitations in constructing appropriate rehabilitation programs after critical illness is the current inability to risk stratify patients. Risk stratification is a fundamental tenet on which many other disciplines devise robust algorithmic treatment approaches to clinical problems. The heterogeneity of critically ill populations is an important barrier that must be addressed to understand differences in functional outcome across different patient groups and the various factors that seem to drive a broad spectrum of outcome. For the sake of discussion and contrast, an enormous difference exists in functional outcome between relatively young survivors of ARDS[1,75] and older chronically critically ill patients,[16] despite the apparent similarities of severity of illness and a protracted ICU length of stay. The young, previously working group with lung injuries had few comorbid disorders,[33] very low mortality after ICU discharge, and a significant, albeit less-than-predicted, improvement in functional status at 1 year, and virtually all returned to independent living. These outcomes are in stark contrast to an older group of chronically critically ill patients with a significant burden of comorbid disease, with a 44% mortality rate at 1 year after ICU discharge and only 11% experiencing a good (ie, alive with no functional dependency) outcome.

Current interventional work focuses on early mobility, which several studies have shown is safe and feasible and alters short-term outcome in those patients who were previously functional.[89–94] It is practical and logical to trial physiotherapy and occupational therapy interventions in those who have a high likelihood of benefit.[92] However, this approach, although important and laudable, will not determine how interventions should be tailored to meet individual needs nor how they should be differentially applied, because almost no guidelines exist on specific patient subgroups. For example, offering these interventions to subpopulations of patients whose muscles and nerves have sustained injury so profound that they have lost any potential for rehabilitation will inappropriately raise expectation. Many models have been proposed for complex rehabilitation after critical illness, but none has focused on how to tailor the program to individual need nor has shown long-term efficacy.[95–98] A recent, multicenter, randomized trial assessing HRQOL in 286 critically ill patients compared outcomes from a nurse-led intensive follow-up program versus standard care at 12 months. No difference was seen in HRQOL on the physical or mental health component scores; however, the nurse-led follow-up program cost significantly more than standard care.[99] Alternatively, a self-help manual with instructions for physical therapy improved 6-month outcomes in physical function assessed using the SF-36 HRQOL instrument, and perhaps patients and families used this guide to tailor recommendations to individual need, although this was not studied explicitly in this trial.[100]

This article has also outlined important neuropsychological disability, and some early work has evaluated potential interventions to improve these outcomes. Jones and colleagues[73] evaluated whether a prospectively collected diary of a patient's ICU stay could reduce the development of new-onset PTSD during convalescence after critical illness. Patients with an ICU stay of more than 72 hours were recruited to the study. Intervention patients received their ICU diary at 1 month after ICU discharge, and assessment of the development of PTSD was made at 3 months. The investigators found an associated decrease of new-onset PTSD in the diary group. These early data are promising, but further understanding of the longer-term effect of the diary intervention is warranted.

SUMMARY

Current ARDS outcomes literature suggests that patients will sustain some degree of neuromuscular, functional, or neuropsychological morbidity as a result of their severe lung injury, and that may not be wholly reversible, even in younger patients who were previously working and highly functional. Pulmonary outcomes are likely to be very good in patients who are younger and have no premorbid pulmonary disease. Some studies suggest that ARDS will interact with underlying pulmonary pathology and that outcomes may be more compromised. Health care costs are high, but younger patients who receive support in transitioning back to work return at an overwhelming rate. Patients with more comorbid illness and premorbid functional disability will have poor longer-term outcomes. Family caregivers of patients with ARDS may acquire new mood disorders that impair their HRQOL and also may modify outcomes in patients surviving lung injury. ICU-acquired weakness represents a major morbidity, and studies on interventions such as early mobility and ICU multidisciplinary interventions are promising, but more work must be performed on risk stratification so that programs can be tailored to individual and family needs.

REFERENCES

1. Herridge MS, Cheung AM, Tansey CM, et al. One-year outcomes in survivors of the acute respiratory distress syndrome. N Engl J Med 2003;348(8):683–93.
2. Cheung AM, Tansey CM, Tomlinson G, et al. Two-year outcomes, health care use, and costs of survivors of acute respiratory distress syndrome. Am J Respir Crit Care Med 2006;174(5):538–44.

3. Angus DC, Musthafa AA, Clermont G, et al. Quality-adjusted survival in the first year after the acute respiratory distress syndrome. Am J Respir Crit Care Med 2001;163(6):1389–94.
4. Weinert CR, Gross CR, Kangas JR, et al. Health-related quality of life after acute lung injury. Am J Respir Crit Care Med 1997;156(4 Pt 1):1120–8.
5. Dowdy DW, Eid MP, Dennison CR, et al. Quality of life after acute respiratory distress syndrome: a meta-analysis. Intensive Care Med 2006;32(8):1115–24.
6. McHugh LG, Milberg JA, Whitcomb ME, et al. Recovery of function in survivors of the acute respiratory distress syndrome. Am J Respir Crit Care Med 1994; 150(1):90–4.
7. Davidson TA, Caldwell ES, Curtis JR, et al. Reduced quality of life in survivors of acute respiratory distress syndrome compared with critically ill control patients. JAMA 1999;281(4):354–60.
8. Orme J Jr, Romney JS, Hopkins RO, et al. Pulmonary function and health-related quality of life in survivors of acute respiratory distress syndrome. Am J Respir Crit Care Med 2003;167(5):690–4.
9. Hopkins RO, Weaver LK, Chan KJ, et al. Quality of life, emotional, and cognitive function following acute respiratory distress syndrome. J Int Neuropsychol Soc 2004;10(7):1005–17.
10. Herridge MS, Tansey CM, Matté A, et al. Canadian Critical Care Trials Group. Functional disability 5 years after acute respiratory distress syndrome. N Engl J Med 2011;364(14):1293–304.
11. Hopkins RO, Weaver LK, Pope D, et al. Neuropsychological sequelae and impaired health status in survivors of severe acute respiratory distress syndrome. Am J Respir Crit Care Med 1999;160(1):50–6.
12. Hopkins RO, Weaver LK, Collingridge D, et al. Two-year cognitive, emotional, and quality-of-life outcomes in acute respiratory distress syndrome. Am J Respir Crit Care Med 2005;171(4):340–7.
13. Kapfhammer HP, Rothenhausler HB, Krauseneck T, et al. Posttraumatic stress disorder and health-related quality of life in long-term survivors of acute respiratory distress syndrome. Am J Psychiatry 2004;161(1):45–52.
14. Rothenhausler HB, Ehrentraut S, Stoll C, et al. The relationship between cognitive performance and employment and health status in long-term survivors of the acute respiratory distress syndrome: results of an exploratory study. Gen Hosp Psychiatry 2001;23(2):90–6.
15. Schelling G, Stoll C, Vogelmeier C, et al. Pulmonary function and health-related quality of life in a sample of long-term survivors of the acute respiratory distress syndrome. Intensive Care Med 2000;26(9):1304–11.
16. Unroe M, Kahn JM, Carson SS, et al. One-year trajectories of care and resource utilization for recipients of prolonged mechanical ventilation: a cohort study. Ann Intern Med 2010;153(3):167–75.
17. Angus DC, Clermont G, Linde-Zwirble WT, et al. Healthcare costs and long-term outcomes after acute respiratory distress syndrome: a phase III trial of inhaled nitric oxide. Crit Care Med 2006;34(12):2883–90.
18. Bernard GR, Artigas A, Brigham KL, et al. The American-European Consensus Conference on ARDS. Definitions, mechanisms, relevant outcomes, and clinical trial coordination. Am J Respir Crit Care Med 1994;149(3 Pt 1):818–24.
19. Rubenfeld GD, Caldwell E, Peabody E, et al. Incidence and outcomes of acute lung injury. N Engl J Med 2005;353(16):1685–93.
20. Ashbaugh DG, Bigelow DB, Petty TL, et al. Acute respiratory distress in adults. Lancet 1967;2(7511):319–23.

21. Ghio AJ, Elliott CG, Crapo RO, et al. Impairment after adult respiratory distress syndrome. An evaluation based on American Thoracic Society recommendations. Am Rev Respir Dis 1989;139(5):1158–62.
22. Elliott CG, Rasmusson BY, Crapo RO, et al. Prediction of pulmonary function abnormalities after adult respiratory distress syndrome (ARDS). Am Rev Respir Dis 1987;135(3):634–8.
23. Suchyta MR, Elliott CG, Jensen RL, et al. Predicting the presence of pulmonary function impairment in adult respiratory distress syndrome survivors. Respiration 1993;60(2):103–8.
24. Heyland DK, Groll D, Caeser M. Survivors of acute respiratory distress syndrome: relationship between pulmonary dysfunction and long-term health-related quality of life. Crit Care Med 2005;33(7):1549–56.
25. Cooper AB, Ferguson ND, Hanly PJ, et al. Long-term follow-up of survivors of acute lung injury: lack of effect of a ventilation strategy to prevent barotrauma. Crit Care Med 1999;27(12):2616–21.
26. Neff TA, Stocker R, Frey HR, et al. Long-term assessment of lung function in survivors of severe ARDS. Chest 2003;123(3):845–53.
27. Masclans JR, Roca O, Munoz X, et al. Quality of life, pulmonary function and tomographic scan abnormalities after an acute respiratory distress syndrome. Chest 2011;139(6):1340–6.
28. Nobauer-Huhmann IM, Eibenberger K, Schaefer-Prokop C, et al. Changes in lung parenchyma after acute respiratory distress syndrome (ARDS): assessment with high-resolution computed tomography. Eur Radiol 2001;11(12):2436–43.
29. de Jonghe B, Lacherade JC, Sharshar T, et al. Intensive care unit-acquired weakness: risk factors and prevention. Crit Care Med 2009;37(Suppl 10):S309–15.
30. Desai SR, Wells AU, Rubens MB, et al. Acute respiratory distress syndrome: CT abnormalities at long-term follow-up. Radiology 1999;210(1):29–35.
31. Linden VB, Lidegran MK, Frisen G, et al. ECMO in ARDS: a long-term follow-up study regarding pulmonary morphology and function and health-related quality of life. Acta Anaesthesiol Scand 2009;53(4):489–95.
32. Levine S, Nguyen T, Taylor N, et al. Rapid disuse atrophy of diaphragm fibers in mechanically ventilated humans. N Engl J Med 2008;358(13):1327–35.
33. De Jonghe B, Sharshar T, Lefaucheur JP, et al. Paresis acquired in the intensive care unit: a prospective multicenter study. JAMA 2002;288(22):2859–67.
34. Iwashyna TJ, Ely EW, Smith DM, et al. Long-term cognitive impairment and functional disability among survivors of severe sepsis. JAMA 2010;304(16):1787–94.
35. Stevens RD, Marshall SA, Cornblath DR, et al. A framework for diagnosing and classifying intensive care unit-acquired weakness. Crit Care Med 2009;37(Suppl 10):S299–308.
36. Bolton CF, Gilbert JJ, Hahn AF, et al. Polyneuropathy in critically ill patients. J Neurol Neurosurg Psychiatry 1984;47(11):1223–31.
37. de Letter MA, Schmitz PI, Visser LH, et al. Risk factors for the development of polyneuropathy and myopathy in critically ill patients. Crit Care Med 2001;29(12):2281–6.
38. Stevens RD, Dowdy DW, Michaels RK, et al. Neuromuscular dysfunction acquired in critical illness: a systematic review. Intensive Care Med 2007;33(11):1876–91.
39. van den BG, Schoonheydt K, Becx P, et al. Insulin therapy protects the central and peripheral nervous system of intensive care patients. Neurology 2005;64(8):1348–53.
40. Pandit L, Agrawal A. Neuromuscular disorders in critical illness. Clin Neurol Neurosurg 2006;108(7):621–7.

41. Latronico N, Fenzi F, Recupero D, et al. Critical illness myopathy and neuropathy. Lancet 1996;347(9015):1579–82.
42. Angel MJ, Bril V, Shannon P, et al. Neuromuscular function in survivors of the acute respiratory distress syndrome. Can J Neurol Sci 2007;34(4):427–32.
43. Campellone JV, Lacomis D, Kramer DJ, et al. Acute myopathy after liver transplantation. Neurology 1998;50(1):46–53.
44. Helliwell TR, Coakley JH, Wagenmakers AJ, et al. Necrotizing myopathy in critically-ill patients. J Pathol 1991;164(4):307–14.
45. Hudson SJ, Brett SJ. Heterotopic ossification—a long-term consequence of prolonged immobility. Crit Care 2006;10(6):174.
46. Adhikari NK, McAndrews MP, Tansey CM, et al. Self-reported symptoms of depression and memory dysfunction in survivors of ARDS. Chest 2009;135(3): 678–87.
47. Christie JD, Biester RC, Taichman DB, et al. Formation and validation of a telephone battery to assess cognitive function in acute respiratory distress syndrome survivors. J Crit Care 2006;21(2):125–32.
48. Duning T, Ellger B. Is hypoglycaemia dangerous? Best Pract Res Clin Anaesthesiol 2009;23(4):473–85.
49. Jones C, Griffiths RD, Slater T, et al. Significant cognitive dysfunction in non-delirious patients identified during and persisting following critical illness. Intensive Care Med 2006;32(6):923–6.
50. Sukantarat KT, Burgess PW, Williamson RC, et al. Prolonged cognitive dysfunction in survivors of critical illness. Anaesthesia 2005;60(9):847–53.
51. van der SM, Dettling DS, Beelen A, et al. Poor functional status immediately after discharge from an intensive care unit. Disabil Rehabil 2008;30(23):1812–8.
52. Hopkins RO, Jackson JC, Wallace CJ. Neurocognitive impairments in ICU patients with prolonged mechanical ventilation [abstract]. Presented at the International Neuropsychological Society 33rd Annual Meeting; 2005.
53. Jackson JC, Gordon SM, Burger C, et al. Acute respiratory distress syndrome and long-term cognitive impairment: a case study [abstract]. Arch Clin Neuropsychol 2003;18(7):688.
54. Al Saidi F, McAndrews MP, Cheung AM, et al. Neuropsychological sequelae in ARDS survivors [abstract]. Am J Respir Crit Care Med 2003;167(7):A737.
55. Suchyta MR, Hopkins RO. The incidence of cognitive dysfunction after ARDS [abstract]. Am J Respir Crit Care Med 2004;169(7):A18.
56. Ehlenbach WJ, Hough CL, Crane PK, et al. Association between acute care and critical illness hospitalization and cognitive function in older adults. JAMA 2010; 303(8):763–70.
57. Davydow DS, Desai SV, Needham DM, et al. Psychiatric morbidity in survivors of the acute respiratory distress syndrome: a systematic review. Psychosom Med 2008;70(4):512–9.
58. Hopkins RO, Key CW, Suchyta MR, et al. Risk factors for depression and anxiety in survivors of acute respiratory distress syndrome. Gen Hosp Psychiatry 2010; 32(2):147–55.
59. Dowdy DW, Bienvenu OJ, Dinglas VD, et al. Are intensive care factors associated with depressive symptoms 6 months after acute lung injury? Crit Care Med 2009;37(5):1702–7.
60. Katon W, Sullivan MD. Depression and chronic medical illness. J Clin Psychiatry 1990;51(Suppl):3–11.
61. Silverstone PH. Prevalence of psychiatric disorders in medical inpatients. J Nerv Ment Dis 1996;184(1):43–51.

62. Davydow DS, Gifford JM, Desai SV, et al. Depression in general intensive care unit survivors: a systematic review. Intensive Care Med 2009;35(5):796–809.
63. Horowitz M, Wilner N, Alvarez W. Impact of Event Scale: a measure of subjective stress. Psychosom Med 1979;41(3):209–18.
64. Schelling G, Stoll C, Haller M, et al. Health-related quality of life and posttraumatic stress disorder in survivors of the acute respiratory distress syndrome. Crit Care Med 1998;26(4):651–9.
65. Davydow DS, Gifford JM, Desai SV, et al. Posttraumatic stress disorder in general intensive care unit survivors: a systematic review. Gen Hosp Psychiatry 2008;30(5):421–34.
66. Cox CE, Docherty SL, Brandon DH, et al. Surviving critical illness: acute respiratory distress syndrome as experienced by patients and their caregivers. Crit Care Med 2009;37(10):2702–8.
67. McCartney JR, Boland RJ. Anxiety and delirium in the intensive care unit. Crit Care Clin 1994;10(4):673–80.
68. Skodol AE. Anxiety in the medically ill: nosology and principles of differential diagnosis. Semin Clin Neuropsychiatry 1999;4(2):64–71.
69. Szokol JW, Vender JS. Anxiety, delirium, and pain in the intensive care unit. Crit Care Clin 2001;17(4):821–42.
70. Kiekkas P, Theodorakopoulou G, Spyratos F, et al. Psychological distress and delusional memories after critical care: a literature review. Int Nurs Rev 2010;57(3):288–96.
71. Myhren H, Ekeberg O, Toien K, et al. Posttraumatic stress, anxiety and depression symptoms in patients during the first year post intensive care unit discharge. Crit Care 2010;14(1):R14.
72. Bienvenu OJ, Neufeld KJ. Post-traumatic stress disorder in medical settings: focus on the critically ill. Curr Psychiatry Rep 2011;13(1):3–9.
73. Jones C, Backman C, Capuzzo M, et al. Intensive care diaries reduce new onset post traumatic stress disorder following critical illness: a randomised, controlled trial. Crit Care 2010;14(5):R168.
74. Ware JE Jr, Kosinski M. SF-36 physical and mental health summary scores: a manual for users of version 1. 2nd edition. Quality Metrics Incorporated; 2005.
75. Dowdy DW, Eid MP, Sedrakyan A, et al. Quality of life in adult survivors of critical illness: a systematic review of the literature. Intensive Care Med 2005;31(5):611–20.
76. Needham DM, Dennison CR, Dowdy DW, et al. Study protocol: the improving care of acute lung injury patients (ICAP) study. Crit Care 2006;10:R9.
77. Valta P, Uusaro A, Nunes S, et al. Acute respiratory distress syndrome: frequency, clinical course, and costs of care. Crit Care Med 1999;27(11):2367–74.
78. Hamel MB, Phillips RS, Davis RB, et al. Outcomes and cost-effectiveness of ventilator support and aggressive care for patients with acute respiratory failure due to pneumonia or acute respiratory distress syndrome. Am J Med 2000;109(8):614–20.
79. Chelluri L, Im KA, Belle SH, et al. Long-term mortality and quality of life after prolonged mechanical ventilation. Crit Care Med 2004;32(1):61–9.
80. Cameron JI, Herridge MS, Tansey CM, et al. Well-being in informal caregivers of survivors of acute respiratory distress syndrome. Crit Care Med 2006;34(1):81–6.
81. Azoulay E, Pochard F, Kentish-Barnes N, et al. Risk of post-traumatic stress symptoms in family members of intensive care unit patients. Am J Respir Crit Care Med 2005;171(9):987–94.

82. Im K, Belle SH, Schulz R, et al. Prevalence and outcomes of caregiving after prolonged (> or = 48 hours) mechanical ventilation in the ICU. Chest 2004; 125(2):597–606.
83. Jones C, Skirrow P, Griffiths RD, et al. Post-traumatic stress disorder-related symptoms in relatives of patients following intensive care. Intensive Care Med 2004;30(3):456–60.
84. Van P, Milbrandt EB, Qin L, et al. Informal caregiver burden among survivors of prolonged mechanical ventilation. Am J Respir Crit Care Med 2007;175(2): 167–73.
85. Foster M, Chaboyer W. Family carers of ICU survivors: a survey of the burden they experience. Scand J Caring Sci 2003;17(3):205–14.
86. Douglas SL, Daly BJ, Kelley CG, et al. Impact of a disease management program upon caregivers of chronically critically ill patients. Chest 2005; 128(6):3925–36.
87. Pochard F, Darmon M, Fassier T, et al. Symptoms of anxiety and depression in family members of intensive care unit patients before discharge or death. A prospective multicenter study. J Crit Care 2005;20(1):90–6.
88. Johnson P, Chaboyer W, Foster M, et al. Caregivers of ICU patients discharged home: what burden do they face? Intensive Crit Care Nurs 2001;17(4):219–27.
89. Needham DM. Mobilizing patients in the intensive care unit: improving neuromuscular weakness and physical function. JAMA 2008;300(14):1685–90.
90. Bailey P, Thomsen GE, Spuhler VJ, et al. Early activity is feasible and safe in respiratory failure patients. Crit Care Med 2007;35(1):139–45.
91. Morris PE, Goad A, Thompson C, et al. Early intensive care unit mobility therapy in the treatment of acute respiratory failure. Crit Care Med 2008;36(8):2238–43.
92. Hopkins RO, Spuhler VJ, Thomsen GE. Transforming ICU culture to facilitate early mobility. Crit Care Clin 2007;23(1):81–96.
93. Schweickert WD, Pohlman MC, Pohlman AS, et al. Early physical and occupational therapy in mechanically ventilated, critically ill patients: a randomised controlled trial. Lancet 2009;373(9678):1874–82.
94. Burtin C, Clerckx B, Robbeets C, et al. Early exercise in critically ill patients enhances short-term functional recovery. Crit Care Med 2009;37(9):2499–505.
95. Rubenfeld GD. Post-hospital case management to improve clinical outcomes in individuals requiring mechanical ventilation. 2009. Available at: http://clinicaltrials.gov/ct2/show/NCT00149513. Accessed March 1, 2001.
96. Daly BJ, Douglas SL, Kelley CG, et al. Trial of a disease management program to reduce hospital readmissions of the chronically critically ill. Chest 2005; 128(2):507–17.
97. Gosselink R, Bott J, Johnson M, et al. Physiotherapy for adult patients with critical illness: recommendations of the European Respiratory Society and European Society of Intensive Care Medicine Task Force on Physiotherapy for Critically Ill Patients. Intensive Care Med 2008;34(7):1188–99.
98. Tan T, Brett SJ, Stokes T. Rehabilitation after critical illness: summary of NICE guidance. BMJ 2009;338:b822.
99. Cuthbertson BH, Rattray J, Campbell MK, et al. The PRaCTICaL study of nurse led, intensive care follow-up programmes for improving long term outcomes from critical illness: a pragmatic randomised controlled trial. BMJ 2009;339: b3723.
100. Jones C, Skirrow P, Griffiths RD, et al. Rehabilitation after critical illness: a randomized, controlled trial. Crit Care Med 2003;31(10):2456–61.

Gene Therapy for ALI/ARDS

Xin Lin, PhD[a], David A. Dean, PhD[b,*]

KEYWORDS

- Gene therapy • Acute lung injury • Viral vectors
- Nonviral vectors

Acute lung injury (ALI) and acute respiratory distress syndrome (ARDS) are life-threatening conditions of acute respiratory failure, which is induced by direct and indirect injury to the lung, such as by pneumonia, sepsis, or trauma. ALI/ARDS has a mortality rate of up to 40% in the United States, leading to 74,500 deaths and 3.6 million hospital days every year.[1] Although many potential therapeutic approaches have been developed to control ALI/ARDS, these treatments have so far proven unable to decrease the mortality of patients with ALI/ARDS. Although laboratories around the world have focused on the disease and uncovered a number of molecular mechanisms involved in its pathogenesis and resolution, translating this into productive treatments has lagged.

Gene therapy is a potentially powerful approach to treat any number of diseases, including ALI/ARDS, but most approaches have serious limitations and thus have hampered the use of this technology in clinical medicine. Gene delivery approaches are based on 2 types of delivery vehicles: those based on viral systems, so-called viral vectors, and those not based on viruses, or nonviral vectors, which are typically plasmid-based. Viral vector systems have been associated with inflammation, immunologic responses, and nonspecificity of cell targeting, despite very high delivery efficiency in the lung. For example, adenovirus appears to be the most widely used vector for pulmonary gene: therapy in the laboratory because of high-efficiency transduction in a variety of target cells and high expression of the delivered genes. However, the use of adenovirus can result in inflammatory responses, which cause cell damage and limit repeated administration. By contrast, much less inflammation and fewer immune responses are generated against nonviral DNA, but the major drawbacks to nonviral gene therapy in the lung are side effects of certain vectors and inefficiency

This project was supported by NIH grants HL81148, HL92801, EB9903, and GM94228.

[a] Department of Pediatrics, School of Medicine and Dentistry, University of Rochester, Rochester, NY, USA

[b] Department of Pediatrics, School of Medicine and Dentistry, University of Rochester, Box 850, 601 Elmwood Avenue, Rochester, NY 14642, USA

* Corresponding author.

E-mail address: david_dean@urmc.rochester.edu

Crit Care Clin 27 (2011) 705–718
doi:10.1016/j.ccc.2011.04.002 criticalcare.theclinics.com
0749-0704/11/$ – see front matter

of gene transfer, often leading to expression that is 10-fold to 1000-fold less than that seen with their viral counterparts.

Although transfer and expression of therapeutic genes to the lung using both viral and nonviral gene therapy technologies have been performed with some success, there is still a long way to go to move this methodology toward clinical use. In this article, we provide an overview of the current status of viral and nonviral gene therapy for ALI/ARDS, focus on issues of mechanism and applications as they influence in vivo gene delivery, and extend the utility of this strategy for future medical treatments.

GENE DELIVERY TO THE LUNG

The lung is a complex organ and can be divided into the conducting large and small airways, including the trachea, bronchi, and bronchioles, and the parenchyma, which consists of gas-exchanging alveolar cells. Gene therapy is notably attractive for many acute and chronic pulmonary diseases. However, with the presence of barriers to lung gene transfer, such as pulmonary architecture, the innate immune system, and immune activation, it is somewhat more difficult and less effective to deliver genes into the parenchyma. As a consequence, many investigations have focused on improving gene transfer to the airway and alveolar epithelium to make it more efficient, less inflammatory, and to have extended duration of expression.[2] To date, a number of viral and nonviral vector systems have been used to deliver transgenes into the lung to treat diverse pulmonary diseases.[3]

Viral Vectors for Gene Delivery to the Lung

Adenovirus, perhaps the most widely used of vectors for lung gene therapy, is a double-stranded DNA virus that is made to be replication-deficient for gene therapy by deletion of essential genes. The major advantages of adenovirus are the high-efficiency transduction seen in dividing and nondividing cells and the very high expression of delivered genes. However, inflammation, immunologic responses, and nonspecificity of cell targeting are just a few of the problems associated with adenovirus vectors. Furthermore, immune responses developed against the viral vector limit the success of repeated administration (thus it can be used only once or twice in an individual for effective gene delivery).[4] Adenovirus can directly deliver genes to the airway and alveolar epithelia and have been the vector of choice for animal models of many pulmonary diseases in the laboratory, but in clinical trials, the vector results in acute inflammation and innate immune responses, limiting effectiveness.[5,6] Further, the receptors for adenovirus reside primarily on the basolateral surface of epithelial cells in the lower airways, making high-level gene transfer dependent on transient barrier dysfunction, which is not desirable in many disease states.[7] Much effort has been directed at making vectors that show reduced host immune reactions to the viral gene products, so “gutless” or “helper-dependent” third-generation adenovirus vectors have been developed to extend expression and limit the initial inflammatory responses to administration.[8] However, the safety issues surrounding this vector may outweigh its superior ability to transfer genes for widespread clinical use.

Another popular viral vector is based on adeno-associated virus (AAV), a nonpathogenic single-stranded DNA virus of the *Dependovirus* genus, which requires a helper virus (typically adenovirus) to complete its lytic life cycle.[9] AAV is attractive because it has shown broad specificity of infection and persistent expression in the lung. The vector appears less inflammatory and elicits weaker immune responses than does adenovirus.[10] Furthermore, Moss and colleagues[11] have demonstrated successful and safe repeated gene transfer of aerosolized AAV to the lungs of humans with cystic fibrosis. However, this vector has been significantly limited for lung gene transfer because of the small cloning capacity of the virus, the difficulty in getting high viral titers during production, and the relatively low efficiency in human trials.

Retroviruses provide prolonged gene expression owing to integration of the virus into the host genome, but require dividing cells for integration and show no transduction in the terminally differentiated, nondividing epithelium.[12] By contrast, lentiviruses, a subclass of retroviruses that are based on HIV (human immunodeficiency virus) and pseudotyped with the vesicular stomatitis virus (VSV) glycoprotein, can efficiently transfer genes to nondividing cells and thus have been developed as gene transfer vectors.[13] But again, similar to adenovirus, these vectors when pseudotyped with VSV glycoprotein demonstrate inefficient gene transfer to cells owing to their receptor being expressed on the basolateral surface of the epithelium in vivo.[14] However, Kobinger and colleagues[15] have shown that efficient transduction of the apical surface of the epithelium can be achieved in the mouse lung using an envelope protein derived from the Zaire strain of Ebola virus to pseudotype lentivirus vectors. In either case of retroviruses or lentiviruses, the necessity for integration to achieve effective levels of gene expression in vivo may also result in activation of oncogenes depending on the site of random integration.

Nonviral Vectors for Gene Delivery to the Lung

To combat inflammatory and immune responses mediated by viral vectors, nonviral vectors are an attractive alternative for gene therapy because of their ability to be repeatedly administered and their generally good safety profile.[16] The primary nonviral vector systems constitute plasmids complexed with cationic lipids as lipoplexes or with polymers, such as diethylaminoethyl-dextran (DEAE-dextran) and polyethylenimine (PEI) to form polyplexes protecting naked DNA from degradation.[17] Lipoplexes have proven to be an attractive tool for gene transfer into cells with respect to simplicity of use, ease of production, and low immunogenicity since their initial development by Felgner and colleagues in 1987.[18,19] However, the results from clinical trials have shown that lipoplexes do indeed generate inflammatory responses, albeit much less than do their viral counterparts, when they are used for gene therapy approaches in the lung.[20,21] This, taken together with their low efficiency for in vivo gene delivery in the lung, has limited their clinical potential. Similarly, the use of DEAE-dextran for gene delivery to the lung has largely been abandoned owing to low levels of gene transfer, cellular toxicity, and lack of biodegradability.[22] PEI has shown some promise to enhance levels of gene transfer. In the presence of PEI, plasmid DNA condenses to form a DNA-PEI complex, which can protect DNA from degradation by serum nucleases during gene transfer to the lung in vivo. Once endocytosed into the cell, PEI induces osmotic swelling to promote endosomal escape and releases DNA into the cytoplasm, so it achieves greater levels of gene transfer to the lung. Unfortunately, PEI has been shown to interfere with transcriptional and translational processes and show mild to moderate toxicity (primarily owing to low molecular weight PEI contaminants) and innate immune responses.[23,24] More recent, and as yet not completely vetted, systems include the use of glycoconjugates, targeting serpin-enzyme complex receptors, and nanoparticle formulations.[25] Some groups have even combined viral vectors with liposomes containing dexamethasone-spermine (DS)/dioleoylphosphatidylethanolamine (DOPE) to improve targeting to the apical airway epithelium in vivo and to attenuate vector-induced inflammation.[26]

The simplest nonviral vectors are naked plasmid DNA in which the specific sequences can uniquely manipulate transgene expression.[27] It is an attractive approach for gene transfer to the lung owing to reduced inflammatory and immune responses compared with liposome or polymer complexes.[28] However, unprotected DNA is susceptible to nuclease degradation and thus it needs to rapidly cross the plasma membrane of target cells in lung tissue.[17] Therefore, the efficiency of gene expression is restricted by the quantity of naked DNA that reaches its target cells. Recent research from our laboratory and others has demonstrated that electroporation can be used to efficiently deliver DNA to various tissues, including the lung, with high-level gene expression and without damage.[29–32] The method is simple, fast, and safe: naked DNA is administered to the lungs of anesthetized animals and a series of 8 consecutive, 10-millisecond square-wave electric pulses is applied to the lungs using electrodes placed on either side of the chest over a 10-second period (**Fig. 1**). The application of electric pulses to the lung transiently opens pores in the cell membrane that allows plasmid DNA to enter the cell.[29] Electroporation leads to safe,

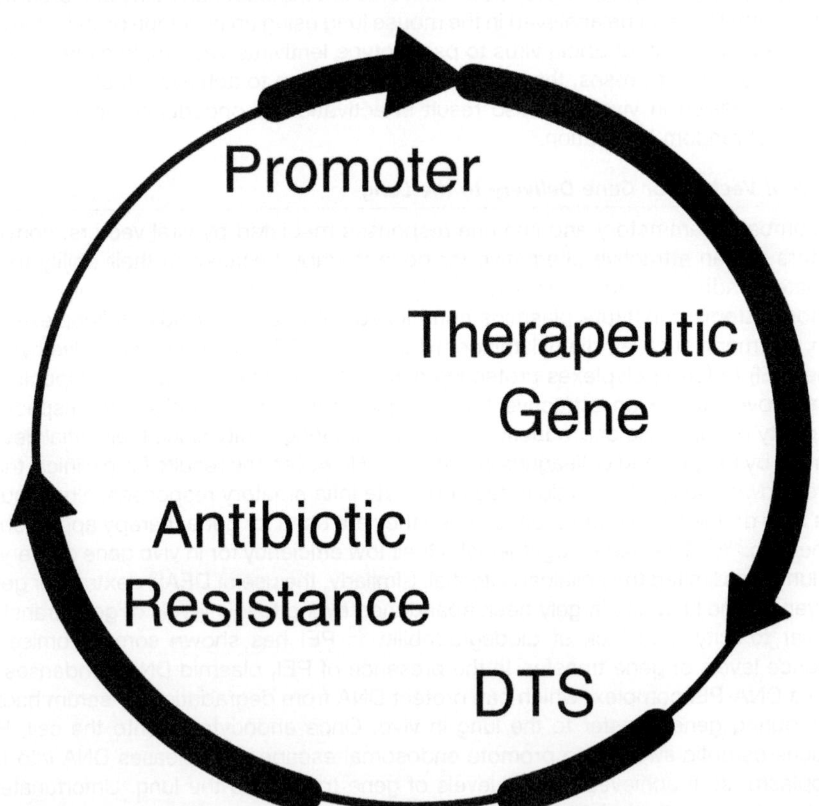

Fig. 1. Common elements of a gene therapy plasmid. A typical plasmid is depicted showing control elements and expressed genes. Promoters that express for a short period of time (eg, the CMViep), a long period of time (eg, the UbC promoter), or in specific cell types (eg, the SP-C promoter for expression in AT2 cells or the CC10 promoter for expression in clara cells) are used to drive expression of the gene of interest. In almost all cases, cDNA for the gene to be expressed is used instead of genomic sequence, thus eliminating all introns to make the gene smaller in size and allow for more efficient expression that does not require mRNA splicing and maturation. A DTS can be included downstream of the transgene to aid in general or cell-specific DNA nuclear import, and an antibiotic resistance gene is carried on the plasmid for maintenance and production of the plasmids in bacteria.

efficient, and reproducible transgene expression in the lung.[28] Besides electroporation, effort has also been made to develop several other physical methods for nonviral gene delivery, including jet injection, the gene gun, hydrodynamic delivery, and sonoporation.[33–36] As yet, their use in the lung has been limited.

Although many investigators have demonstrated that DNA can be directly delivered to the lung to express genes for short periods, an effective delivery system should be able to express a transferred gene for long-term periods at therapeutic levels and with specificity of cell targeting if desired. To date, we and others have used electroporation to noninvasively deliver plasmid DNA into the lung parenchyma and have shown either short-term (1 to 7 days using the cytomegalovirus [CMV] immediate early promoter/enhancer) or long-term (<30 days using the ubiquitin [UbC] promoter) transgene expression.[31,37,38] Thus, by choosing the appropriate promoters, the duration of expression can be well controlled (**Fig. 2**). As for controlling the distribution of gene expression, electroporation is unlike all other gene-delivery approaches in that delivery is not restricted to the surface layer of cells with which the vector comes into contact. Rather, it has the ability to transfer the nonviral vector across the epithelial barrier and into subepithelial cells below, reaching interstitial fibroblasts, airway and vascular smooth muscle cells, and even endothelial cells following DNA administration via the airways.[31] Despite the ability to transfer genes to all cell types within

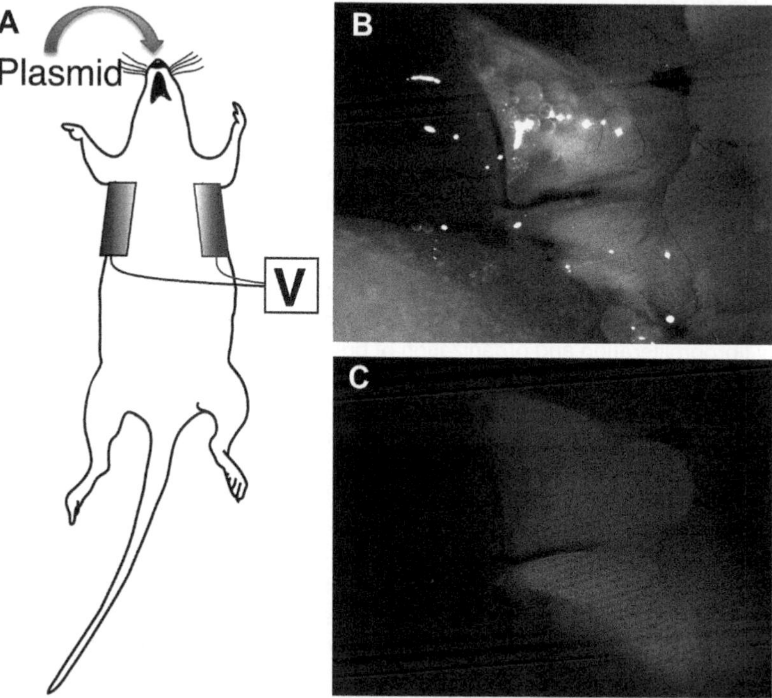

Fig. 2. In vivo pulmonary electroporation. (*A*) In vivo plasmid delivery and electroporation for the lungs showing endotracheal tube and electrodes. (*B, C*) GFP-β1 expressing plasmids (600 μg) were administered to the lungs and electroporated (200 V/cm, 8 pulses at 10 μsec each). Three days later, the lungs were visualized in situ (*B*) and GFP-β1 expression was detected by fluorescence microscopy (*C*). (*Adapted from* Machado-Aranda D, Adir Y, Young JL, et al. Gene transfer of the Na^+,K^+-ATPase beta1 subunit using electroporation increases lung liquid clearance. Am J Respir Crit Care Med 2005;171:204–11; with permission.)

a tissue, it is often very desirable, especially in the lung, to limit gene delivery and expression to specific cell targets. We have used 2 approaches to restrict delivery and expression to specific cell types in the lung: use of cell-specific promoters to drive expression only in desired cells (ie, the smooth muscle gamma actin promoter for expression in smooth muscle cells) and the use of cell-specific DNA nuclear targeting sequences to limit delivery of plasmids to the nuclei of desired cell types. A number of years ago, our laboratory demonstrated that plasmids can gain entry into the nuclei of nondividing cells only if they carry unique DNA sequences termed DNA nuclear targeting sequences (DTS).[39–41] These sequences interact with cytoplasmically localized transcription factors and the protein nuclear import machinery to traffic the plasmid-protein complex into the nucleus through the nuclear pore complex. Several such sequences that act in all cell types have been identified. Further, a number of sequences that act in specific cell types, because they bind cell-specific transcription factors that are expressed only in those cells, have also been identified. For example, we have demonstrated that a sequence within the human surfactant protein C (SP-C) promoter is able to mediate nuclear localization of plasmid DNA specifically in type II alveolar epithelial (AT2) cells but not in other cell types both in cultured cells and in the mouse lung.[42] More recently, we have identified additional DTS that restrict plasmid delivery to multiple cell types in the lung, including smooth muscle cells,[43–45] endothelial cells,[46] and type I alveolar epithelial cells, all potential targets for gene therapy for ALI/ARDS and other lung diseases.

GENE THERAPY FOR ALI/ARDS

ALI and ARDS are clinically characterized by acute hypoxemic respiratory failure, caused by direct injury, including viral or bacterial infections, gastric aspiration, trauma, and hyperoxia, and indirect injury to the lung, such as in sepsis. ALI/ARDS is subdivided into the acute exudative phase and the later fibroproliferative phase.[47] The exudative phase of ALI/ARDS is initially characterized by disruption of the alveolar-capillary interface and leakage of protein-rich edema fluid into the interstitium and alveolar space, followed by extensive release of multiple inflammatory cytokines and chemokines and neutrophil infiltration. The later phase of ALI/ARDS is characterized by fibroproliferation and organization of previously deposited exudates. Over the past 20 years, the feasibility of using gene transfer to treat ALI/ARDS has been demonstrated using a variety of viral and nonviral vectors to deliver various transgenes to the lung in multiple animal models, although none have moved to clinical trials.

Gene Therapy for Improved Alveolar Fluid Clearance

ALI/ARDS is characterized by abnormal accumulation of protein-rich edema fluid in the alveolar spaces, caused by increased movement of fluid from the capillaries to the lung interstitium, and decreased fluid transport out of alveolar air spaces.[48] Injury to the alveolar epithelium plays an important role in the pathogenesis of increased alveolar fluid because 99% of the surface area of lung is composed of the alveolar epithelium, which is the major site for the removal of excess alveolar fluid.[49] Therefore, treatments to improve alveolar epithelial function might become one of the key therapeutic strategies to accelerate recovery and decrease the mortality of patients with ALI/ARDS.

The alveolar epithelial monolayer consists of flat type I alveolar epithelial (AT1) cells, which comprise approximately 90% of the alveolar surface area, and cuboidal type II alveolar epithelial (AT2) cells, which produce surfactant proteins, vectorially transport ions, and act as progenitor cells to regenerate the epithelium after injury. The presence of multiple ion transporters, including the epithelial Na^+ channel (ENaC), the Na^+, K^+

transporting adenosine-5′-triphosphatase (Na^+, K^+-ATPase), the cystic fibrosis transmembrane conductance regulator (CFTR), and several K^+ channels in both AT1 and AT2 cells, creates a transepithelial osmotic gradient formed by the active movement of Na^+, which is needed for the transit of edema fluid from the alveolar airspace. It is well accepted that alveolar fluid clearance is driven by sodium transport entering the alveolar epithelial cell via ENaC on the apical surface and then being pumped out by the Na^+, K^+-ATPase within the basolateral surface into the interstitium and the pulmonary circulation.[50] Studies have demonstrated that overexpression of genes such as ENaC and Na^+, K^+-ATPase regulated by β-adrenergic receptor or cAMP can enhance alveolar active transport to clear pulmonary edema.[37,51–53] For gene transfer to be useful, it is necessary to transduce the alveolar epithelium. Both viral and nonviral approaches for the overexpression of Na^+, K^+-ATPase and CFTR channels in the lung as well as the delivery of keratinocyte growth factor and hemoxygenase-1 to the lung have been tested with the aim of increasing alveolar fluid clearance. Gene therapy may prove to be an important alternative for the treatment and prevention of pulmonary edema by restoring alveolar epithelial function.

It has been demonstrated previously that transfer of the α2-subunit or β1-subunit of Na^+, K^+-ATPase using recombinant adenoviruses can increase Na^+, K^+-ATPase expression and alveolar fluid clearance function in normal rat lungs and in rat lungs injured by ventilation.[54–57] Factor and colleagues[58] showed that adenovirus-mediated gene transfer of the Na^+, K^+-ATPase β1-subunit to the alveolar epithelium improved alveolar fluid clearance in rat models of ALI induced by ventilation, acutely elevated left atrial pressure,[59] and hyperoxia.[55] Similarly, Qiao and colleagues[60] demonstrated that lentivirus-mediated gene transfer of the β1, not α1, subunit of the Na^+, K^+-ATPase to rat primary alveolar epithelial cells can augment the activity of the Na^+, K^+-ATPase, indicating augmentation of alveolar fluid clearance. Adenoviruses were able to transfer genes to the pulmonary epithelium after hyperoxia-mediated acute lung injury as efficiently as they could in healthy rat lungs, a prerequisite for any potential treatment option that would have to be given to patients with preexisting disease.[61] In addition, adenovirus-mediated transfer of the β2-adrenergic receptor gene to rat lungs enhanced their sensitivity to catecholamines and resulted in increases in both ENaC and Na^+, K^+-ATPase expression, leading to increased alveolar fluid clearance.[52,62,63] Transfer of CFTR gene by adenovirus to the alveolar epithelium of normal rats and mice accelerated alveolar fluid clearance owing to increased expression and function of components of the active Na^+ transport machinery as well.[64] Taking a different approach to alter endogenous expression of ion channels, another group showed that adenoviral overexpression of superoxide dismutase could prevent the hypoxia-mediated decrease in alveolar fluid reabsorption attributable to decreased Na^+, K^+-ATPase levels at the membrane (as hypoxia normally inhibits Na^+, K^+-ATPase activity, preventing production of reactive oxygen species and accumulation by gene transfer of superoxide dismutase abrogated the effects of hypoxia).[65]

However, a drawback to all these in vivo viral vector studies is that the effects of gene transfer on protection from injury (none tested whether gene therapy could be used to treat existing ALI/ARDS) could only be measured experimentally 7 days after gene delivery because of the induction of inflammatory responses by the viral vector. In other words, use of these viral vectors caused profound inflammatory responses in healthy animals; using similar vectors to treat what is largely an inflammatory disease could trip the balance to endanger animals or patients with preexisting disease. As such, the use of viral vectors for ALI/ARDS may not be the most promising approach, and the much less inflammatory nonviral approaches may be better suited for this disease.

By contrast, the liposome-DNA complexes were primarily thought to induce weaker immunologic responses than viral vectors. Indeed, Eric Alton's group showed that liposome-mediated gene transfer of α-subunits and β-subunits of the Na^+, K^+-ATPase can protect from subsequent thiourea-induced pulmonary edema in mice caused by increased Na^+, K^+-ATPase activity.[66] In this study, very little inflammation was noted following delivery of the plasmid-liposome complexes. Another approach to upregulate edema clearance has been to use growth factors. Keratinocyte growth factor (KGF) is a growth factor that has been shown to be an AT2 mitogen and can increase active ion transport in the lung through transcriptional upregulation of the Na^+, K^+-ATPase. Work from Alton's group has shown that gene transfer of KGF using liposomes into mouse lungs protected animals from oleic acid–induced lung injury, albeit much less than administration of recombinant protein itself, suggesting that the efficacy of gene delivery is still not optimal.[67] In support of this, the use of adenovirus to transfer KGF resulted in greater levels of KGF expression, significant proliferation of AT2 cells, and greater protection in a hyperoxia model of ALI.[68] Research from our laboratory and others has demonstrated that electroporation can be used to effectively deliver "naked" DNA to living animal lungs with no damage and high-level gene expression.[29,31,45,69,70] Indeed, after electroporation-mediated transfer of β1-subunit of Na^+, K^+-ATPase to the lungs of healthy rats, alveolar fluid clearance rates can be increased almost twofold, similar to using adenovirus expressing the same gene.[37] More recently, we have also shown that transfer of genes encoding the α-subunit and/or β-subunit of the Na^+, K^+-ATPase using electroporation not only protects from subsequent endotoxin-induced lung injury in mice, but also can be used to treat previously injured lungs with existing pulmonary edema and neutrophil infiltrates by upregulating mechanisms of pulmonary edema clearance (**Fig. 3**).[51] Not only were rates of alveolar fluid clearance increased in lipopolysaccharide (LPS)-treated mice at the height of injury when plasmids expressing the Na^+, K^+-ATPase subunit genes were delivered by electroporation, but the number of infiltrating neutrophils and alveolar macrophages were decreased in these treated animals and the lungs appeared less injured by histology (**Fig. 4**).[51]

Gene Therapy Targeted at Sepsis and Pulmonary Inflammation

The development of ALI results from both direct insults to the lung such as pneumonia, aspiration, or lung contusion, as well as from indirect pulmonary insults such as extrapulmonary sepsis, trauma, and shock. Consequently, indirect treatment of ALI could be achieved by gene therapy approaches to limit or prevent these insults. Pneumonia is common, resulting from a variety of causes, including infection with bacteria, virus, and fungi and can contribute to the morbidity and mortality associated with ALI/ARDS. Multiple cytokines and chemokines are released during infections resulting in acute respiratory syndromes, such as hemophagocytic syndrome and lymphoid depletion. It is possible that these elevated levels of cytokines and chemokines are associated with increased severity of pneumonia and subsequent ALI. Gene therapy may be a powerful method to deliver cytokines and chemokines to the lung to modulate the inflammatory environment to treat pneumonia and the ensuing ALI.

A number of groups have used gene delivery to overexpress various cytokines and chemokines in the lung to directly attenuate inflammation caused by infection. These include the anti-inflammatory cytokines interleukin (IL)-10,[71] interferon protein-10 (IP-10),[72] IL-12,[73] and transforming growth factor beta-1 (TGF-β1).[74] Despite being transferred with adenoviral vectors that can exacerbate the inflammatory response, delivery of all of these anti-inflammatory cytokines has improved survival in mice and reduced inflammation, as predicted. Several other less obvious approaches

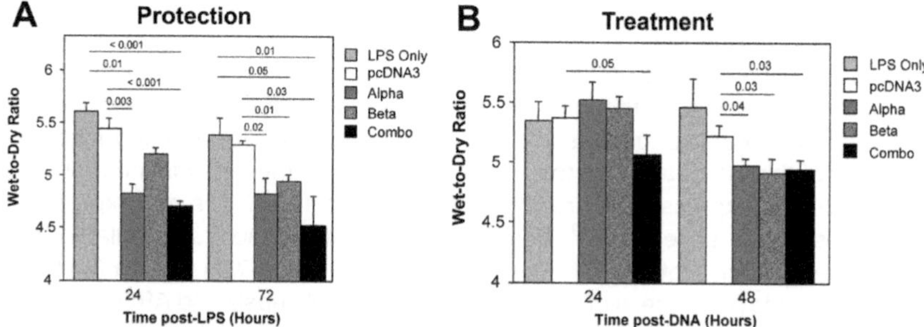

Fig. 3. Electroporation-mediated gene transfer of subunits of the Na^{+}, K^{+}-ATPase can both protect from subsequent LPS-induced lung injury and reverse preexisting LPS-induced lung injury. (*A*) Protection studies. One hundred µg of plasmid in 50 µL was administered intratracheally to mice by electroporation. One day later, LPS (4 mg/kg) was administered to the lungs and 24 or 27 hours after this, lungs were removed for wet-to-dry ratio analysis (mean ± sem; n = 5). (*B*) Treatment studies. LPS (4 mg/kg) was administered intratracheally to Balb/c mice, and 1 day later 100 µg of plasmid was delivered to the lungs by electroporation. Twenty-four or 48 hours later, lungs were removed for gravimetric analysis. Wet-to-dry ratios are shown as mean ± SEM (n = 5). Statistical analysis was by nonparametric Mann-Whitney *U* test. (*Adapted from* Mutlu GM, Machado-Aranda D, Norton JE, et al. Electroporation mediated gene transfer of the Na^{+}, K^{+}-ATPase rescues endotoxin-induced lung injury. Am J Respir Crit Care Med 2007;176:582–90; with permission.)

have also been taken to limit inflammation or control immune responses in the lung in response to infection. For example, one group used 4-1BB ligand (4-1BBL) to protect from lung injury caused by influenza infection in the lung.[75] The 4-1BBL binds to 4-1BB (CD137), a member of the tumor necrosis factor receptor family expressed on activated T cells that is rapidly upregulated on T cells following viral infection. Binding and signaling of 4-1BBL leads to increased T-cell expansion, and T-cell trafficking to and retention in the lungs. Gene transfer of 4-1BBL in a mouse influenza infection model showed greater control of the infection and reduced lung injury. Another approach has been to use hemoxygenase-1 (HO-1) to modulate neutrophil activity. Although the main function of HO-1 is to regulate heme metabolism, evidence

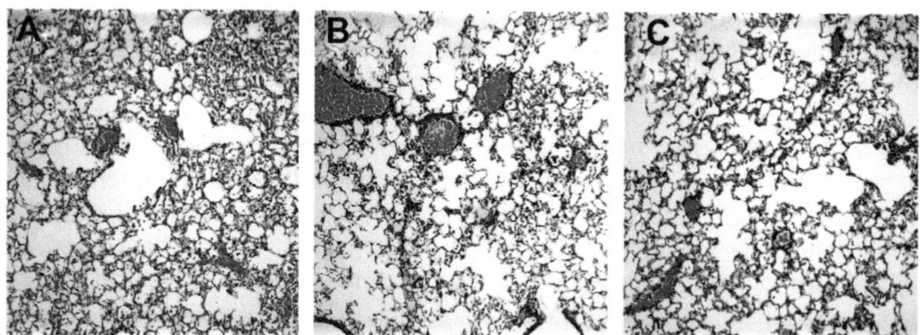

Fig. 4. Electroporation-mediated gene transfer of the Na^{+}, K^{+}-ATPase shows reduced pulmonary infiltrates in LPS-injured lungs. LPS (4 mg/kg) was administered intratracheally to Balb/c mice, and 1 day later 100 µg of plasmid was delivered to the lungs by electroporation. Forty-eight hours later, lungs were removed and processed for histology using hematoxylin and eosin staining. (*A*) LPS only. (*B*) LPS followed by pCMV-β1. (*C*) LPS followed by a mixture of pCMV-α1 and pCMV-β1 (50 µg of each). Magnification 100×.

suggests that the enzyme is also involved in controlling infiltration of neutrophils into the injured lung and in the resolution of inflammation by modulating apoptotic cell death and cytokine expression. Consequently, several groups have delivered HO-1 expressing adenoviruses to the lungs in both pneumonia and hyperoxia models and have shown significant reductions in inflammation and subsequent lung injury.[76–78] At least part of this effect appears to be mediated through the anti-inflammatory cytokine IL-10, whose expression is greatly upregulated when HO-1 is overexpressed.[78] Finally, Weiss and colleagues[79] demonstrated that adenovirus-mediated gene delivery of heat shock protein-70 to the pulmonary epithelium can protect from cecal ligation and double puncture, a clinically relevant model of sepsis and ARDS-mediated lung injury in mice.

As alluded to previously, although a number of studies indicate that viral vectors are promising candidates for gene therapy to control these direct or indirect pulmonary infections, inflammation can actually be accelerated by the viral vector systems carrying the desired transgenes. Therefore, major efforts have been directed toward developing nonviral vectors for these purposes. For example, the β-defensin-2 delivered to rat lungs by polyethylenimine can effectively inhibit *Pseudomonas aeruginosa* infection in the lung.[80] However, certain nonviral lipid or polymer formulations can also induce varying levels of inflammatory cytokines, and their efficiency of gene transfer remains low. Recently, electroporation has gained increasing attention for development of nonviral gene therapies and vaccines. Using skeletal muscle as bioreactors, it has been shown that vaccines can be delivered by electroporation to protect from bacteria-induced or virus-induced pneumonia.[81,82] Taken together, these nonviral approaches may indeed show great promise for treating pulmonary infections leading to and/or resulting from ALI/ARDS as long as gene transfer efficiencies are improved.

SUMMARY

Extensive research on ALI/ARDS, using animal models and humans, has revealed a variety of molecular mechanisms that contribute directly and indirectly to the pathogenesis of these diseases. Consequently, the opportunities for the use of gene therapy are great. It is likely that gene therapy will become a novel therapeutic approach in clinical medicine for treating a variety of inherited and acquired lung diseases in the near future, if concerns for safety and high-level gene expression are kept in balance. Although the technology is rapidly evolving, the limitation in development of gene therapy for ALI/ARDS is not at the level of the understanding of molecular mechanisms of the disease but rather at the level of drug-delivery technology. Improved vectors and delivery systems that are nontoxic and noninflammatory, allow repeated dosing, produce therapeutic levels of gene product, and that do so in specific cells are needed. Although each technology may address one or more of these problems, none to date have solved all of them. It is likely that combinations of approaches will be used for successful treatment. With the development of these more efficient gene therapy approaches, the first clinical use of therapeutic gene therapy shown to be safe and efficacious for treatment of ALI/ARDS is not far off.

REFERENCES

1. Rubenfeld GD, Caldwell E, Peabody E, et al. Incidence and outcomes of acute lung injury. N Engl J Med 2005;353(16):1685–93.
2. Kolb M, Martin G, Medina M, et al. Gene therapy for pulmonary diseases. Chest 2006;130(3):879–84.

3. Geiger J, Aneja MK, Rudolph C. Vectors for pulmonary gene therapy. Int J Pharm 2010;390(1):84–8.
4. Kushwah R, Cao H, Hu J. Potential of helper-dependent adenoviral vectors in modulating airway innate immunity. Cell Mol Immunol 2007;4(2):81–9.
5. Muruve DA. The innate immune response to adenovirus vectors. Hum Gene Ther 2004;15(12):1157–66.
6. Sakurai H, Kawabata K, Sakurai F, et al. Innate immune response induced by gene delivery vectors. Int J Pharm 2008;354(1/2):9–15.
7. Grubb BR, Pickles RJ, Ye H, et al. Inefficient gene transfer by adenovirus vector to cystic fibrosis airway epithelia of mice and humans. Nature 1994;371(6500):802–6.
8. Koehler DR, Martin B, Corey M, et al. Readministration of helper-dependent adenovirus to mouse lung. Gene Ther 2006;13(9):773–80.
9. Conway JE, Zolotukhin S, Muzyczka N, et al. Recombinant adeno-associated virus type 2 replication and packaging is entirely supported by a herpes simplex virus type 1 amplicon expressing Rep and Cap. J Virol 1997;71(11):8780–9.
10. Tal J. Adeno-associated virus-based vectors in gene therapy. J Biomed Sci 2000;7(4):279–91.
11. Moss RB, Rodman D, Spencer LT, et al. Repeated adeno-associated virus serotype 2 aerosol-mediated cystic fibrosis transmembrane regulator gene transfer to the lungs of patients with cystic fibrosis: a multicenter, double-blind, placebo-controlled trial. Chest 2004;125(2):509–21.
12. Engelhardt JF, Yankaskas JR, Wilson JM. In vivo retroviral gene transfer into human bronchial epithelia of xenografts. J Clin Invest 1992;90(6):2598–607.
13. Trono D. Lentiviral vectors: turning a deadly foe into a therapeutic agent. Gene Ther 2000;7(1):20–3.
14. Pickles RJ. Physical and biological barriers to viral vector-mediated delivery of genes to the airway epithelium. Proc Am Thorac Soc 2004;1(4):302–8.
15. Kobinger GP, Weiner DJ, Yu QC, et al. Filovirus-pseudotyped lentiviral vector can efficiently and stably transduce airway epithelia in vivo. Nat Biotechnol 2001;19(3):225–30.
16. Lam AP, Dean DA. Progress and prospects: nuclear import of nonviral vectors. Gene Ther 2010;17(4):439–47.
17. Miller AM, Dean DA. Tissue-specific and transcription factor-mediated nuclear entry of DNA. Adv Drug Deliv Rev 2009;61(7/8):603–13.
18. Felgner PL, Gadek TR, Holm M, et al. Lipofection: a highly efficient, lipid-mediated DNA-transfection procedure. Proc Natl Acad Sci U S A 1987;84(21):7413–7.
19. Liu Y, Liggitt D, Zhong W, et al. Cationic liposome-mediated intravenous gene delivery. J Biol Chem 1995;270(42):24864–70.
20. Caplen NJ, Alton EW, Middleton PG, et al. Liposome-mediated CFTR gene transfer to the nasal epithelium of patients with cystic fibrosis. Nat Med 1995;1(1):39–46.
21. Gill DR, Southern KW, Mofford KA, et al. A placebo-controlled study of liposome-mediated gene transfer to the nasal epithelium of patients with cystic fibrosis. Gene Ther 1997;4(3):199–209.
22. De Smedt SC, Demeester J, Hennink WE. Cationic polymer-based gene delivery systems. Pharm Res 2000;17(2):113–26.
23. Godbey WT, Wu KK, Mikos AG. Poly(ethylenimine)-mediated gene delivery affects endothelial cell function and viability. Biomaterials 2001;22(5):471–80.
24. Chollet P, Favrot MC, Hurbin A, et al. Side-effects of a systemic injection of linear polyethylenimine-DNA complexes. J Gene Med 2002;4(1):84–91.

25. Davis PB, Cooper MJ. Vectors for airway gene delivery. AAPS J 2007;9(1):E11–7.
26. Price A, Limberis M, Gruneich JA, et al. Targeting viral-mediated transduction to the lung airway epithelium with the anti-inflammatory cationic lipid dexamethasone-spermine. Mol Ther 2005;12(3):502–9.
27. Herweijer H, Wolff JA. Progress and prospects: naked DNA gene transfer and therapy. Gene Ther 2003;10(6):453–8.
28. Zhou R, Norton JE, Zhang N, et al. Electroporation-mediated transfer of plasmids to the lung results in reduced TLR9 signaling and inflammation. Gene Ther 2007; 14(9):775–80.
29. Somiari S, Glasspool-Malone J, Drabick JJ, et al. Theory and in vivo application of electroporative gene delivery. Mol Ther 2000;2(3):178–87.
30. Conwell CC, Huang L. Recent advances in non-viral gene delivery. Adv Genet 2005;53PA:1–18.
31. Dean DA, Machado-Aranda D, Blair-Parks K, et al. Electroporation as a method for high-level non-viral gene transfer to the lung. Gene Ther 2003;10(18): 1608–15.
32. Zhou R, Norton JE, Dean DA. Electroporation-mediated gene delivery to the lungs. Methods Mol Biol 2008;423:233–47.
33. Walther W, Siegel R, Kobelt D, et al. Novel jet-injection technology for nonviral intratumoral gene transfer in patients with melanoma and breast cancer. Clin Cancer Res 2008;14(22):7545–53.
34. Goudy KS, Wang B, Tisch R. Gene gun-mediated DNA vaccination enhances antigen-specific immunotherapy at a late preclinical stage of type 1 diabetes in nonobese diabetic mice. Clin Immunol 2008;129(1):49–57.
35. Suda T, Liu D. Hydrodynamic gene delivery: its principles and applications. Mol Ther 2007;15(12):2063–9.
36. Sheyn D, Kimelman-Bleich N, Pelled G, et al. Ultrasound-based nonviral gene delivery induces bone formation in vivo. Gene Ther 2008;15(4):257–66.
37. Machado-Aranda D, Adir Y, Young JL, et al. Gene transfer of the Na+, K+-ATPase beta1 subunit using electroporation increases lung liquid clearance. Am J Respir Crit Care Med 2005;171(3):204–11.
38. Gazdhar A, Bilici M, Pierog J, et al. In vivo electroporation and ubiquitin promoter—a protocol for sustained gene expression in the lung. J Gene Med 2006;8(7):910–8.
39. Dean DA. Import of plasmid DNA into the nucleus is sequence specific. Exp Cell Res 1997;230:293–302.
40. Dean DA, Dean BS, Muller S, et al. Sequence requirements for plasmid nuclear entry. Exp Cell Res 1999;253:713–22.
41. Dean DA, Strong DD, Zimmer WE. Nuclear entry of nonviral vectors. Gene Ther 2005;12(11):881–90.
42. Degiulio JV, Kaufman CD, Dean DA. The SP-C promoter facilitates alveolar type II epithelial cell–specific plasmid nuclear import and gene expression. Gene Ther 2010;17(4):541–9.
43. Miller AM, Dean DA. Cell-specific nuclear import of plasmid DNA in smooth muscle requires tissue-specific transcription factors and DNA sequences. Gene Ther 2008;15(15):1107–15.
44. Vacik J, Dean BS, Zimmer WE, et al. Cell-specific nuclear import of plasmid DNA. Gene Ther 1999;6:1006–14.
45. Young JL, Zimmer WE, Dean DA. Smooth muscle-specific gene delivery in the vasculature based on restriction of DNA nuclear import. Exp Biol Med (Maywood) 2008;233(7):840–8.

46. Dean DA. Nucleocytoplasmic trafficking. In: Mahato RI, editor. Pharmaceutical perspectives of nucleic acid-based therapeutics. London: Harwood Academic Publishers; 2002. p. 229–60.
47. Raghavendran K, Pryhuber GS, Chess PR, et al. Pharmacotherapy of acute lung injury and acute respiratory distress syndrome. Curr Med Chem 2008;15(19): 1911–24.
48. Liu KD, Matthay MA. Advances in critical care for the nephrologist: acute lung injury/ARDS. Clin J Am Soc Nephrol 2008;3(2):578–86.
49. Mutlu GM, Sznajder JI. Mechanisms of pulmonary edema clearance. Am J Physiol Lung Cell Mol Physiol 2005;289(5):L685–95.
50. Budinger GR, Sznajder JI. The alveolar-epithelial barrier: a target for potential therapy [abstract ix]. Clin Chest Med 2006;27(4):655–69.
51. Mutlu GM, Machado-Aranda D, Norton JE, et al. Electroporation-mediated gene transfer of the Na+, K+ -ATPase rescues endotoxin-induced lung injury. Am J Respir Crit Care Med 2007;176(6):582–90.
52. Mutlu GM, Dumasius V, Burhop J, et al. Upregulation of alveolar epithelial active Na+ transport is dependent on beta2-adrenergic receptor signaling. Circ Res 2004;94(8):1091–100.
53. Snyder PM. Liddle's syndrome mutations disrupt cAMP-mediated translocation of the epithelial Na(+) channel to the cell surface. J Clin Invest 2000;105(1):45–53.
54. Factor P, Saldias F, Ridge K, et al. Augmentation of lung liquid clearance via adenovirus-mediated transfer of a Na, K-ATPase beta1 subunit gene. J Clin Invest 1998;102(7):1421–30.
55. Factor P, Dumasius V, Saldias F, et al. Adenovirus-mediated transfer of an Na+/K+-ATPase beta1 subunit gene improves alveolar fluid clearance and survival in hyperoxic rats. Hum Gene Ther 2000;11(16):2231–42.
56. Ridge KM, Olivera WG, Saldias F, et al. Alveolar type 1 cells express the alpha2 Na, K-ATPase, which contributes to lung liquid clearance. Circ Res 2003;92(4):453–60.
57. Adir Y, Welch LC, Dumasius V, et al. Overexpression of the Na-K-ATPase alpha2-subunit improves lung liquid clearance during ventilation-induced lung injury. Am J Physiol Lung Cell Mol Physiol 2008;294(6):L1233–7.
58. Adir Y, Factor P, Dumasius V, et al. Na, K-ATPase gene transfer increases liquid clearance during ventilation-induced lung injury. Am J Respir Crit Care Med 2003;168(12):1445–8.
59. Azzam ZS, Dumasius V, Saldias FJ, et al. Na, K-ATPase overexpression improves alveolar fluid clearance in a rat model of elevated left atrial pressure. Circulation 2002;105(4):497–501.
60. Qiao R, Zhou B, Harboe-Schmidt E, et al. Subunit-specific coordinate upregulation of sodium pump activity in alveolar epithelial cells by lentivirus-mediated gene transfer. Hum Gene Ther 2004;15(5):457–68.
61. Factor P, Mendez M, Mutlu GM, et al. Acute hyperoxic lung injury does not impede adenoviral-mediated alveolar gene transfer. Am J Respir Crit Care Med 2002;165(4):521–6.
62. Dumasius V, Jameel M, Burhop J, et al. In vivo timing of onset of transgene expression following adenoviral-mediated gene transfer. Virology 2003;308(2):243–9.
63. Dumasius V, Sznajder JI, Azzam ZS, et al. beta(2)-adrenergic receptor overexpression increases alveolar fluid clearance and responsiveness to endogenous catecholamines in rats. Circ Res 2001;89(10):907–14.
64. Mutlu GM, Adir Y, Jameel M, et al. Interdependency of beta-adrenergic receptors and CFTR in regulation of alveolar active Na+ transport. Circ Res 2005;96(9): 999–1005.

65. Litvan J, Briva A, Wilson MS, et al. Beta-adrenergic receptor stimulation and adenoviral overexpression of superoxide dismutase prevent the hypoxia-mediated decrease in Na, K-ATPase and alveolar fluid reabsorption. J Biol Chem 2006;281(29):19892–8.
66. Stern M, Ulrich K, Robinson C, et al. Pretreatment with cationic lipid-mediated transfer of the Na+K+-ATPase pump in a mouse model in vivo augments resolution of high permeability pulmonary oedema. Gene Ther 2000;7(11):960–6.
67. Ulrich K, Stern M, Goddard ME, et al. Keratinocyte growth factor therapy in murine oleic acid-induced acute lung injury. Am J Physiol Lung Cell Mol Physiol 2005;288(6):L1179–92.
68. Baba Y, Yazawa T, Kanegae Y, et al. Keratinocyte growth factor gene transduction ameliorates acute lung injury and mortality in mice. Hum Gene Ther 2007;18(2): 130–41.
69. Dean DA. Electroporation of the vasculature and the lung. DNA Cell Biol 2003; 22(12):797–806.
70. Favard C, Dean DS, Rols MP. Electrotransfer as a non viral method of gene delivery. Curr Gene Ther 2007;7(1):67–77.
71. Buff SM, Yu H, McCall JN, et al. IL-10 delivery by AAV5 vector attenuates inflammation in mice with *Pseudomonas* pneumonia. Gene Ther 2010;17(5):567–76.
72. McAllister F, Ruan S, Steele C, et al. CXCR3 and IFN protein-10 in Pneumocystis pneumonia. J Immunol 2006;177(3):1846–54.
73. Ruan S, McKinley L, Zheng M, et al. Interleukin-12 and host defense against murine Pneumocystis pneumonia. Infect Immun 2008;76(5):2130–7.
74. Mora BN, Boasquevisque CH, Boglione M, et al. Transforming growth factor-beta1 gene transfer ameliorates acute lung allograft rejection. J Thorac Cardiovasc Surg 2000;119(5):913–20.
75. Lin GH, Sedgmen BJ, Moraes TJ, et al. Endogenous 4-1BB ligand plays a critical role in protection from influenza-induced disease. J Immunol 2009;182(2):934–47.
76. Otterbein LE, Kolls JK, Mantell LL, et al. Exogenous administration of heme oxygenase-1 by gene transfer provides protection against hyperoxia-induced lung injury. J Clin Invest 1999;103(7):1047–54.
77. Hashiba T, Suzuki M, Nagashima Y, et al. Adenovirus-mediated transfer of heme oxygenase-1 cDNA attenuates severe lung injury induced by the influenza virus in mice. Gene Ther 2001;8(19):1499–507.
78. Inoue S, Suzuki M, Nagashima Y, et al. Transfer of heme oxygenase 1 cDNA by a replication-deficient adenovirus enhances interleukin 10 production from alveolar macrophages that attenuates lipopolysaccharide-induced acute lung injury in mice. Hum Gene Ther 2001;12(8):967–79.
79. Weiss YG, Maloyan A, Tazelaar J, et al. Adenoviral transfer of HSP-70 into pulmonary epithelium ameliorates experimental acute respiratory distress syndrome. J Clin Invest 2002;110(6):801–6.
80. Hu Q, Zuo P, Shao B, et al. Administration of nonviral gene vector encoding rat beta-defensin-2 ameliorates chronic *Pseudomonas aeruginosa* lung infection in rats. J Gene Med 2010;12(3):276–86.
81. Thacker EL, Holtkamp DJ, Khan AS, et al. Plasmid-mediated growth hormone-releasing hormone efficacy in reducing disease associated with *Mycoplasma hyopneumoniae* and porcine reproductive and respiratory syndrome virus infection. J Anim Sci 2006;84(3):733–42.
82. Saha S, Takeshita F, Sasaki S, et al. Multivalent DNA vaccine protects mice against pulmonary infection caused by *Pseudomonas aeruginosa*. Vaccine 2006;24(37–39):6240–9.

Mesenchymal Stem Cells and Acute Lung Injury

Jeffrey E. Gotts, MD, PhD*, Michael A. Matthay, MD

KEYWORDS

• Acute lung injury • ALI • Adult respiratory distress syndrome
• ARDS • Mesenchymal stem cells • MSC

Acute respiratory distress syndrome (ARDS) was first recognized in the 1960s[1] as a clinical syndrome of severe acute respiratory failure presenting with hypoxemia and bilateral pulmonary infiltrates, most often in the setting of pneumonia, sepsis, or major trauma. The distinction between acute lung injury (ALI) and ARDS relates to the severity of hypoxemia, with the former having a Pao_2/Fio_2 of less than 300, and the latter with a Pao_2/Fio_2 of less than 200. The pathogenesis of ALI/ARDS involves lung endothelial injury, alveolar epithelial injury, and the accumulation of protein-rich fluid and cellular debris in the alveolar space (for recent review see Matthay and Zemans[2]). In 2005, approximately 200,000 patients in the United States developed ALI/ARDS, with an estimated mortality of 40%.[3] In the era of lung protective ventilation, mortality has declined to approximately 25%.[4] However, of the broad array of pharmacologic therapies evaluated in clinical trials to date, including inhaled surfactant, nitric oxide, prostacyclins, glucocorticoids, ketoconazole, antioxidants, β-agonists, and pentoxifylline, none has proved effective, and none can be currently recommended as standard therapy for ALI.[5] Some may have value as rescue therapies.[6] It is possible that the lack of efficacy with pharmacologic therapies is in part caused by the late stage at which therapy is initiated, as well as the heterogeneity of ALI, with different pathophysiologic cascades predominating in ALI caused by trauma versus infectious causes of ALI.[7] Given these challenges, and with severe pathologic changes at the level of the alveolus in ALI, it seems increasingly unlikely that any single molecule will prove sufficient to reverse the course of this syndrome rapidly enough to provide substantial clinical benefit.

Financial disclosure: the authors have nothing to disclose.
Departments of Medicine Anesthesiology, The Cardiovascular Research Institute, University of California, 505 Parnassus Avenue, Moffitt Hospital, Room M-917, San Francisco, CA 94143-0624, USA
* Corresponding author. Division of Pulmonary and Critical Care Medicine, UCSF, 505 Parnassus Avenue, M1087, Box 0111, San Francisco, CA 94143-0111.
E-mail address: jeffrey.gotts@ucsf.edu

Crit Care Clin 27 (2011) 719–733
doi:10.1016/j.ccc.2011.04.004 **criticalcare.theclinics.com**
0749-0704/11/$ – see front matter

A potential strategy to circumvent these difficulties involves cell-based therapies. Given the ability of some cells to produce dozens of active molecules that can potentially modulate inflammatory cascades at multiple levels as well as enhance repair, it is conceivable that such therapies would prove more successful than single molecules. A steadily enlarging body of evidence from preclinical studies of lung injury, sepsis, and other disease states indicates that one ideal candidate may be the mesenchymal stem cell.

MESENCHYMAL STEM CELLS: GENERAL PROPERTIES

Mesenchymal stem cells (MSCs) are multipotent, self-renewing cells initially isolated from bone marrow that can differentiate into muscle, bone, fat, fibroblasts, and cartilage. They were first described in the late 1960s[8] when it was discovered that a fraction of cells from whole bone marrow adhered to plastic. These cells were spindlelike, formed colonies, could reconstitute a hematopoietic environment, and could regenerate bone tissue in serial transplants, showing their ability to self-renew. Initially termed colony-forming unit–fibroblastic (CFU-F), these cells were later referred to as marrow stromal cells, and ultimately were labeled mesenchymal stem cells by Caplan and colleagues.[9] The lack of specific cell markers has slowed their in vivo characterization. For example, it is still not known whether MSCs originate from the mesoderm, from the neuroepithelium, or from different sources at progressive developmental stages as a recent study has suggested.[10] It is now generally accepted that MSCs or MSC-like cells can be isolated not just from bone marrow but also from fat, umbilical cord blood, placental tissue, tendons, and skeletal muscle.[11–15] In the absence of cell-specific markers, the following criteria have been put forth by the International Society of Cellular Therapy[16]: (1) adherence to plastic; (2) expression of CD105, CD73, and CD90; lack of expression of CD45, CD34, CD14, CD11b, CD79α, CD19, and human leukocyte antigen (HLA) II; and (3) ability to differentiate into osteoblasts, adipocytes, and chondroblasts in vitro.

Based on their differentiation capacity, researchers have studied these cells for their potential to repair damaged musculoskeletal tissues. However, MSCs are now known to possess multiple other properties that have galvanized the scientific community. MSCs expanded in vitro home to sites of tissue damage.[17,18] Although a full review of their properties is beyond the scope of this article, some are considered briefly here. MSCs produce a wide variety of molecules, including hematopoietic factors, chemokines, and angiogenic factors.[19] Given their presence in the bone marrow, it is not surprising that they have potent immunomodulatory effects. Generally, they shift the immune response toward tolerant, antiinflammatory phenotypes.[20] They mostly lack major histocompatibility complex class II antigens, and consequently can evade immune destruction following allogeneic, or even xenogeneic, transplant. For this reason, MSCs have been developed as vectors for gene therapy, and to help induce tolerance in allogeneic bone marrow transplantation.[21] MSCs have been found to have beneficial effects in preclinical models of diseases, ranging from Crohn disease[22] to traumatic brain injury.[23] In the last decade, several investigators have reported that exogenously administered MSCs can mitigate several types of lung disease in a variety of animal models.

MSCs IN LUNG DISEASE

Bleomycin exposure has previously been developed as a model of fibrotic lung disease in mice.[24,25] Ortiz and colleages[26] isolated murine MSCs and administered them intravenously immediately or 7 days following bleomycin injury. They found that exogenous MSCs could be found in areas of bleomycin-induced lung injury, and that these cells appeared to acquire characteristics of epithelial cells. Mice treated with MSCs immediately following bleomycin exposure also had significantly reduced collagen deposition, and reduced expression of matrix metalloproteinases 2 and 9. The degree of the antiinflammatory effects was striking compared with the low levels of lung engraftment. In subsequent work,[27] this group reported that MSC in vivo administration blocks the bleomycin-induced increase in interleukin (IL)-1α. Rojas and colleagues[28] administered bleomycin to mice with or without preceding busulfan-induced myelosuppression. Myelosuppression enhanced the initial injury and was associated with reduced survival. However, myelosuppressed mice that received green fluorescent protein (GFP)-tagged MSCs 6 hours after bleomycin injury had improved survival, an effect that was associated with engraftment of GFP-positive cells that expressed markers of fibroblasts, myofibroblasts, as well as type I and type II alveolar epithelial cells. Similarly, Moodley and colleagues[29] derived MSCs from umbilical cord tissue and infused them intravenously following nasal bleomycin in mice. MSCs were identified 2 weeks later in inflamed portions of the lung. MSCs reduced collagen concentration as well as Smad2 phosphorylation, suggesting that these cells had antifibrotic properties.

In a model of bronchopulmonary dysplasia, Chang and colleagues[30] delivered MSCs intratracheally in postnatal rats exposed to prolonged hyperoxia. The MSCs significantly reduced apoptosis, myeloperoxidase activity, and collagen deposition, as well as the inflammatory molecules IL-6, tumor necrosis factor (TNF)-α, and transforming growth factor-β. Furthermore, a few of the MSCs differentiated into type II alveolar epithelial cells, although as in many such studies, at a low level. In similar studies with postnatal rats exposed to prolonged hyperoxia, van Haaften and colleagues[31] reported that intratracheal MSCs improved survival and exercise tolerance, and decreased alveolar and vascular lung injury, as well as pulmonary hypertension, in a neonatal model of lung injury.

MSCs delivered intratracheally reduced pulmonary hypertension induced by monocrotaline in rats, and improved measures of vascular endothelial function.[32] In a rat model of emphysema induced by radiation and papain, Zhen and colleagues[33] reported that MSC administration reduced emphysematous changes. In addition, MSCs differentiated into type II alveolar epithelial cells. Thus, MSCs have therapeutic effects in several models of lung disease. Because of their antiinflammatory properties, they would be especially well suited to mitigating the lung damage in ALI.

MSCs IN ANIMAL MODELS OF ALI AND SEPSIS: EVIDENCE OF BENEFICIAL EFFECTS

Lipopolysaccharide (LPS) has been widely used to produce ALI in animal models. When given by the airway, LPS triggers a large influx of polymorphonuclear neutrophil leukocytes (PMNs) into the airspaces that peaks at around 48 hours and is associated with increased microvascular permeability.[34] Several investigators have studied the properties of MSCs in LPS-induced models of ALI (**Table 1**). Yamada and colleagues[35] delivered LPS intranasally and showed that MSCs were increased in peripheral blood 4 hours later. They next subjected irradiated mice with bone marrow reconstituted from GFP transgenic donors to intranasal LPS, and showed abundant GFP-positive cells in the lungs 3 weeks later. Some of these cells expressed cytokeratin, a marker of epithelial cells, whereas others expressed CD34, a marker of endothelial cells. These results suggested that endogenous MSCs might play an important role in repairing inflammatory damage following LPS. Following sublethal irradiation to induce bone marrow suppression, intranasal LPS produced a similar pattern of

Table 1
MSCs in models of ALI

Reference	Injury Model	MSCs Given	Beneficial Effects	Increased	Decreased	Other
Gupta et al[38]	Intratracheal LPS in mice	Intratracheally, 4 h after LPS; Sac at 24 and 48 h	↓Lung edema ↓Lung hemorrhage ↓BAL protein ↓Mortality	IL-10	MIP-2, TNF-α	No significant engraftment
Xu et al[37]	Intraperitoneal LPS in mice	Intravenously, 1 h after LPS; Sac at 6 h, 24 h, 48 h, and 14 d	↓Lung PMNs ↓Lung edema	—	IFN-γ, IL-1β, MIP-1α, KC	No significant engraftment
Mei et al[40]	Cecal ligation and puncture in mice	Intravenously 6 h after CLP; Sac at 28 h	↓BAL cell counts ↓BAL albumin ↓Lung edema and inflammation ↓Kidney injury ↓Mortality	—	IL-6, IL-1β, IL-10, KC, JE, CCL5	Microarray analysis: downregulation of inflammatory genetic pathways; enhanced bacterial clearance
Németh et al[41]	Cecal ligation and puncture in mice	Intravenously 24 h before or 1 h after CLP; Sac at 1 and 4 d	↓Kidney injury ↓Transaminases ↓Splenic apoptosis ↓Mortality ↓Tissue myeloperoxidase	IL-10, PGE2	TNF-α and IL-6	In vitro MSCs reprogram monocytes/macrophages to secrete IL-10
Krasnodembskaya et al[39]	Intratracheal *E coli* in mice	Intratracheally 4 hours after *E coli*; Sac at 18 h	↓BAL neutrophils ↓BAL protein	—	MIP-2	MSC-produced LL-37 decreases bacterial growth in vitro and BAL bacterial growth in vivo

Abbreviations: CLP, cecal ligation and puncture; IL, interleukin; LPS, lipopolysaccharide; MIP, macrophage inflammatory protein; PGE2, prostaglandin E2; PMN, polymorphonuclear neutrophil leukocytes; TNF, tumor necrosis factor.

histologic damage and bronchoalveolar lavage (BAL) neutrophilia but, at 1 week, large lesions that appeared emphysematous were noted. These lesions could be prevented by marrow reconstitution, suggesting that the absence of endogenous MSCs may have compromised normal repair processes.

Mei and colleagues[36] infused MSCs intravenously 30 minutes after intratracheal LPS, showing a significant reduction in BAL total cell and neutrophil counts 3 days later. Histologic analysis confirmed a marked decrease in inflammatory infiltrates, interalveolar septal thickening, and interstitial edema. Using fluorescent tags for MSCs, these researchers showed many labeled cells in the lungs of both LPS-injured and control animals 15 minutes after cell infusion, with a few labeled cells persisting at 3 days.

Xu and colleagues[37] used intraperitoneal LPS at 1 mg/kg (a dose that causes minimal mortality), and 1 hour later infused MSCs or fibroblasts intravenously. Histologic analysis revealed that MSCs, but not fibroblasts, significantly reduced lung neutrophils at 6, 24, and 48 hours. Seeking to model a more realistic clinical time course and a more critical illness, Gupta and colleagues[38] administered MSCs intratracheally to mice 4 hours following intratracheal administration of 5 mg/kg LPS, a dose that produces significant mortality. MSC-treated mice had improved survival relative to PBS-treated mice: 80% versus 42% at 48 hours, and 64% versus 18% at 72 hours. MSC reduced the severity of lung injury as measured by excess lung water, wet/dry ratio, and BAL protein concentration. Histologic analysis at 48 hours revealed less hemorrhage and edema. Nonviable MSCs and fibroblasts did not replicate this effect, suggesting undifferentiated, viable MSCs were required to ameliorate LPS-induced ALI. Recent work from Krasnodembskaya and colleagues[39] extended this work in a model of *Escherichia coli* pneumonia. *E coli* were administered to mice intratracheally. Four hours later, these mice were treated with intratracheal MSCs, PBS, or fibroblasts. MSCs substantially reduced lung inflammation, as measured by BAL neutrophil count.

Mei and colleagues[40] studied a cecal ligation and puncture (CLP) model of sepsis in mice. Six hours following CLP, MSCs or saline were infused intravenously. All mice received daily broad-spectrum antibiotics. The investigators found that MSC-treated mice had decreased BAL cell counts and albumin. Histology confirmed reduced inflammatory lung infiltrates and interstitial edema at 28 hours. The therapeutic benefit of MSCs was not confined to the lungs, because MSC-treated mice had reduced apoptotic kidney cells and improved serum creatinine. CLP results in severe systemic injury, as shown by 45% mortality at 28 hours. MSC treatment improved mortality by 50% at this time point.

Nemeth and colleagues[41] administered intravenous (IV) MSCs or control cells (heat-killed MSCs or skin fibroblasts) 24 hours before or 1 hour after CLP in mice. All mice received subcutaneous isotonic fluid and broad-spectrum antibiotics. They showed a substantial survival benefit for MSCs (with both administration times) at 4 days. MSCs from multiple different strains of mice provided an equivalent survival benefit for the C57BL/6 recipients. MSC-treated mice also had lower serum creatinine and kidney tubular injury scores, improved hepatic glycogen storage, and reduced transaminases, amylase, and splenic apoptosis, suggesting multiple beneficial systemic effects. Most of these effects were observed in mice treated with MSCs 24 hours before CLP.

MSCs IN ANIMAL MODELS OF ALI AND SEPSIS: POTENTIAL MECHANISMS

In the last several years, investigators have examined how MSCs may exert their therapeutic effects in models of ALI and sepsis, and have discovered an increasing number of potential mechanisms (**Fig. 1**). It is helpful first to consider the processes governing the production and removal of alveolar edema fluid.

Endothelial Permeability, Epithelial Permeability, and Alveolar Fluid Clearance

Edema accumulates in the alveoli through some combination of increased permeability to protein of the endothelial and epithelial barriers, and reduced (or insufficient) alveolar fluid clearance (AFC). Several groups have reported that MSCs reduce the increase in endothelial permeability associated with ALI. BAL albumin and protein are commonly used as markers of lung endothelial permeability, although they reflect a combination of endothelial and epithelial permeability. Mei and colleagues[36] found that BAL albumin, total protein, and immunoglobulin M (IgM) were increased 3 days following intratracheal LPS. This increase was attenuated by MSCs given intravenously 30 minutes after the injury. Angiopoietin-1 (Ang-1) may help maintain adult

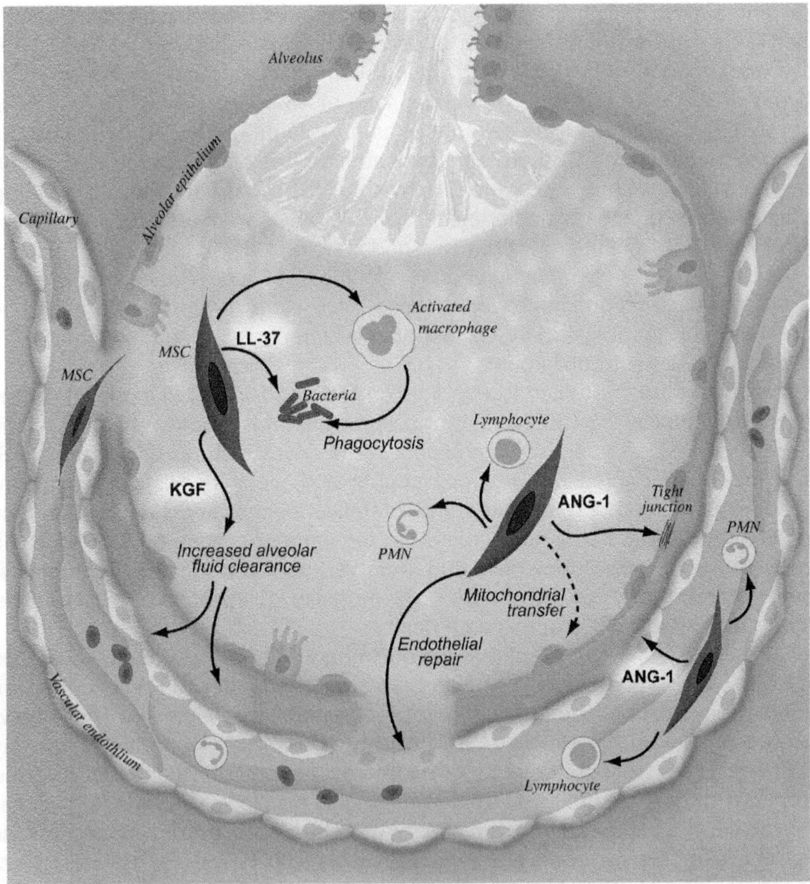

Fig. 1. Beneficial effects of MSCs in ALI. Protein-rich edema fluid and inflammatory cells fill an injured alveolus after endothelial and epithelial injury. MSCs exert immunomodulatory effects on neutrophils, lymphocytes, and macrophages; assist in repair of the injured epithelial and endothelial barriers; improve alveolar fluid clearance; and secrete several molecules including the antibacterial peptide LL-37, angiopoietin-1 (Ang-1), and keratinocyte growth factor (KGF).

vascular endothelial cells in a quiescent state, and Ang-1 has been shown to reduce permeability and promote endothelial cell survival.[42–44] Mei and colleagues[36] reported that MSCs engineered to produce Ang-1 further reduced BAL protein, albumin, and IgM to levels in uninjured mice. They reasoned that Ang-1 acted on the vascular endothelium following delivery of MSCs into the pulmonary circulation, diminishing inflammatory cell influx and reducing plasma protein leakage into the alveolar space. In a similar set of experiments, Xu and colleagues[45] showed that MSCs overexpressing Ang-1 delivered intravenously on the first of 7 days of nebulized LPS reduced BAL protein 7 and 14 later. More recently, Mei and colleagues[40] reported that IV infusion of MSCs 6 hours following CLP reduced BAL protein and albumin 28 hours following injury, suggesting that MSCs reduce the endothelial permeability associated with sepsis as well. This finding was further supported by the work of Nemeth and colleagues.[41] These researchers showed that, 24 hours following CLP in mice, Evans blue dye leakage was reduced by IV MSC administration in multiple organs, including the lung, liver, and kidney. Krasnodembskaya and colleagues[39] tested the effects of MSC administration in a more biologically relevant model of pneumonia. They reported that mice given live *E coli* intratracheally had increased BAL protein 18 hours later, and that BAL protein was significantly decreased by intratracheal delivery of MSCs (but not fibroblasts) 4 hours after the injury.

As indicated earlier, measurements of BAL protein provide an estimate of the combined changes in lung endothelial permeability, epithelial permeability, and AFC. The alveolar epithelium normally forms a tighter barrier than the endothelium, and its loss of integrity in ALI is of great significance. It had previously been shown that pulmonary edema fluid from patients with ALI increased epithelial protein permeability in primary cultures of human alveolar type II (ATII) cells grown on a semipermeable membrane with an air-liquid interface.[46] Fang and colleagues[47] sought to study the effect of MSCs on the alveolar epithelium using this model. When exposed to a potent mixture of inflammatory cytokines (cytomix, composed of IL-1β, TNF-α, and interferon [IFN]-γ), protein permeability across the epithelial layer increased by approximately 500%. However, when cocultured with allogeneic MSCs (in the lower compartment of a Transwell system, precluding cell contact), protein permeability was reduced to control levels. Ang-1, shown in several in vivo studies to augment the beneficial effect of MSCs (discussed earlier), was not produced by ATII cells at baseline or in response to cytomix. However, MSCs secreted Ang-1, and appeared to augment its production in response to cytomix. When Ang-1 production was blocked by siRNA, MSCs no longer prevented cytomix-induced increased epithelial permeability. However, the effect was restored by the addition of recombinant Ang-1. In an additional series of experiments, Ang-1 acted on epithelial cells through a Tie-2 receptor mechanism involving NF-κB to prevent the formation of actin stress fibers and maintain the localization of claudin-18, a key tight junction protein, at the cell periphery. These findings suggest that MSCs, acting in part through angiopoietin, improve the critical barrier function of the alveolar epithelium in the inflammatory milieu of ALI.

AFC is the capacity of the epithelium of the lung to remove alveolar fluid in pulmonary edema of any cause, and impaired AFC is associated with worsened outcomes in ALI/ARDS.[48,49] Many conditions can reduce AFC, including high tidal volume ventilation, live bacteria, acid instillation, and proinflammatory cytokines.[50–54] Gupta and colleagues[38] found that intratracheal MSCs 4 hours after LPS reduced excess lung water, but did not distinguish between changes in formation of fluid (via increased endothelial and epithelial permeability) and changes in AFC. Lee and colleagues[55] developed an ex vivo perfused human lung preparation, and tested the effects of allogeneic MSCs following intrabronchial administration of LPS. In this model, LPS resulted in a marked decrease in AFC, from approximately 20% per hour to near 0% per hour, an effect that required the presence of blood in the perfusate, suggesting that blood elements such as PMNs, monocytes, and platelets were required for the injurious effect of LPS. Instillation of fibroblasts into the injured lung 1 hour after LPS had no effect on AFC. However, instillation of human MSCs or their conditioned medium normalized AFC to baseline levels. This effect appeared to be modulated in part by keratinocyte growth factor (KGF), because siRNA for KGF reduced the therapeutic effect of MSCs on AFC by 80%. Thus, MSCs seem to improve both endothelial/epithelial permeability and AFC in multiple models of ALI.

Engraftment

Although MSCs were initially noted to differentiate into bone, fat, muscle, and cartilage,[56] researchers discovered in the late 1990s that, in certain conditions, these cells could develop a nonmesodermal phenotype.[57,58] Kotton and colleagues[59] showed that labeled MSCs incorporated into lung tissue following bleomycin injury and developed morphologic and molecular characteristics of type I pneumocytes. Xu and colleagues[37] noted large numbers of labeled MSCs in the lung parenchyma 24 hours following IP LPS and IV MSC infusion. However, 2 weeks later, few labeled cells remained, suggesting that the substantial presence of MSCs in the lung is a transient phenomenon following ALI. Gupta and colleagues[38] found scattered labeled MSCs at 24 and 48 hours following IT LPS and MSC delivery, with less than 5% engraftment. Xu and colleagues[45] treated mice daily for 7 days with nebulized LPS, infusing GFP-labeled MSCs on the first day. In some animals, MSCs were also engineered to express Ang-1, the ligand for Tie-2 known to decrease endothelial permeability. Fourteen days after infusion, labeled cells were seen in the lung (reported 9% engraftment with MSCs and 16% with MSC–Ang-1), although the engrafted cells were not further characterized. Taken together, the data suggest that MSC differentiation into mature lung cell types following ALI may occur at low levels but is unlikely to produce much of their beneficial effect.

Immunomodulation

MSCs were first recognized to have potent immunomodulatory effects based on their ability to engraft and differentiate following xenogeneic transplantation.[60] MSCs have since been shown to suppress many functions of naive and memory T cells, B cells, natural killer (NK) cells, and the differentiation and function of monocytes.[61–63] In many models of ALI, MSC administration results in altered signaling related to immune cell activation and recruitment. In their intratracheal LPS model, Gupta and colleagues[38] reported that intratracheal MSCs reduced BAL levels of the proinflammatory cytokines TNF-α and macrophage inflammatory protein (MIP)-2 as well as plasma levels of MIP-2. There was a corresponding increase in the antiinflammatory cytokines IL-10, IL-1ra, and IL-13. Furthermore, the addition of MSCs to LPS-stimulated macrophages in vitro reduced the level of TNF-α, an effect that persisted in the presence of a Transwell that prevented contact between the cell types. These findings suggest that the administration of MSCs in a model of ALI shifts the injured lung milieu from proinflammatory to antiinflammatory, in part through effects of soluble mediators on macrophages.

Xu and colleagues[37] showed that IV MSCs moderated the LPS-induced increase in serum proinflammatory IFN-γ, IL-1β, MIP-1α, and KC (murine homolog of IL-8). In their CLP model, Nemeth and colleagues[41] reported that IV MSCs reduced serum TNF-α and IL-6 but increased IL-10 24 hours after injury. They also found that MSCs reduced myeloperoxidase in the liver and kidneys of LPS-treated mice, suggesting less neutrophil invasion and associated organ damage. They then performed a series of experiments to help elucidate the molecular signaling driving these effects. MSCs improved survival in mice genetically lacking mature T and B cells, and in mice depleted of NK cells. Next they depleted mice of monocytes and macrophages and found that the MSCs were no longer effective, suggesting that these were the cells through which MSCs exert their beneficial effects. In vitro, MSCs were shown to increase cyclooxygenase-2 (COX2) expression and activity within 5 hours of LPS stimulation, followed by increased levels of prostaglandin E2 (PGE2), effects that were abolished in MSCs taken from TLR4 knockout mice or in the presence of antibodies to TNF-α. MSCs were then cultured with macrophages, and the addition of LPS was found to increase IL-10. In a series of experiments, this effect was shown to depend on TLR4, MyD88 (required for NF-κB activation by TLR4), TNF-α, and TNF receptor-1. In additional experiments, they showed that the macrophages responded to PGE2 via EP2 and EP4 receptors. Thus they concluded that MSCs activated by LPS reprogram macrophages to secrete IL-10, and that this reduces neutrophil migration into tissues and helps mitigate tissue damage.

Mei and colleagues[40] reported that, 28 hours following CLP, mice treated with IV MSCs (given 6 hours after injury) had diminished serum levels of the proinflammatory cytokines, IL-6, IL-1β, KC, JE (murine homolog of MCP-1), and chemokine ligand 5 (CCL5; murine homolog of RANTES [regulated on activation, normal T expressed and secreted]). Serum IL-10 was also decreased by MSCs in this model, in contrast with the previous study by Nemeth and colleagues[41] It is unclear why IL-10 was increased in one model of CLP and decreased in another, but this may relate to technical differences such as the timing of MSC administration relative to injury or the number of cells infused. As became more clear following a gene expression analysis in this model (discussed later), it seems likely that MSC administration simultaneously modulates several inflammatory pathways rather than acting through any single mediator.

Antibacterial Effects

It had been puzzling that MSCs could have such potent antiinflammatory effects and yet lead to robust improvements in survival following sepsis induced by live bacteria. Some exciting recent experiments suggest that this seems to be caused in part by MSCs ability to reduce the bacterial burden. As described earlier, Mei and colleagues[40] gave IV MSCs 6 hours following CLP and found a significant improvement in survival. They compared bacterial CFU from the spleen 28 hours after injury, and found that MSC treatment reduced mean CFU by an order of magnitude. Next they isolated total cells or the CD11b+ fraction (monocytes/macrophages and neutrophils) of cells from the peritoneal space and spleens of mice 24 hours after CLP. They showed that both the total cell population and the CD11b+ fraction had increased phagocytic capacity for gram-negative and gram-positive aerobic bacteria following MSC treatment. Additional experiments suggested that MSCs themselves infrequently engaged in phagocytosis, which suggested that they must indirectly modulate the host's phagocytes. In a gene expression analysis of splenic tissue 28 hours after CLP, MSC treatment downregulated genes involved in inflammatory pathways such as IL-6, IL-1, the IL-1 receptor, and IL-10. Conversely, MSCs tended to upregulate genes involved in phagocytosis.

Krasnodembskaya and colleagues[39] recently reported that MSCs possess additional antimicrobial properties. These researchers first showed that MSCs (compared with fibroblasts) reduced the growth of *E coli* in vitro. MSC-conditioned medium had no effect on gram-negative bacterial growth unless the cells had previously been stimulated with *E coli*, suggesting that this induced them to produce an antibacterial substance. They next screened the media of bacteria-stimulated MSCs for known antimicrobial peptides and proteins, and found significant quantities of human cathelicidin (LL-37). Synthetic LL-37 reduced the growth of *E coli* and *Pseudomonas aeruginosa* and, when incubated with a blocking antibody for LL-37, the conditioned medium of bacterial-stimulated MSCs lost its antibacterial effect. When mice were given *E coli* intratracheally and then treated with MSCs 4 hours later, both lung homogenates and BAL showed more than an order of magnitude reduction in bacterial counts. This reduction was largely prevented by coadministration of a neutralizing antibody to LL-37. That BAL neutrophil counts were similarly reduced by MSC treatments suggested that improved bacterial clearance was not dependent on this cell type. In addition, the BAL from MSC-treated mice itself inhibited bacterial growth. Taken together, the results suggest that MSCs both exert direct effects on bacteria and positively modulate the host's phagocytic capacity. Future experiments should help clarify the precise cellular and molecular pathways of phagocytic augmentation, and may identify additional direct antibacterial effects.

Other Possible Mechanisms

Several recent studies have also revealed entirely new mechanisms of interaction between MSCs and tissue cells. Spees and colleagues[64] depleted functional mitochondria in A549 cells using ethidium bromide to mutate mitochondrial DNA. When subsequently cultured with MSCs, the A549 cells acquired functional mitochondria whose DNA matched that of the MSCs. Time-lapse microscopy showed that MSCs develop extensions of their cytoplasm toward the A549 cells through which mitochondria subsequently streamed. This report did not establish the ultrastructural mechanism of mitochondrial transfer. More recently, Plotnikov and colleagues[65] showed in vitro mitochondrial transfer from MSCs to cardiac myocytes. Electron microscopy revealed extremely thin structures termed nanotubes, through which the mitochondria appeared to travel. Whether the mitochondria travel by vesicles, nanotubes, or some other mechanism, the observation that MSCs can rescue energetically compromised cells by directly transferring their mitochondria suggests another potential beneficial role in vivo, because mitochondrial compromise is a common feature of many models of organ injury.

Microvesicles (MV) are vesicles/exosomes released by multiple types of cells, including stem cells, and have recently been recognized to be an important mechanism of communication.[66,67] Embryonic stem cells have been shown to reprogram hematopoietic progenitors by mRNAs carried in microvesicles.[68] MSCs seem to release microvesicles as well. Bruno and colleagues[69] showed that MSC-derived microvesicles increased proliferation of kidney tubular epithelial cells in vitro, and made them resistant to apoptosis in response to serum deprivation or administration of vincristine and *cis*-platinum. Next, they showed that MSCs or their microvesicles, when given to severe combined immunodeficient mice, had similar protective effects against acute kidney injury caused by glycerol. RNase abolished the positive effect of microvesicles in vitro and in vivo, suggesting that the effect was caused by MSC-derived RNAs. Gene chip analysis of MSC microvesicles revealed mRNAs associated with transcription, proliferation, and immune cell regulation. More recent work from this same group has shown that MSC-derived microvesicles contain microRNAs as well.[70] What role microvesicles or mitochondrial transfer may play in the beneficial effects of MSCs in models of ALI remains to be determined.

FUTURE STUDIES

Much about MSC biology remains to be discovered. These cells are known to exert a wide range of effects through an impressive and growing array of mechanisms. Future work should help clarify the relative contributions of engraftment, immunomodulation, antibacterial effects, mitochondrial transfer, and microvesicular transfer of genetic information. Some additional basic questions remain. The lack of reliable cell surface markers for these cells has significantly limited in vivo study. There is no knockout mouse for MSCs, no MSC-specific promoters or immunohistochemical markers, and this has left open the question of where MSCs can be found outside the bone marrow, with some groups suggesting that they may be equivalent to pericytes, which line most vascular elements in the body.[71,72] Although the spectrum of beneficial effects from exogenous MSC administration is impressive, there is little sense of how native MSCs respond to injury, or whether there are ways to augment these responses, short of supplying them exogenously, with potential risks to patients. It is also important to know how much of their beneficial effects in vivo depend on paracrine factors and cell contact–independent pathways versus cell contact–dependent mechanisms.

There has been enough promising preclinical data in a variety of disease states to initiate human clinical trials. MSCs are currently being studied in acute myocardial infarction, dilated cardiomyopathy, Crohn disease, chronic obstructive pulmonary disease, stroke, multiple sclerosis, acute graft-versus-host disease, type I diabetes mellitus, diabetic foot ulcer, cirrhosis, and immune reconstitution syndrome in human immunodeficiency virus (http://clinicaltrials.gov). The safety record for these cells has been reassuring to date.[73] However, there have not yet been any clinical trials of MSCs in ALI or sepsis, despite the promising work outlined in this article. It is likely that this will change soon. The spectrum of possible MSC-based therapies for ALI includes both targeted intrapulmonary and IV administration, as well as any number of genetic modifications to these versatile cells. Further discussion on possible clinical trials can be found in a recent review.[74]

ACKNOWLEDGMENTS

We thank Diana Lim for her excellent work in preparing Fig. 1.

REFERENCES

1. Ashbaugh DG, Bigelow DB, Petty TL, et al. Acute respiratory distress in adults. Lancet 1967;2(7511):319–23.
2. Matthay MA, Zemans RL. The acute respiratory distress syndrome: pathogenesis and treatment. Annu Rev Pathol 2010. Available at: http://www.ncbi.nlm.nih.gov/pubmed/20936936. Accessed November 3, 2010.
3. Rubenfeld GD, Caldwell E, Peabody E, et al. Incidence and outcomes of acute lung injury. N Engl J Med 2005;353(16):1685–93.
4. Wheeler AP, Bernard GR, Thompson BT, et al. Pulmonary-artery versus central venous catheter to guide treatment of acute lung injury. N Engl J Med 2006;354(21):2213–24.
5. Cepkova M, Matthay MA. Pharmacotherapy of acute lung injury and the acute respiratory distress syndrome. J Intensive Care Med 2006;21(3):119–43.
6. Diaz JV, Brower R, Calfee CS, et al. Therapeutic strategies for severe acute lung injury. Crit Care Med 2010;38(8):1644–50.

7. Calfee CS, Eisner MD, Ware LB, et al. Trauma-associated lung injury differs clinically and biologically from acute lung injury due to other clinical disorders. Crit Care Med 2007;35(10):2243–50.
8. Friedenstein AJ, Petrakova KV, Kurolesova AI, et al. Heterotopic of bone marrow. Analysis of precursor cells for osteogenic and hematopoietic tissues. Transplantation 1968;6(2):230–47.
9. Caplan AI. Adult mesenchymal stem cells for tissue engineering versus regenerative medicine. J Cell Physiol 2007;213(2):341–7.
10. Takashima Y, Era T, Nakao K, et al. Neuroepithelial cells supply an initial transient wave of MSC differentiation. Cell 2007;129(7):1377–88.
11. Bi Y, Ehirchiou D, Kilts TM, et al. Identification of tendon stem/progenitor cells and the role of the extracellular matrix in their niche. Nat Med 2007;13(10): 1219–27.
12. Bieback K, Klüter H. Mesenchymal stromal cells from umbilical cord blood. Curr Stem Cell Res Ther 2007;2(4):310–23.
13. Crisan M, Yap S, Casteilla L, et al. A perivascular origin for mesenchymal stem cells in multiple human organs. Cell Stem Cell 2008;3(3):301–13.
14. Igura K, Zhang X, Takahashi K, et al. Isolation and characterization of mesenchymal progenitor cells from chorionic villi of human placenta. Cytotherapy 2004;6(6):543–53.
15. Xu Y, Malladi P, Wagner DR, et al. Adipose-derived mesenchymal cells as a potential cell source for skeletal regeneration. Curr Opin Mol Ther 2005;7(4): 300–5.
16. Dominici M, Le Blanc K, Mueller I, et al. Minimal criteria for defining multipotent mesenchymal stromal cells. The International Society for Cellular Therapy position statement. Cytotherapy 2006;8(4):315–7.
17. Mansilla E, Marin GH, Sturla F, et al. Human mesenchymal stem cells are tolerized by mice and improve skin and spinal cord injuries. Transplant Proc 2005;37(1): 292–4.
18. Ries C, Egea V, Karow M, et al. MMP-2, MT1-MMP, and TIMP-2 are essential for the invasive capacity of human mesenchymal stem cells: differential regulation by inflammatory cytokines. Blood 2007;109(9):4055–63.
19. Kode JA, Mukherjee S, Joglekar MV, et al. Mesenchymal stem cells: immunobiology and role in immunomodulation and tissue regeneration. Cytotherapy 2009; 11(4):377–91.
20. Ghannam S, Bouffi C, Djouad F, et al. Immunosuppression by mesenchymal stem cells: mechanisms and clinical applications. Stem Cell Res Ther 2010;1(1):2.
21. Le Blanc K, Rasmusson I, Sundberg B, et al. Treatment of severe acute graft-versus-host disease with third party haploidentical mesenchymal stem cells. Lancet 2004;363(9419):1439–41.
22. Valcz G, Krenács T, Sipos F, et al. The role of the bone marrow derived mesenchymal stem cells in colonic epithelial regeneration. Pathol Oncol Res 2010. Available at: http://www.ncbi.nlm.nih.gov/pubmed/20405350. Accessed October 30, 2010.
23. Harting MT, Jimenez F, Xue H, et al. Intravenous mesenchymal stem cell therapy for traumatic brain injury. J Neurosurg 2009;110(6):1189–97.
24. Bowden DH. Unraveling pulmonary fibrosis: the bleomycin model. Lab Invest 1984;50(5):487–8.
25. Harrison JH, Lazo JS. High dose continuous infusion of bleomycin in mice: a new model for drug-induced pulmonary fibrosis. J Pharmacol Exp Ther 1987;243(3): 1185–94.

26. Ortiz LA, Gambelli F, McBride C, et al. Mesenchymal stem cell engraftment in lung is enhanced in response to bleomycin exposure and ameliorates its fibrotic effects. Proc Natl Acad Sci U S A 2003;100(14):8407–11.
27. Ortiz LA, Dutreil M, Fattman C, et al. Interleukin 1 receptor antagonist mediates the antiinflammatory and antifibrotic effect of mesenchymal stem cells during lung injury. Proc Natl Acad Sci U S A 2007;104(26):11002–7.
28. Rojas M, Xu J, Woods CR, et al. Bone marrow-derived mesenchymal stem cells in repair of the injured lung. Am J Respir Cell Mol Biol 2005;33(2):145–52.
29. Moodley Y, Atienza D, Manuelpillai U, et al. Human umbilical cord mesenchymal stem cells reduce fibrosis of bleomycin-induced lung injury. Am J Pathol 2009; 175(1):303–13.
30. Chang YS, Oh W, Choi SJ, et al. Human umbilical cord blood-derived mesenchymal stem cells attenuate hyperoxia-induced lung injury in neonatal rats. Cell Transplant 2009;18(8):869–86.
31. van Haaften T, Byrne R, Bonnet S, et al. Airway delivery of mesenchymal stem cells prevents arrested alveolar growth in neonatal lung injury in rats. Am J Respir Crit Care Med 2009;180(11):1131–42.
32. Baber SR, Deng W, Master RG, et al. Intratracheal mesenchymal stem cell administration attenuates monocrotaline-induced pulmonary hypertension and endothelial dysfunction. Am J Physiol Heart Circ Physiol 2007;292(2):H1120–8.
33. Zhen G, Liu H, Gu N, et al. Mesenchymal stem cells transplantation protects against rat pulmonary emphysema. Front Biosci 2008;13:3415–22.
34. Chignard M, Balloy V. Neutrophil recruitment and increased permeability during acute lung injury induced by lipopolysaccharide. Am J Physiol Lung Cell Mol Physiol 2000;279(6):L1083–90.
35. Yamada M, Kubo H, Kobayashi S, et al. Bone marrow-derived progenitor cells are important for lung repair after lipopolysaccharide-induced lung injury. J Immunol 2004;172(2):1266–72.
36. Mei SH, McCarter SD, Deng Y, et al. Prevention of LPS-induced acute lung injury in mice by mesenchymal stem cells overexpressing angiopoietin 1. PLoS Med 2007;4(9):e269.
37. Xu J, Woods CR, Mora AL, et al. Prevention of endotoxin-induced systemic response by bone marrow-derived mesenchymal stem cells in mice. Am J Physiol Lung Cell Mol Physiol 2007;293(1):L131–41.
38. Gupta N, Su X, Popov B, et al. Intrapulmonary delivery of bone marrow-derived mesenchymal stem cells improves survival and attenuates endotoxin-induced acute lung injury in mice. J Immunol 2007;179(3):1855–63.
39. Krasnodembskaya A, Song Y, Fang X, et al. Antibacterial effect of human mesenchymal stem cells is mediated in part from secretion of the antimicrobial peptide LL-37. Stem cells. 2010. Available at: http://www.ncbi.nlm.nih.gov/pubmed/20945332. Accessed October 30, 2010.
40. Mei SH, Haitsma JJ, Dos Santos CC, et al. Mesenchymal stem cells reduce inflammation while enhancing bacterial clearance and improving survival in sepsis. Am J Respir Crit Care Med 2010;182(8):1047–57.
41. Németh K, Leelahavanichkul A, Yuen PS, et al. Bone marrow stromal cells attenuate sepsis via prostaglandin E(2)-dependent reprogramming of host macrophages to increase their interleukin-10 production. Nat Med 2009;15(1):42–9.
42. Papapetropoulos A, García-Cardeña G, Dengler TJ, et al. Direct actions of angiopoietin-1 on human endothelium: evidence for network stabilization, cell survival, and interaction with other angiogenic growth factors. Lab Invest 1999; 79(2):213–23.

43. Thurston G, Suri C, Smith K, et al. Leakage-resistant blood vessels in mice transgenically overexpressing angiopoietin-1. Science 1999;286(5449):2511–4.
44. Thurston G, Rudge JS, Ioffe E, et al. Angiopoietin-1 protects the adult vasculature against plasma leakage. Nat Med 2000;6(4):460–3.
45. Xu J, Qu J, Cao L, et al. Mesenchymal stem cell-based angiopoietin-1 gene therapy for acute lung injury induced by lipopolysaccharide in mice. J Pathol 2008;214(4):472–81.
46. Lee JW, Fang X, Dolganov G, et al. Acute lung injury edema fluid decreases net fluid transport across human alveolar epithelial type II cells. J Biol Chem 2007; 282(33):24109–19.
47. Fang X, Neyrinck AP, Matthay MA, et al. Allogeneic human mesenchymal stem cells restore epithelial protein permeability in cultured human alveolar type II cells by secretion of angiopoietin-1. J Biol Chem 2010;285(34):26211–22.
48. Matthay MA, Wiener-Kronish JP. Intact epithelial barrier function is critical for the resolution of alveolar edema in humans. Am Rev Respir Dis 1990;142(6 Pt 1): 1250–7.
49. Ware LB, Matthay MA. Alveolar fluid clearance is impaired in the majority of patients with acute lung injury and the acute respiratory distress syndrome. Am J Respir Crit Care Med 2001;163(6):1376–83.
50. Dagenais A, Fréchette R, Yamagata Y, et al. Downregulation of ENaC activity and expression by TNF-alpha in alveolar epithelial cells. Am J Physiol Lung Cell Mol Physiol 2004;286(2):L301–11.
51. Frank JA, Pittet J, Lee H, et al. High tidal volume ventilation induces NOS2 and impairs cAMP- dependent air space fluid clearance. Am J Physiol Lung Cell Mol Physiol 2003;284(5):L791–8.
52. Frank J, Roux J, Kawakatsu H, et al. Transforming growth factor-beta1 decreases expression of the epithelial sodium channel alphaENaC and alveolar epithelial vectorial sodium and fluid transport via an ERK1/2-dependent mechanism. J Biol Chem 2003;278(45):43939–50.
53. Roux J, Kawakatsu H, Gartland B, et al. Interleukin-1beta decreases expression of the epithelial sodium channel alpha-subunit in alveolar epithelial cells via a p38 MAPK-dependent signaling pathway. J Biol Chem 2005;280(19):18579–89.
54. Folkesson HG, Matthay MA. Alveolar epithelial ion and fluid transport: recent progress. Am J Respir Cell Mol Biol 2006;35(1):10–9.
55. Lee JW, Fang X, Gupta N, et al. Allogeneic human mesenchymal stem cells for treatment of *E. coli* endotoxin-induced acute lung injury in the ex vivo perfused human lung. Proc Natl Acad Sci U S A 2009;106(38):16357–62.
56. Prockop DJ. Marrow stromal cells as stem cells for nonhematopoietic tissues. Science 1997;276(5309):71–4.
57. Krause DS, Theise ND, Collector MI, et al. Multi-organ, multi-lineage engraftment by a single bone marrow-derived stem cell. Cell 2001;105(3):369–77.
58. Kopen GC, Prockop DJ, Phinney DG. Marrow stromal cells migrate throughout forebrain and cerebellum, and they differentiate into astrocytes after injection into neonatal mouse brains. Proc Natl Acad Sci U S A 1999;96(19):10711–6.
59. Kotton DN, Ma BY, Cardoso WV, et al. Bone marrow-derived cells as progenitors of lung alveolar epithelium. Development 2001;128(24):5181–8.
60. Liechty KW, MacKenzie TC, Shaaban AF, et al. Human mesenchymal stem cells engraft and demonstrate site-specific differentiation after in utero transplantation in sheep. Nat Med 2000;6(11):1282–6.
61. Aggarwal S, Pittenger MF. Human mesenchymal stem cells modulate allogeneic immune cell responses. Blood 2005;105(4):1815–22.

62. Corcione A, Benvenuto F, Ferretti E, et al. Human mesenchymal stem cells modulate B-cell functions. Blood 2006;107(1):367–72.
63. Glennie S, Soeiro I, Dyson PJ, et al. Bone marrow mesenchymal stem cells induce division arrest anergy of activated T cells. Blood 2005;105(7):2821–7.
64. Spees JL, Olson SD, Whitney MJ, et al. Mitochondrial transfer between cells can rescue aerobic respiration. Proc Natl Acad Sci U S A 2006;103(5):1283–8.
65. Plotnikov EY, Khryapenkova TG, Vasileva AK, et al. Cell-to-cell cross-talk between mesenchymal stem cells and cardiomyocytes in co-culture. J Cell Mol Med 2008; 12(5A):1622–31.
66. Schorey JS, Bhatnagar S. Exosome function: from tumor immunology to pathogen biology. Traffic 2008;9(6):871–81.
67. Deregibus MC, Cantaluppi V, Calogero R, et al. Endothelial progenitor cell derived microvesicles activate an angiogenic program in endothelial cells by a horizontal transfer of mRNA. Blood 2007;110(7):2440–8.
68. Ratajczak J, Miekus K, Kucia M, et al. Embryonic stem cell-derived microvesicles reprogram hematopoietic progenitors: evidence for horizontal transfer of mRNA and protein delivery. Leukemia 2006;20(5):847–56.
69. Bruno S, Grange C, Deregibus MC, et al. Mesenchymal stem cell-derived microvesicles protect against acute tubular injury. J Am Soc Nephrol 2009;20(5): 1053–67.
70. Collino F, Deregibus MC, Bruno S, et al. Microvesicles derived from adult human bone marrow and tissue specific mesenchymal stem cells shuttle selected pattern of miRNAs. PLoS One 2010;5(7):e11803.
71. Meirelles LD, Fontes AM, Covas DT, et al. Mechanisms involved in the therapeutic properties of mesenchymal stem cells. Cytokine Growth Factor Rev 2009;20(5/6): 419–27.
72. Feng J, Mantesso A, Sharpe PT. Perivascular cells as mesenchymal stem cells. Expert Opin Biol Ther 2010;10(10):1441–51.
73. Hare JM, Traverse JH, Henry TD, et al. A randomized, double-blind, placebo-controlled, dose-escalation study of intravenous adult human mesenchymal stem cells (prochymal) after acute myocardial infarction. J Am Coll Cardiol 2009;54(24):2277–86.
74. Matthay MA, Thompson BT, Read EJ, et al. Therapeutic potential of mesenchymal stem cells for severe acute lung injury. Chest 2010;138(4):965–72.

Experimental Models and Emerging Hypotheses for Acute Lung Injury

Thomas R. Martin, MD*, Gustavo Matute-Bello, MD

KEYWORDS

• Lung injury • Animal model • Respiratory distress

Acute lung injury (ALI), and its more severe form, acute respiratory distress syndrome (ARDS), are syndromes of acute hypoxemic respiratory failure resulting from a variety of direct and indirect injuries to the gas exchange parenchyma of the lungs. The clinical syndrome is characterized by critical hypoxemia (partial pressure of oxygen in arterial blood/fraction of inspired oxygen <300 for ALI and <200 for ARDS), bilateral pulmonary infiltrates suggesting edema, no clinical or measured evidence of cardiac failure, and no other explanation for these findings. Pulmonary or nonpulmonary infections with sepsis are the most common causes of ALI and ARDS, although gastric aspiration, massive transfusions, trauma, and other factors contribute.[1] The diversity of causes and the stereotyped physiologic and pathologic responses have made modeling human ALI and ARDS difficult, but new themes are evolving from experimental studies, some of which are reviewed in this article.

Most of what is known about the pathology of ALI and ARDS comes from the studies of patients who have died, although a limited number of patients have undergone open lung biopsy (**Fig. 1**). The pathologic changes include an early phase of diffuse alveolar damage, with an increase in endothelial permeability, evidence of intravascular thrombi, severe epithelial injury with denudation of alveolar wall basement membranes, accumulation of protein and fibrin-rich alveolar infiltrates in the airspaces, and abundant alveolar neutrophilic infiltrates. If patients survive, these changes progress for days to a repair phase, characterized by hyaline membrane formation, transition from neutrophilic to mononuclear infiltrates, and the appearance of intra-alveolar and

Supported in part by a research grant from the Department of Veterans Affairs and grants HL081764 (to TRM) and HL083044 (to GMB) from the National Institutes of Health.

Medical Research Service, Division of Pulmonary and Critical Care Medicine, Department of Medicine, VA Puget Sound Medical Center, University of Washington School of Medicine, Seattle, WA, USA

* Corresponding author. Hospital and Specialty Medicine, 111CHF, VA Puget Sound Medical Center, 1660 South Columbian Way, Seattle, WA 98108.

E-mail address: trmartin@u.washington.edu

Crit Care Clin 27 (2011) 735–752

doi:10.1016/j.ccc.2011.05.013

0749-0704/11/$ – see front matter. Published by Elsevier Inc.

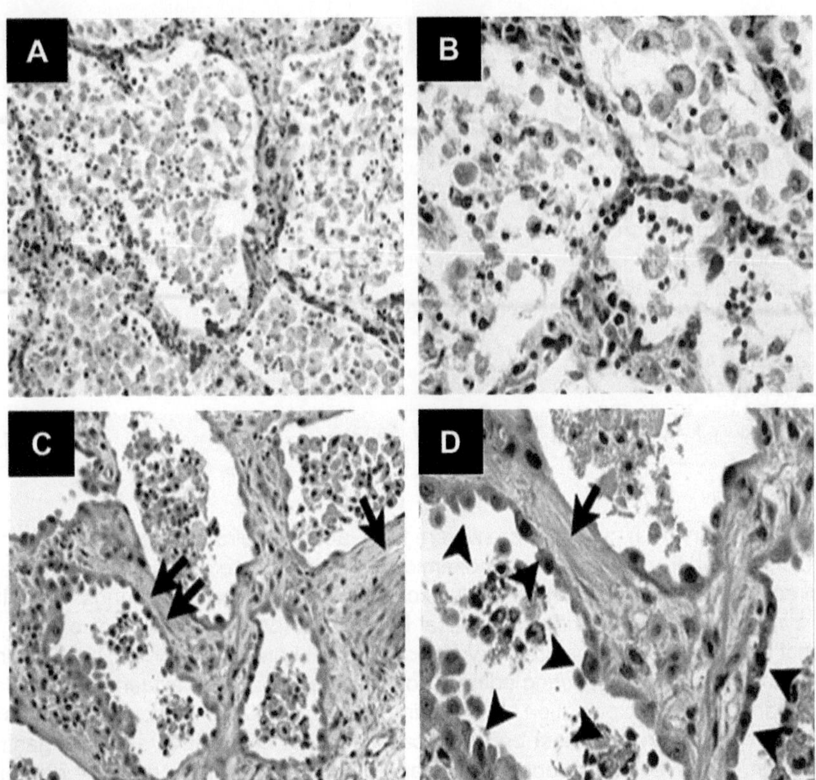

Fig. 1. ALI in humans. Photomicrographs of the lungs of 2 different patients with ALI, stained with hematoxylin and eosin. (*A, B*) Acute phase. Alveolar spaces are filled with a mixed neutrophilic and monocytic infiltrate and alveolar wall capillaries are congested. Alveolar hemorrhage is visible. (*C, D*) Later phase. Fibroproliferative response with collagen deposition in alveolar walls (*arrows*). Alveolar walls are lined with cuboidal epithelial cells that are proliferating type II pneumocytes. (*From* Matute-Bello G, Frevert CW, Martin TR. Animal models of acute lung injury. Am J Physiol Lung Cell Mol Physiol 2008;295:L381; with permission.)

interstitial fibrosis. Patients who survive often have persistent hypoxemia and restrictive ventilatory defects, but both of these abnormalities improve with time after hospital discharge. Neuromuscular weakness, rather than respiratory insufficiency, is the most important cause of long-term disability in survivors of ALI and ARDS.[2,3]

The causative factors that precipitate ALI can be grouped broadly into direct and indirect factors. Direct factors include bacterial and viral infections in the lungs and aspiration of gastric contents, all of which cause direct injury to the airway and alveolar epithelium and other structures in the airspaces. Indirect factors include systemic infections, which cause the sepsis syndrome, blood transfusions, and the effects of systemic medications and illicit drugs. This dual paradigm is plausible, even though clinical studies do not show major differences in outcomes in patients with direct versus indirect ALI.

A major overall theme emerging from clinical studies is that humans are inherently variable in their responses to the stimuli that cause ALI. Although investigators planning clinical trials strive to enroll uniform patient populations, clinicians recognize that patients with seemingly similar stimuli, for example pneumococcal bacteremia, vary a great deal in the clinical severity of their disease. Studies of how normal people respond to the common bacterial stimulus, gram-negative lipopolysaccharide (LPS), show differences of more than 2 orders of magnitude in cytokine responses in whole blood.[4] Studies of normal humans who were high or low responders to bacterial products identified a polymorphism in the Toll-like receptor (TLR)1 that marked high cytokine responses to gram-positive bacterial peptidoglycan.[5] This polymorphism was more common in critically ill patients with gram-positive sepsis who died. Thus, studying variability in innate immune responses in the normal population can provide important insights about disease susceptibility in critically ill patients.

MODELING ARDS: THE ROLE OF ANIMAL MODELS

Modeling the acute and chronic pathologic changes of ALI to understand the cellular and molecular pathogenesis has been a significant challenge from the time that ARDS was first described in humans.[6,7] Many different animal models have been used and each has advantages and disadvantages.[8] The ideal animal model would include an acute inflammatory response with an increase in microvascular and alveolar epithelial permeability, neutrophil influx into the alveolar spaces, and protein and fibrin-rich alveolar exudates in the acute phase. This response would be followed by an organization phase with an increase in alveolar mononuclear cells and interstitial lymphocytes, and a repair phase with proliferating type II pneumocytes and fibroblasts, and accumulation of interstitial and alveolar fibrin. These changes would be accompanied by acute hypoxemia and a decrease in lung compliance, along with measurable changes in systemic organ function. Ideally, the animal would be treated with mechanical ventilation to simulate the primary treatment applied to patients with ALI. These changes would evolve for several days, and surviving animals would be amenable to longer-term outcome studies to assess persistent changes in lung function and systemic organ function, particularly in the neuromuscular system.

Only large animal models permit studies in ventilated animals over time, such as ventilated and tracheostomized primates, dogs, sheep, or pigs. Such models are extremely expensive, because of the need to create an animal intensive care unit, and molecular reagents for large animals are limited. Short-term studies in mice, rats, and rabbits have been useful in studying individual pathways, but the ability to generalize results to humans is limited.[8] Nevertheless, if the characteristics of the animal model are well known and the results are interpreted with appropriate caution, animal studies can provide focused evaluations of key physiologic and molecular pathways, and can be used to develop new hypotheses to test in humans.

Aside from size, important physiologic and immunologic differences exist among animal species (**Table 1**). Pulmonary intravascular macrophages (PIMs) are prominent in the pulmonary microcirculation of sheep, pigs, goats, cattle, and horses. In these animals, intravascular particles, including microbes, are more likely to localize in the pulmonary microcirculation and stimulate local intravascular inflammatory responses. Dogs, rodents, rabbits, nonhuman primates, and humans have few PIMs, and intravascular particles localize to macrophages in liver and spleen.[9] Depletion of PIMs in sheep reduced lung injury from intravenous LPS.[10] The nitric oxide (NO) pathway promotes vasodilation and microbial killing, and important species differences exist in NO production.[11] Inducible nitric oxide synthase is prominent in rodents, and NO production is an important microbial killing mechanism in murine macrophages. Human macrophages produce far less NO unless they are suitably activated, typically by interferon-γ.[12–14] Nevertheless, the NO products, nitrate and nitrite, and evidence

Table 1
Unique characteristics of animal species relevant to modeling lung injury

Animal	Identity with Human TLR4 HVR (%)	Pulmonary Intravascular Macrophages	LPS Sensitivity	Nitric Oxide Production
Human	100	No	Intermediate	+
NHP	95	No	Intermediate	+
Pig	ND	Yes	High	++
Dog	ND	No	Low	++
Sheep	ND	Yes	High	++
Rabbit	57	No	Intermediate	++
Rat	48	No	Low	+++
Mouse	48	No	Low	+++

Abbreviations: HVR, hypervariable region of TLR4; ND, not determined; NH, nonhuman primate.
From Matute-Bello G, Frevert CW, Martin TR. Animal models of acute lung injury. Am J Physiol Lung Cell Mol Physiol 2008;295:L381; with permission.

of nitration of intracellular proteins are detectable in the bronchoalveolar lavage fluid and alveolar macrophages of humans with ALI,[15] suggesting that NO-dependent reactions are important in ALI. Bacterial recognition pathways via TLRs also differ among species,[16] and divergent forms of TLR4 recognize different LPS structures,[17] which could contribute to the known variation in LPS sensitivity among different species.

EMERGING THEMES FROM ANIMAL MODELS AND EXPERIMENTAL STUDIES

Interactions Between Stretch and Innate Immunity

One important theme in clinical and experimental ALI is that activation of innate immunity adversely affects the lung's response to mechanical stretch. Patients with normal lungs, such as those with neuromuscular diseases, can be ventilated with large tidal volumes exceeding 10 mL/kg without causing injury. Experimental studies show that, at normal tidal volumes, the alveolar walls in rodent lungs fold and unfold, whereas alveolar walls do not begin to stretch until lung volumes exceed about 40% of total lung capacity.[18] In contrast, the effective alveolar volume of injured lungs is much lower than normal, owing to large areas of alveolar filling and collapse. In this case, the use of normal tidal volumes results in stretching of the walls of the open alveolar units. Experimental studies in a variety of systems show that activation of innate immunity pathways through TLR4 and other TLRs triggers acute inflammation and an increase in alveolar epithelial permeability. When human alveolar macrophages are exposed to cyclic pressure, cotreatment with LPS causes a marked accentuation of cytokine responses.[19] Pretreatment of rats with intravenous LPS accentuated cytokine and inflammatory responses when the lungs were ventilated ex vivo.[20] Mechanical ventilation and intravenous LPS have synergistic effects on lung inflammation at moderate tidal volumes via activation of complex transcriptional pathways.[21–23] In addition to direct pulmonary effects, mechanical ventilation and intravenous LPS interact to cause systemic organ dysfunction, which is relevant for the pathogenesis of multiorgan failure.[24] This seems to occur in part by enhancement of GADD45-mediated signaling pathways in the lungs.[22] The GADD45-γ isoform activates a MAPK kinase kinase (MEKK4), leading to activation of p38 MAP kinase and Jun kinase (JNK), resulting in enhanced cytokine production. Mechanical stretch also causes upregulation of CD14 in rabbit lungs, and increased sensitivity of alveolar macrophages to LPS ex vivo.[25] Because CD14 is a key coreceptor for LPS with TLR4, increased expression of CD14 provides a mechanism for synergy between LPS and larger tidal volume ventilation. In studies of ventilated mice, Smith and colleagues[26] have found that this synergism between innate immunity and mechanical stretch seems to be acquired with age, because it does not occur in 3-week-old mice but is reproducibly present in 12-week-old mice.

Other activators of innate immunity are also present in the lungs of patients with ALI. A series of studies have shown that endogenous products generated by injury and inflammatory responses cause sterile inflammation when bacterial products are absent.[27] These products, termed alarmins or danger-associated molecular patterns (DAMPs), include matrix molecules, hyaluronan, the nuclear protein HMGB1, oxidized phospholipids, and other factors that are present in normal lungs and released into the airspaces as a result of injury or inflammation.[28–31] These endogenous products activate TLR4 and other TLRs, initiating inflammation in the same manner as LPS and other bacterial products. By implication, these endogenous molecules should also synergize with mechanical stretch to intensify injury in the lungs. One of the primary suggestions from this line of research is that interrupting the synergistic interactions between innate immunity and mechanical stretch in the lungs would be a strategy to limit the onset or severity of ALI in humans.

The Fate of the Alveolar Epithelium in ALI

Death of the alveolar epithelium in ALI can occur by either necrosis or apoptosis. The classic studies of Bachofen and Weibel[32] examining lungs of patients who died with ALI showed evidence of widespread alveolar epithelial injury, in addition to alveolar hyaline membranes, microvascular injury, and thrombosis. Experimental studies have shown that high distending pressures caused by mechanical ventilation lead directly to disruption and necrosis of the alveolar epithelium in rats.[33,34] In addition, type III bacterial exotoxins, such as pseudomonas ExoU and ExoS, cause direct lysis of the alveolar epithelium and other cells by attacking the cell membrane.[35,36] Disruption of the alveolar epithelium by mechanical stretch can be treated by reducing the ventilator tidal volume, and is likely to explain, in part, the major success of the initial ARDS network trial of low-tidal-volume ventilation in ALI.[37] Because necrosis cannot be regulated by manipulating cellular pathways, strategies to minimize necrosis must aim at prevention by lowering tidal volume and eradicating bacterial infection.

Apoptosis is a regulated form of cell death that has an essential role in development and repair. An important theme from experimental studies is that cell death pathways are activated in the lungs of patients with ALI and are likely to contribute to alveolar epithelial death.[38] Apoptosis is mediated by a family of death receptors, principally the tumor necrosis factor (TNF) receptors (TNFR1 and TNFR2) and the Fas receptor. TNFα is not abundant in bronchoalveolar lavage (BAL) fluid of patients with ALI, and the concentrations of the soluble TNF receptors far exceeds the concentrations of free TNFα, suggesting that TNF activity that exists is localized to lung tissues.[39,40] The Fas receptor is present on the alveolar and airway epithelium,[41] and biologically active soluble Fas ligand (sFasL) is detectable in the airspaces of patients with ALI.[42,43] In experimental studies, activation of the Fas receptor in the lungs of mice causes alveolar epithelial apoptosis, and increased epithelial permeability and alveolar hemorrhage in rabbits.[44,45] In mice and rabbits, activation of Fas also causes inflammation, with production of interleukin (IL)-8 and other acute inflammatory cytokines. Repeated activation of Fas in mice causes acute inflammation, an acute increase in alveolar epithelial permeability, and delayed fibrosis, which is dependent on macrophage metalloelastase, MMP-12.[46] Studies with chimeric animals have shown that

Fas on nonmyeloid cells of the lungs is required for apoptosis and inflammation to occur in response to Fas activation.[47]

The sFasL molecule is released from cell membranes via the action of membrane MMP-7.[48,49] Like TNFα, sFasL multimerizes in aqueous solution and the multimeric form clusters Fas receptors in the cell membrane. Clustered Fas molecules recruit caspase-8 molecules to the intracellular portions of the Fas molecules to form the death-inducing complex (DISC). Caspase-8 clusters are autocatalytic, yielding cleaved caspase-8, which initiates caspase cascades that lead to fragmentation of nuclear DNA and cellular apoptosis. The biologic activity of sFasL depends on the structure of the N-terminal sequence of the molecule, and the state of aggregation.[50] Oxidation of key methionine residues promotes aggregation of sFasL in solution and enhances biologic activity. Free MMP-7 cleaves the stalk region and reduces biologic activity, so that the intensity of the oxidizing environment and the concentration of soluble MMP-7 regulate the biologic activity of sFasL in vivo.[50] Mice lacking an active Fas receptor (*lpr* mice) have reduced lung inflammation when undergoing large-volume mechanical ventilation. Inactivation of Fas signaling in normal mice using siRNA technology reduced secondary lung injury in response to hemorrhagic shock and cecal ligation and puncture, suggesting that the Fas pathway in the lungs connects systemic responses with alveolar inflammation and epithelial injury.[51,52]

These and other data support the theme that Fas-mediated alveoli epithelial apoptosis is likely to be important in the acute lung injury process in humans, which in turn suggests that a strategy to inhibit apoptosis in the lungs might be useful in limiting the severity of ALI in humans. Apoptosis is also important in the resolution of injury,[53] and tissue repair processes are initiated at the onset of ALI in humans,[54,55] so any strategy modulating cellular apoptosis would have to be focused on the early phase of ALI to avoid interfering with normal repair in the lungs.

TGFβ as a Key Mediator of ALI

Transforming growth factor β (TGFβ) is a pleuripotent cytokine that has a key role in tissue homeostasis. A latent form of TGFβ is activated when bound by the integrin α-v-β 6 in lungs and skin.[56] Mice lacking the a-v-b 6 integrin were protected from lung injury following intratracheal bleomycin, and mice treated with an anti-TGFβ construct were protected from lung injury caused by bleomycin or LPS. TGFβ enhanced epithelial permeability in vitro in part by depleting intracellular glutathione.[57] A subsequent study showed that TGFβ1 reduced expression of the epithelial sodium channel (ENaC), and reduced sodium and water transport across rat and human type II alveolar epithelial cells and reduced amiloride sensitive sodium transport in intact rat lungs at a low dose that did not affect alveolar epithelial permeability.[58] These animal studies suggest that TGFβ activation in the lungs of patients with ALI could be a mechanism that contributes to epithelial injury and impairs sodium and water transport out of the alveolar spaces. Strategies to inhibit TGFβ transiently might be considered in humans with ALI.

Networks and Complexity

Animal models of ALI and ARDS have been used primarily to study single pathways involved in lung injury, but treatments designed to inhibit single pathways have been unsuccessful in patients with sepsis, as well as ALI. Advances in proteomics and genomics technologies have enabled investigators to appreciate the complexity of ALI in humans as well as in animal models. In humans, analysis of proteins in human BAL fluid shows the complexity of protein networks at the onset of ALI and the changes that occur over time.[59] Key nodes in these networks identify central proteins, which could provide targets for new treatments. In addition, proteomics analysis identified the unsuspected importance of the nonprotein, β-estradiol, as a node in major protein networks. Gene array technology illustrated the complexity of mRNA networks in a canine model of ventilator-induced lung injury.[60] Genes involved in inflammation and immune responses, cell proliferation, adhesion, signaling, and apoptosis were activated in the lungs, and major regional differences were noted between dependent and nondependent areas. This approach provided additional support for the role of apoptosis pathways in ALI. Genomic approaches have also been used to study the complexity of transcriptional responses in mice treated with mechanical ventilation with or without systemic LPS.[23] Integrating gene expression profiling with gene ontology and promoter analysis enabled the construction of a regulatory map of important processes in the lungs of ventilated animals in the presence or absence of LPS as a simultaneous activator of innate immunity (**Fig. 2**). Differentially expressed biologic modules included those related to defense responses, immune responses, and oxidoreductase activity. The gene regulatory network included transcription factors such as IFN-stimulated response element IRF-7 and Sp1 (**Table 2**). Studies such as these highlight the complexity of the lung responses in experimental animals with ALI, and set the stage for strategies that address multiple pathways simultaneously or sequentially in critically ill humans.

New Understanding of Specific Risk Factors for ALI

Animal models have provided a new understanding of several risk factors for ALI, including the pathogenesis of ALI following gastric aspiration and the transfusion of blood products, and the roles of chronic alcohol use and fever. Aspiration of gastric contents exposes the airway and alveolar environment to a complex mixture of acid, particulates, and oropharyngeal bacteria and bacterial products. The classic model of acid aspiration in animals involves intratracheal instillation of acid, typically pH 1.5. This acid causes ALI and inflammation with production of IL-8 and other proinflammatory cytokines. However, humans are routinely treated with H-2 antagonists and/or proton pump inhibitors, so that the pH of gastric acid is typically much higher in patients, and less acidic solutions do not injure the lungs of animals. Bregeon and colleagues[61] sampled gastric juice from critically ill patients and studied proinflammatory activity using a validated target cell assay. The gastric juice from critically ill patients had more proinflammatory activity than was detected in gastric juice of ventilated control patients. The samples with high proinflammatory activity in vitro caused intense lung inflammation in the lungs of ventilated rabbits, which was dependent on IL-1β activity in the gastric juice and independent of pH and particulate matter. This finding helps to explain the intense, and often transient, inflammatory responses associated with gastric aspiration in patients who are treated with antacid regimens.

Transfusions of red blood cells, platelets, and other high volume plasma blood products are known to be associated with transfusion reactions, which can lead to severe transfusion-associated lung injury (TRALI).[62] Animal models show that a priming event, such as administration of intravenous or intratracheal LPS, is usually required for lung injury, consistent with the observation that TRALI is more common in humans with critical illness. Interactions between antibodies, leukocytes, and platelets are typically involved, and lipid mediators in plasma also have been implicated. In one model, passive infusion of anti–MHC-1 antibodies led to TRALI that was dependent on the Fc-γ receptor, neutrophils, and platelets.[63,64] Mice raised in a barrier facility were less susceptible, and pretreating the mice with either intravenous or intratracheal LPS restored susceptibility. Studies with chimeric mice showed that the functional TLR4 on leukocytes was required for this effect, which increases trapping of

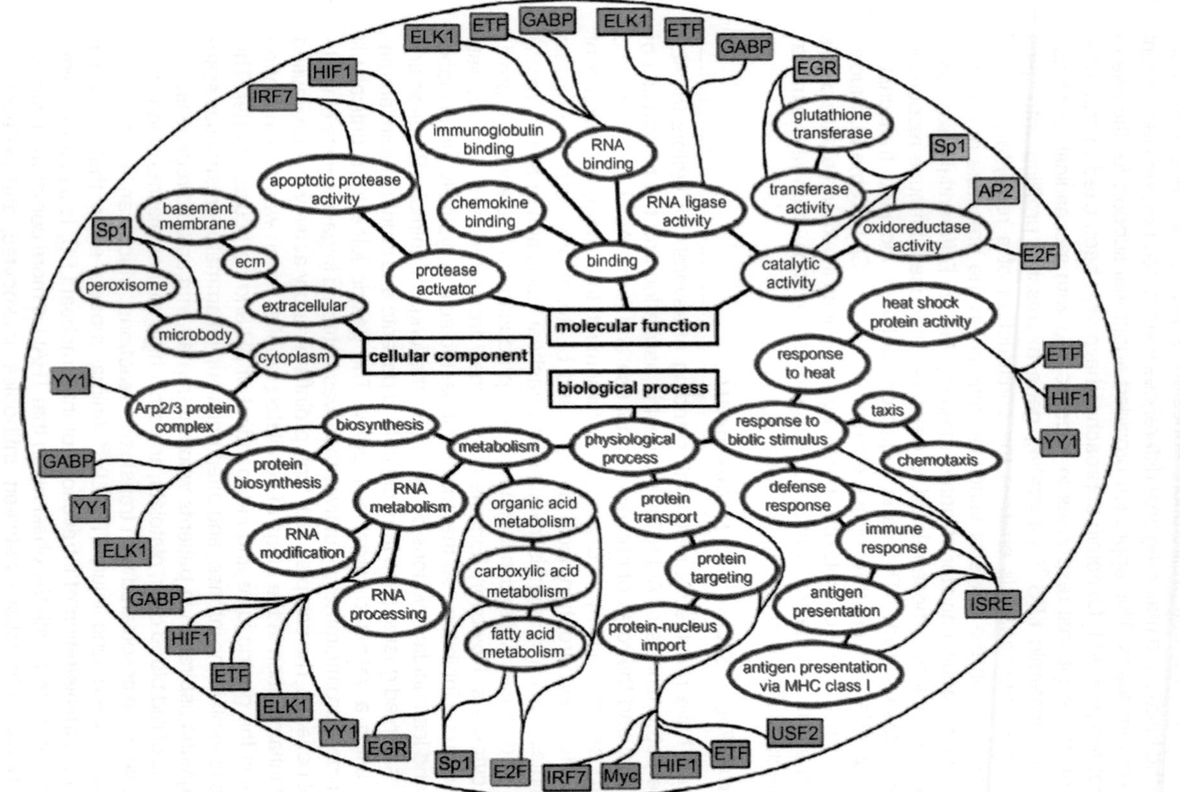

Fig. 2. Important processes and transcription factors identified during ALI in mice treated with intratracheal LPS and mechanical ventilation. Overrepresented biologic modules among upregulated (*red ovals*) and downregulated (*blue ovals*) genes are organized based on their gene ontology annotations and are assigned to 1 of 3 groups: molecular function, cellular components, and biologic processes. Putative transcription factors regulating genes within these modules are shown in the periphery. (*From* Gharib SA, Liles WC, Matute-Bello G, et al. Computational identification of key biologic modules and transcription factors in acute lung injury. Am J Respir Crit Care Med 2006;173:657; with permission.)

polymorphonuclear leukocytes in the lung microcirculation and superoxide production in response to stimuli. Thus, there seems to be a key role for activation of innate immunity via TLR4, and perhaps other TLRs, in enhancing susceptibility to TRALI.

Animal and clinical studies have contributed to understanding the mechanisms by which chronic alcohol ingestion increases susceptibility to lung injury.[65,66] Rats fed a high-alcohol diet (36% of total calories) develop glutathione depletion in the epithelial lining fluid of the lungs and reduced sodium and water transport in vivo.[67] Glutathione is a major intracellular pathway for capturing oxidant species, and glutathione depletion renders the lungs and other tissues susceptible to oxidative injury. Glutathione is depleted in type II pneumocytes from rats fed high-alcohol diets, and type II monolayers have increased permeability to high-molecular-weight solutes.[68,69] These experimental observations parallel findings in clinically stable people who ingest alcohol on a chronic basis, who have reduced concentrations of glutathione in the alveolar epithelial lining fluid and have increased susceptibility to lung injury.[70]

Fever is a beneficial host response to bacterial and other infections, but many patients with ALI who are treated with antibiotic regimens do not have overt bacterial infection in the lungs.[71] Fever improves outcome in mice with peritonitis and in other models of infection,[72] but fever also worsens the response of the lungs to hyperoxia and localized klebsiella infections, in part by enhancing neutrophil recruitment.[73,74] Lipke and colleagues[75] found that fever has dramatic effects on innate immunity in the lungs, because the induction of fever in mice treated with low doses of LPS to stimulate TLR4 causes a dramatic increase in mortality, which is associated with the induction of apoptosis pathways in the lungs. These findings will drive better clinical studies of the effects of fever in patients who do not have major microbial infections.

Stem Cells in Lung Injury

One of the most interesting themes from animal studies is that mesenchymal stem cells can modulate ALI. Mesenchymal stem cells (MSC) are a population of progenitor cells with the ability to self-renew in an undifferentiated state and differentiate into mesenchymal tissues, such as bone, fat, smooth muscle, or collagen.[76] MSC have been known to exist in the mononuclear cell fraction of bone marrow, as defined by density gradient centrifugation.[77] The International Society for Cellular Therapy has proposed the following criteria to define multipotent stromal mesenchymal cells: (1) adhesion to plastic; (2) expression of CD105, CD73, and CD90, and lack of expression of CD45, CD34, CD14 or CD11b, CD79a or CD19, and HLA-DR surface molecules; and (3) ability to differentiate into osteoblasts, adipocytes, and chondroblasts in vitro.[78]

Initial studies investigating the role of bone marrow–derived MSC (BM-MSC) in pulmonary fibrosis focused on the hypothesis that BM-MSC could be protective by regenerating injured lung tissue. In a seminal study, Ortiz and colleagues[79] found that bleomycin-induced lung injury was decreased in C57BL/6 mice receiving intravenous injections of BM-MSC purified from bleomycin-resistant BALB/c mice, compared with mice receiving no BM-MSC. The protective effect occurred only when the BM-MSC were given immediately after the bleomycin challenge, but not when the cells were administered 7 days after bleomycin. Subsequent studies suggested that bleomycin induces mobilization of BM-MSC from the bone marrow, and possible migration into the lungs.[80,81] Some of these studies suggest that the BM-MSC engraft in the lungs and can differentiate into a variety of cell types.[81] However, subsequent studies have shown that, although engraftment can occur, it is rare and the physiologic significance remains uncertain.[82–84] Despite significant engraftment, MSC administration in a variety of injury models is associated with a decrease in the expression of several inflammatory cytokines, showing that the BM-MSC are

Table 2
Enriched putative transcription factors among differentially expressed genes during mechanical ventilation (MV), LPS, and MV+LPS relative to untreated animals

MV vs Control		LPS vs Control		MV+LPS vs Control	
Transcription Factor	*P* Value	Transcription Factor	*P* Value	Transcription Factor	*P* Value
Overrepresented Putative Transcription Factors Among Differentially Upregulated Genes					
ETF	4.62×10^{-17}	ISRE	8.03×10^{-16}	ETF	1.29×10^{-11}
E2F	5.36×10^{-12}	cRel	8.51×10^{-11}	ISRE	2.48×10^{-8}
Nrf1	1.12×10^{-9}	IRF	3.69×10^{-10}	NF–B	2.43×10^{-7}
CREB	3.64×10^{-8}	NFκB	1.26×10^{-9}	cRel	3.84×10^{-7}
HIF1	1.35×10^{-6}	ICSBP	1.08×10^{-7}	CREB	8.01×10^{-7}
—	—	PU.1	4.91×10^{-6}	IRF-7	1.92×10^{-6}
—	—	—	—	ATF	2.05×10^{-6}
Overrepresented Putative Transcription Factors Among Differentially Downregulated Genes					
Sp1	3.01×10^{-6}	Sp1	8.38×10^{-17}	Sp1	5.16×10^{-26}
NF-Y	8.17×10^{-5}	E2F	1.96×10^{-14}	E2F	1.18×10^{-21}
—	—	NF-Y	1.96×10^{-7}	EGR	1.30×10^{-9}
—	—	AP2	2.31×10^{-6}	ZF5	1.78×10^{-9}
—	—	—	—	AP2	2.99×10^{-9}
—	—	—	—	NF-Y	4.16×10^{-9}

From Gharib SA, Liles WC, Matute-Bello G, et al. Computational identification of key biologic modules and transcription factors in acute lung injury. Am J Respir Crit Care Med 2006;173:656; with permission.

able to modulate the inflammatory response. Gupta and colleagues[85] confirmed the immunomodulatory properties of BM-MSC in vivo by finding that direct intratracheal instillation of BM-MSC attenuates LPS-induced lung injury by mechanisms involving a paracrine effect unrelated to tissue regeneration. Later studies by Ortiz and colleagues[86] suggested that the protective effect of BM-MSC on bleomycin-induced lung injury is largely related to the ability of BM-MSC to release the IL-1β receptor antagonist (IL-1RA). Since then, several studies have shown that BM-MSCs can attenuate injury in different experimental animal models.[87] Thus, BM-MSCs attenuate lung injury by immunomodulation, and most studies published thus far suggest a protective role. The role of MSC in lung inflammation and fibrosis is the subject of a separate review.[88]

Resolution of ALI

Human studies have shown that repair processes are initiated almost as soon as ALI begins. Markers of collagen production, reflecting activation of repair processes, are detectable at the onset of ALI.[54,55] A great deal of work has been devoted to determining how neutrophils and their products are cleared from inflamed lungs. Isolated neutrophils rapidly undergo apoptosis in vitro, but the lung fluids of patients with ALI delay neutrophil apoptosis by a mechanism involving G-CSF and GM-CSF in lung fluids.[89] Apoptotic neutrophils are rapidly ingested by macrophages in the airspaces, via recognition of phosphatidyl serine, calreticulin, and other structures expressed on the surface of apoptotic leukocytes.[90–92] Neutrophil myeloperoxidase and other debris are identifiable in alveolar macrophages recovered from the BAL fluid of patients with ALI.[89] The mechanisms that control the uptake and clearance of leukocytes and other cells undergoing necrosis or other nonapoptotic cell death are less well understood.

A new theme from animal studies is that lymphocytes also have an important role in the resolution of ALI. Studies with Rag-1$^{-/-}$ mice, which lack mature B and T cells, showed that resolution of LPS-induced lung inflammation was markedly delayed.[93] Mortality was higher in the Rag-1$^{-/-}$ mice, and they remained clinically ill for a longer period of time than similarly treated C57BL/6 mice. Reconstitution of the Rag-1$^{-/-}$ mice with regulatory T cells expressing the IL-1α receptor and the FoxP3 transcription factor (Tregs), improved the resolution of lung injury. Tregs increased with time after the onset of LPS-induced lung inflammation in normal mice, and transfer of Tregs into Rag-1$^{-/-}$ mice increased lung levels of TGFβ and enhanced neutrophil apoptosis. Following these animal studies, the investigators found that Tregs were detectable by flow cytometry in lung lavage fluids of patients with ALI. Manipulation of regulatory T cells might offer an approach to enhancing the repair of ALI.

Viruses and ALI

A consistent theme from animal studies is that the clinical manifestations of viral infections in the lungs reflect the primary sites of infection in the lungs. Adenoviruses infect primarily the airway epithelium via receptors on the basolateral surface of airway epithelial cells. This feature made replication-deficient adenoviral vectors attractive for gene therapy in the lungs. Adenoviral infections are characterized by bronchopneumonia, which can be severe, leading to acute respiratory failure. Studies in nonhuman primates showed that the severe acute respiratory syndrome (SARS) virus attacks alveolar type II cells, and SARS is associated with diffuse lung injury reflecting alveolar epithelial damage.[94,95] By contrast, the hantavirus is found in lung microvascular endothelial cells and causes widespread lung edema soon after onset of the infection.

An additional theme from animal studies is that viral infections also enhance the sensitivity of the lungs to mechanical ventilation. Bem and colleagues[96] found that mice infected with mouse pneumovirus to simulate respiratory syncytial virus (RSV) infection in children and then subjected to mechanical ventilation had much more severe lung inflammatory and injury responses than mice infected with pneumovirus alone, or mice treated with mechanical ventilation alone. The infected mice had increased cytokine production, increased alveolar epithelial permeability, and activation of apoptosis pathways. This suggests that the key treatment of children with severe RSV infection, mechanical ventilation, can worsen the response of the lungs to the underlying viral infection. Viruses stimulate innate immunity by interacting with TLR3 on the surface of macrophages and other cells. These and other findings support the conclusion that activation of innate immunity via several different TLRs has a synergistic effect with mechanical ventilation on lung injury.

Lung Injury in Children

One of the themes from clinical studies is that ALI is less frequent and less severe in children than adults even though mortality in unselected children with ALI is approximately 20%.[1,97] Children have lungs that are still developing, and children typically have fewer comorbidities than adults with ALI. Nevertheless, a new theme from animal studies is that the interactions between the mechanical ventilator and the lungs of children might be different than in adults. Smith and colleagues[26] compared the pulmonary responses of juvenile (3 weeks old, 5–7 g) and adult (16 weeks old, 25–30 g) mice in a model in which the mice were treated with intratracheal LPS, then subjected to mechanical ventilation for 2 or 4 hours. The adult mice had a synergistic increase in lung inflammation and protein permeability, as compared with animals treated with LPS alone, or mechanical ventilation alone. In contrast, a synergistic interaction between LPS treatment and mechanical ventilation was not found in the juvenile mice. This finding suggests that the adverse interactions between innate immunity and mechanical stretch increase with age. Microarray studies showed that there were major differences in clusters of genes activated in the juvenile and adult lungs in response to LPS and mechanical ventilation and suggested pathways that might be responsible for the different responses of juveniles and adults. Alvira and colleagues[98] treated neonatal and adult mice with intraperitoneal LPS and found that lung inflammation and apoptosis occurred in adult but not neonatal mice. This finding was associated with persistent activation of NF-κB p65/p50 heterodimers in the neonates, whereas in the adults there was initial activation of NF-κB p65/p50 followed by sustained activation of NF-κB p50/p50 homodimers. Developmental differences in NF-κB activation could influence the severity or outcome of pulmonary infections, or the pulmonary response to mechanical ventilation. These studies comparing infant and adult animals could provide a much better perspective on the mechanisms that account for protection from ALI in children and increased susceptibility in adults.

SUMMARY

ALI is an important clinical problem that affects more than 200,000 people per year in the United States. Animal models have been useful in studying individual pathways involved in pathogenesis and new ideas for treatment. No single animal model mimics all of the clinical features of ALI in humans, and each animal model has unique features that affect responses to treatment. Nevertheless, many themes have emerged from animal models that provide valuable insight about lung injury in humans. Studies of innate immunity have shown that innate immunity is triggered not only by microbial products but also by endogenous byproducts of tissue damage and inflammation that can drive inflammation even in the absence of microbial products in tissue. Variability in host innate immune responses accounts for a great deal of variability in the clinical manifestations of ALI. Innate immunity and mechanical stretch have important synergistic interactions in adults that accentuate ALI. These synergistic interactions seem to be acquired with age and are much less pronounced in juvenile animals. Apoptosis pathways are important in clearance of bacteria from the lungs, and also in causing injury and death to alveolar epithelial cells, enhancing permeability edema. Animal models have highlighted the complexity of ALI in humans, by showing the multiplicity of pathways activated by microbial products, mechanical stretch, and the combination. Analysis of protein networks has identified unexpected components that link key protein pathways in the lungs. New light has been shed on clinical risk factors for ALI, such as gastric aspiration, blood product transfusion, alcohol excess, and fever. Stem cell biology has been extended to ALI with the finding of unexpected paracrine effects of MSC in reducing the severity of ALI. New ideas about the resolution of ALI have derived from studies of the clearance of apoptotic cells in the lungs, and the role of regulatory lymphocytes in recovery from lung inflammation and injury. Progress is being made, but strong links between the laboratory and the critical care bedside are still needed to translate new ideas from laboratory studies into clinical treatments that will lessen the severity and improve the outcome from ALI.

REFERENCES

1. Rubenfeld GD, Caldwell E, Peabody E, et al. Incidence and outcomes of acute lung injury. N Engl J Med 2005;353:1685–93.
2. Herridge MS, Cheung AM, Tansey CM, et al. One-year outcomes in survivors of the acute respiratory distress syndrome. N Engl J Med 2003;348:683–93.
3. Herridge MS, Tansey CM, Matte A, et al. Functional disability 5 years after acute respiratory distress syndrome. N Engl J Med 2011;364:1293–304.
4. Wurfel MM, Park WY, Radella F, et al. Identification of high and low responders to lipopolysaccharide in normal subjects: an unbiased approach to identify modulators of innate immunity. J Immunol 2005;175:2570–8.
5. Wurfel MM, Gordon AC, Holden TD, et al. Toll-like receptor 1 polymorphisms affect innate immune responses and outcomes in sepsis. Am J Respir Crit Care Med 2008;178:710–20.
6. Ashbaugh DG, Bigelow DB, Petty TL, et al. Acute respiratory distress in adults. Lancet 1967;2:319–23.
7. Petty TL, Ashbaugh DG. The adult respiratory distress syndrome. Clinical features and factors influencing prognosis and principles of management. Chest 1971;60:233–9.
8. Matute-Bello G, Frevert CW, Martin TR. Animal models of acute lung injury. Am J Physiol Lung Cell Mol Physiol 2008;295:L379–99.
9. Brain JD, Molina RM, deCamp MM, et al. Pulmonary intravascular macrophages: their contribution to the mononuclear phagocyte system in 13 species. Am J Physiol 1999;276:L146–54.
10. Sone Y, Serikov VB, Staub NC Sr. Intravascular macrophage depletion attenuates endotoxin lung injury in anesthetized sheep. J Appl Physiol 1999;87:1354–9.
11. Schneemann M, Schoedon G. Species differences in macrophage NO production are important. Nat Immunol 2002;3:102.
12. Schneemann M, Schoedon G, Hofer S, et al. Nitric oxide synthase is not a constituent of the antimicrobial armature of human mononuclear phagocytes. J Infect Dis 1993;167:1358–63.

13. Panaro MA, Acquafredda A, Lisi S, et al. Inducible nitric oxide synthase and nitric oxide production in *Leishmania infantum*-infected human macrophages stimulated with interferon-gamma and bacterial lipopolysaccharide. Int J Clin Lab Res 1999;29:122–7.
14. Nicolson S, da Gloria Bonecini-Almeida M, Lapa e Silva JR, et al. Inducible nitric oxide synthase in pulmonary alveolar macrophages from patients with tuberculosis. J Exp Med 1996;183:2293–302.
15. Sittipunt C, Steinberg KP, Ruzinski JT, et al. Nitric oxide and nitrotyrosine in the lungs of patients with acute respiratory distress syndrome. Am J Respir Crit Care Med 2001;163:503–10.
16. Rehli M. Of mice and men: species variations of Toll-like receptor expression. Trends Immunol 2002;23:375–8.
17. Hajjar AM, Ernst RK, Tsai JH, et al. Human Toll-like receptor 4 recognizes host-specific LPS modifications. Nat Immunol 2002;3:354–9.
18. Tschumperlin DJ, Margulies SS. Alveolar epithelial surface area-volume relationship in isolated rat lungs. J Appl Physiol 1999;86:2026–33.
19. Pugin J, Dunn I, Jolliet P, et al. Activation of human macrophages by mechanical ventilation in vitro. Am J Physiol 1999;275:L1040–50.
20. Tremblay L, Valenza F, Ribeiro SP, et al. Injurious ventilatory strategies increase cytokines and cfos mRNA expression in an isolated rat lung model. J Clin Invest 1997;5:944–52.
21. Altemeier WA, Matute-Bello G, Frevert CW, et al. Mechanical ventilation with moderate tidal volumes synergistically increases lung cytokine response to systemic endotoxin. Am J Physiol Lung Cell Mol Physiol 2004;287:L533–42.
22. Altemeier WA, Matute-Bello G, Gharib SA, et al. Modulation of lipopolysaccharide-induced gene transcription and promotion of lung injury by mechanical ventilation. J Immunol 2005;175:3369–76.
23. Gharib SA, Liles WC, Matute-Bello G, et al. Computational identification of key biologic modules and transcription factors in acute lung injury. Am J Respir Crit Care Med 2006;173:653–8.
24. O'Mahony DS, Liles WC, Altemeier WA, et al. Mechanical ventilation interacts with endotoxemia to induce extrapulmonary organ dysfunction. Crit Care 2006;10:R136.
25. Moriyama K, Ishizaka A, Nakamura M, et al. Enhancement of the endotoxin recognition pathway by ventilation with a large tidal volume in rabbits. Am J Physiol Lung Cell Mol Physiol 2003;286(6):L1114–21.
26. Smith LS, Gharib SA, Frevert CW, et al. Effects of age on the synergistic interactions between lipopolysaccharide and mechanical ventilation in mice. Am J Respir Cell Mol Biol 2009;43(4):475–86.
27. Oppenheim JJ, Tewary P, de la Rosa G, et al. Alarmins initiate host defense. Adv Exp Med Biol 2007;601:185–94.
28. Noble PW, Jiang D. Matrix regulation of lung injury, inflammation, and repair: the role of innate immunity. Proc Am Thorac Soc 2006;3:401–4.
29. Abraham E, Arcaroli J, Carmody A, et al. HMG-1 as a mediator of acute lung inflammation. J Immunol 2000;165:2950–4.
30. Yu M, Wang H, Ding A, et al. HMGB1 signals through toll-like receptor (TLR) 4 and TLR2. Shock 2006;26:174–9.
31. Imai Y, Slutsky AS, Penninger JM. Identification of oxidative stress and Toll like receptor 4 signaling as a key pathway of acute lung injury. Cell 2008;133(2):235–49.
32. Bachofen A, Weibel ER. Structural alterations of lung parenchyma in the adult respiratory distress syndrome. Clin Chest Med 1982;3:35–56.

33. Dreyfuss D, Saumon G. Ventilator-induced lung injury: lessons from experimental studies. Am J Respir Crit Care Med 1998;157:294–323.
34. Dreyfuss D, Soler P, Basset G, et al. High inflation pressure pulmonary edema. Respective effects of high airway pressure, high tidal volume, and positive end-expiratory pressure. Am Rev Respir Dis 1988;137:1159–64.
35. Kudoh I, Wiener-Kronish JP, Hashimoto W, et al. Exoproduct secretions of *Pseudomonas aeruginosa* strains influence severity of alveolar epithelial injury. Am J Physiol 1994;267:L551–6.
36. Kurahashi K, Kajikawa O, Sawa T, et al. Pathogenesis of septic shock in *Pseudomonas aeruginosa* pneumonia. J Clin Invest 1999;104:743–50.
37. NIH ARDSNet Group. Ventilation with lower tidal volumes as compared with traditional tidal volumes for acute lung injury and the acute respiratory distress syndrome. The Acute Respiratory Distress Syndrome Network. N Engl J Med 2000;342:1301–8.
38. Fine A, Janssen-Heininger Y, Soultanakis RP, et al. Apoptosis in lung pathophysiology. Am J Physiol Lung Cell Mol Physiol 2000;279:L423–7.
39. Park WY, Goodman RB, Steinberg KP, et al. Cytokine balance in the lungs of patients with acute respiratory distress syndrome. Am J Respir Crit Care Med 2001;164:1896–903.
40. Armstrong L, Thickett DR, Christie SJ, et al. Increased expression of functionally active membrane-associated tumor necrosis factor in acute respiratory distress syndrome. Am J Respir Cell Mol Biol 2000;22:68–74.
41. Fine A, Anderson NL, Rothstein TL, et al. Fas expression in pulmonary alveolar type II cells. Am J Physiol 1997;273:L64–71.
42. Matute-Bello G, Liles WC, Steinberg KP, et al. Soluble Fas-ligand induces epithelial cell apoptosis in humans with acute lung injury (ARDS). J Immunol 1999;163:2217–25.
43. Albertine KH, Soulier MF, Wang Z, et al. Fas and fas ligand are up-regulated in pulmonary edema fluid and lung tissue of patients with acute lung injury and the acute respiratory distress syndrome. Am J Pathol 2002;161:1783–96.
44. Matute-Bello G, Winn RK, Jonas M, et al. Activation of Fas (CD95) induces lung injury and apoptosis of type I and II pneumocytes in mice. Am J Respir Crit Care Med 1999;159:A697.
45. Matute-Bello G, Liles WC, Frevert CW, et al. Recombinant human Fas ligand induces alveolar epithelial cell apoptosis and lung injury in rabbits. Am J Physiol Lung Cell Mol Physiol 2001;281:L328–35.
46. Matute-Bello G, Wurfel MM, Lee JS, et al. Essential role of MMP-12 in Fas-induced lung fibrosis. Am J Respir Cell Mol Biol 2007;37:210–21.
47. Matute-Bello G, Lee JS, Liles WC, et al. Fas-mediated acute lung injury requires membrane Fas expression on non-myeloid cells of the lungs [abstract]. Am J Respir Crit Care Med 2004;169:A875.
48. Powell WC, Fingleton B, Wilson CL, et al. The metalloproteinase matrilysin proteolytically generates active soluble Fas ligand and potentiates epithelial cell apoptosis. Curr Biol 1999;9:1441–7.
49. Vargo-Gogola T, Crawford HC, Fingleton B, et al. Identification of novel matrix metalloproteinase-7 (matrilysin) cleavage sites in murine and human Fas ligand. Arch Biochem Biophys 2002;408:155–61.
50. Herrero R, Kajikawa O, Matute-Bello G, et al. The biological activity of FasL in human and mouse lungs is determined by the structure of its stalk region. J Clin Invest 2011;121:1174–90.

51. Perl M, Chung CS, Lomas-Neira J, et al. Silencing of Fas, but not caspase-8, in lung epithelial cells ameliorates pulmonary apoptosis, inflammation, and neutrophil influx after hemorrhagic shock and sepsis. Am J Pathol 2005;167:1545–59.
52. Perl M, Chung CS, Perl U, et al. Fas-induced pulmonary apoptosis and inflammation during indirect acute lung injury. Am J Respir Crit Care Med 2007;176:591–601.
53. Bardales RH, Xie SS, Schaefer RF, et al. Apoptosis is a major pathway responsible for the resolution of Type II pneumocytes in acute lung injury. Am J Pathol 1996;149:845–52.
54. Clark JG, Milberg JA, Steinberg KP, et al. Type III procollagen peptide in the adult respiratory distress syndrome: association of increased peptide levels in bronchoalveolar lavage fluid with increased risk for death. Ann Intern Med 1995; 122:17–23.
55. Chesnutt AN, Matthay MA, Tibayan FA, et al. Early detection of type III procollagen peptide in acute lung injury: pathogenetic and prognostic significance. Am J Respir Crit Care Med 1997;156:840–5.
56. Munger JS, Huang X, Kawakatsu H, et al. The integrin alpha v beta 6 binds and activates latent TGF beta 1: a mechanism for regulating pulmonary inflammation and fibrosis. Cell 1999;96:319–28.
57. Pittet JF, Griffiths MJ, Geiser T, et al. TGF-beta is a critical mediator of acute lung injury. J Clin Invest 2001;107:1537–44.
58. Frank J, Roux J, Kawakatsu H, et al. Transforming growth factor-beta1 decreases expression of the epithelial sodium channel alphaENaC and alveolar epithelial vectorial sodium and fluid transport via an ERK1/2-dependent mechanism. J Biol Chem 2003;278:43939–50.
59. Chang DW, Hayashi S, Gharib SA, et al. Proteomic and computational analysis of bronchoalveolar proteins during the course of the acute respiratory distress syndrome. Am J Respir Crit Care Med 2008;178:701–9.
60. Simon BA, Easley RB, Grigoryev DN, et al. Microarray analysis of regional cellular responses to local mechanical stress in acute lung injury. Am J Physiol Lung Cell Mol Physiol 2006;291:L851–61.
61. Bregeon F, Papazian L, Delpierre S, et al. Role of proinflammatory activity contained in gastric juice from ICU patients to induce lung injury in a rabbit aspiration model. Crit Care Med 2008;36(12):3205–12.
62. Looney MR, Gilliss BM, Matthay MA. Pathophysiology of transfusion-related acute lung injury. Curr Opin Hematol 2010;17:418–23.
63. Looney MR, Su X, Van Ziffle JA, et al. Neutrophils and their Fc gamma receptors are essential in a mouse model of transfusion-related acute lung injury. J Clin Invest 2006;116:1615–23.
64. Looney MR, Nguyen JX, Hu Y, et al. Platelet depletion and aspirin treatment protect mice in a two-event model of transfusion-related acute lung injury. J Clin Invest 2009;119:3450–61.
65. Moss M, Parsons PE, Steinberg KP, et al. Chronic alcohol abuse is associated with an increased incidence of acute respiratory distress syndrome and severity of multiple organ dysfunction in patients with septic shock. Crit Care Med 2003; 31:869–77.
66. Joshi PC, Guidot DM. The alcoholic lung: epidemiology, pathophysiology, and potential therapies. Am J Physiol Lung Cell Mol Physiol 2007;292:L813–23.
67. Guidot DM, Modelska K, Lois M, et al. Ethanol ingestion via glutathione depletion impairs alveolar epithelial barrier function in rats. Am J Physiol Lung Cell Mol Physiol 2000;279:L127–35.

68. Brown LA, Harris FL, Bechara R, et al. Effect of chronic ethanol ingestion on alveolar type II cell: glutathione and inflammatory mediator-induced apoptosis. Alcohol Clin Exp Res 2001;25:1078–85.
69. Brown LA, Harris FL, Guidot DM. Chronic ethanol ingestion potentiates TNF-alpha-mediated oxidative stress and apoptosis in rat type II cells. Am J Physiol Lung Cell Mol Physiol 2001;281:L377–86.
70. Moss M, Guidot DM, Wong-Lambertina M, et al. The effects of chronic alcohol abuse on pulmonary glutathione homeostasis. Am J Respir Crit Care Med 2000;161:414–9.
71. Sutherland KR, Steinberg KP, Maunder RJ, et al. Pulmonary infection during the acute respiratory distress syndrome (ARDS). Am J Respir Crit Care Med 1995; 152:550–6.
72. Jiang Q, Cross AS, Singh IS, et al. Febrile core temperature is essential for optimal host defense in bacterial peritonitis. Infect Immun 2000;68:1265–70.
73. Hasday JD, Garrison A, Singh IS, et al. Febrile-range hyperthermia augments pulmonary neutrophil recruitment and amplifies pulmonary oxygen toxicity. Am J Pathol 2003;162:2005–17.
74. Rice P, Martin E, He JR, et al. Febrile-range hyperthermia augments neutrophil accumulation and enhances lung injury in experimental gram-negative bacterial pneumonia. J Immunol 2005;174:3676–85.
75. Lipke AB, Matute-Bello G, Herrero R, et al. Febrile-range hyperthermia augments lipopolysaccharide-induced lung injury by a mechanism of enhanced alveolar epithelial apoptosis. J Immunol 2010;184:3801–13.
76. Pereira RF, Halford KW, O'Hara MD, et al. Cultured adherent cells from marrow can serve as long-lasting precursor cells for bone, cartilage, and lung in irradiated mice. Proc Natl Acad Sci U S A 1995;92:4857–61.
77. Colter DC, Class R, DiGirolamo CM, et al. Rapid expansion of recycling stem cells in cultures of plastic-adherent cells from human bone marrow. Proc Natl Acad Sci U S A 2000;97:3213–8.
78. Dominici M, Le BK, Mueller I, et al. Minimal criteria for defining multipotent mesenchymal stromal cells. The International Society for Cellular Therapy position statement. Cytotherapy 2006;8:315–7.
79. Ortiz LA, Gambelli F, McBride C, et al. Mesenchymal stem cell engraftment in lung is enhanced in response to bleomycin exposure and ameliorates its fibrotic effects. Proc Natl Acad Sci U S A 2003;100:8407–11.
80. Xu J, Mora A, Shim H, et al. Role of the SDF-1/CXCR4 axis in the pathogenesis of lung injury and fibrosis. Am J Respir Cell Mol Biol 2007;37:291–9.
81. Rojas M, Xu J, Woods CR, et al. Bone marrow-derived mesenchymal stem cells in repair of the injured lung. Am J Respir Cell Mol Biol 2005;33:145–52.
82. Kotton DN, Fabian AJ, Mulligan RC. Failure of bone marrow to reconstitute lung epithelium. Am J Respir Cell Mol Biol 2005;33:328–34.
83. Loi R, Beckett T, Goncz KK, et al. Limited restoration of cystic fibrosis lung epithelium in vivo with adult bone marrow-derived cells. Am J Respir Crit Care Med 2006;173:171–9.
84. Sueblinvong V, Loi R, Eisenhauer PL, et al. Derivation of lung epithelium from human cord blood-derived mesenchymal stem cells. Am J Respir Crit Care Med 2008;177:701–11.
85. Gupta N, Su X, Popov B, et al. Intrapulmonary delivery of bone marrow-derived mesenchymal stem cells improves survival and attenuates endotoxin-induced acute lung injury in mice. J Immunol 2007;179:1855–63.

86. Ortiz LA, Dutreil M, Fattman C, et al. Interleukin 1 receptor antagonist mediates the antiinflammatory and antifibrotic effect of mesenchymal stem cells during lung injury. Proc Natl Acad Sci U S A 2007;104:11002–7.
87. Sueblinvong V, Weiss DJ. Stem cells and cell therapy approaches in lung biology and diseases. Transl Res 2010;156:188–205.
88. Weiss DJ, Kolls JK, Ortiz LA, et al. Stem cells and cell therapies in lung biology and lung diseases. Proc Am Thorac Soc 2008;5:637–67.
89. Matute-Bello G, Liles WC, Radella F, et al. Modulation of neutrophil apoptosis by granulocyte colony-stimulating factor and granulocyte/macrophage colony-stimulating factor during the course of acute respiratory distress syndrome. Crit Care Med 2000;28:1–7.
90. Henson PM, Tuder RM. Apoptosis in the lung: induction, clearance and detection. Am J Physiol Lung Cell Mol Physiol 2008;294(4):L601–11.
91. Gardai SJ, Bratton DL, Ogden CA, et al. Recognition ligands on apoptotic cells: a perspective. J Leukoc Biol 2006;79:896–903.
92. Nakanishi Y, Henson PM, Shiratsuchi A. Pattern recognition in phagocytic clearance of altered self. Adv Exp Med Biol 2009;653:129–38.
93. D'Alessio FR, Tsushima K, Aggarwal NR, et al. CD4+CD25+Foxp3 + Tregs resolve experimental lung injury in mice and are present in humans with acute lung injury. J Clin Invest 2009;119:2898–913.
94. Kuiken T, Fouchier RA, Schutten M, et al. Newly discovered coronavirus as the primary cause of severe acute respiratory syndrome. Lancet 2003;362:263–70.
95. Franks TJ, Chong PY, Chui P, et al. Lung pathology of severe acute respiratory syndrome (SARS): a study of 8 autopsy cases from Singapore. Hum Pathol 2003;34:743–8.
96. Bem RA, van Woensel JB, Bos AP, et al. Mechanical ventilation enhances lung inflammation and caspase activity in a model of mouse pneumovirus infection. Am J Physiol Lung Cell Mol Physiol 2009;296:L46–56.
97. Flori HR, Glidden DV, Rutherford GW, et al. Pediatric acute lung injury: prospective evaluation of risk factors associated with mortality. Am J Respir Crit Care Med 2005;171:995–1001.
98. Alvira CM, Abate A, Yang G, et al. Nuclear factor-kappaB activation in neonatal mouse lung protects against lipopolysaccharide-induced inflammation. Am J Respir Crit Care Med 2007;175:805–15.

Index

Note: Page numbers of article titles are in **boldface** type.

Crit Care Clin 27 (2011) 753–764
doi:10.1016/S0749-0704(11)00042-X
critical care.theclinics.com
0749-0704/11/$ – see front matter

H

I

N

O

R

S

T

U

V

Moving?

Make sure your subscription moves with you!

To notify us of your new address, find your **Clinics Account Number** (located on your mailing label above your name), and contact customer service at:

Email: journalscustomerservice-usa@elsevier.com

800-654-2452 (subscribers in the U.S. & Canada)
314-447-8871 (subscribers outside of the U.S. & Canada)

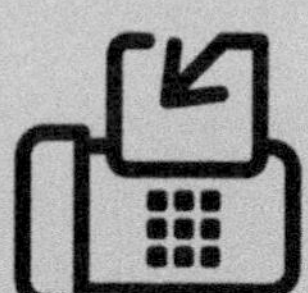

Fax number: 314-447-8029

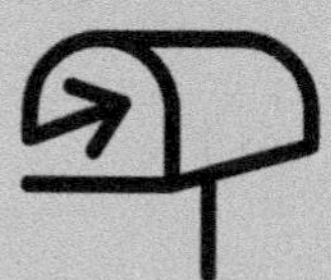

Elsevier Health Sciences Division
Subscription Customer Service
3251 Riverport Lane
Maryland Heights, MO 63043

*To ensure uninterrupted delivery of your subscription, please notify us at least 4 weeks in advance of move.

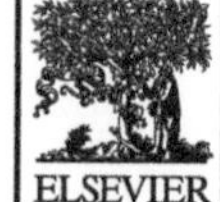